Man and Woman

Karl Wrage, M.D.

Man and Woman

THE BASICS OF SEX AND MARRIAGE

Translated by
STANLEY S. B. GILDER

Illustrated by
GERHARD KAPITZKE

FORTRESS PRESS PHILADELPHIA

This book is a translation of *Mann und Frau. Grundfragen der Geschlechterbeziehung*, copyright © 1966 by Gütersloher Verlagshaus Gerd Mohn in Gütersloh, Germany.

Copyright © 1969 by William Collins Sons & Co. Ltd., London and Fortress Press, Philadelphia. All Rights Reserved.

Library of Congress Catalog Card Number 72-78986

Printed in Great Britain
by Collins Clear-Type Press
London and Glasgow

Contents

Preface   9

I

DEVELOPMENT AND EDUCATION OF THE TWO SEXES

Man and Woman in Society   13
   Social forms · Plurality of functions (roles) · Marriage and family in society

Sex Education in Childhood   19
   Education and Instruction   19
   Obstacles to sex education · Early questions on sex · Incorrect approaches to education · Concept of one's own sex · Naming the sex organs · Familiarity with sex · Nudity in the family · Sharing in mother's new pregnancy · The attitude of the parents towards the new pregnancy · Modesty and nudity · Children in the parents' bedroom · Consequences of erroneous sex education in childhood
   Bases of Sex Education   35
   Shaping of conscience · Striving for contact · Striving for possession · Striving for status · Striving for love and tenderness · Striving for physical sexual satisfaction and erotic sexual relationships
   Answering Children's Questions   48
   The first questions · Questions before and at puberty · Influences outside the home

Puberty and Adolescence   54
   Development and Education before and at Puberty   54
   Emotional tensions in puberty · Informed education · Physical maturation · Development of sexual drive · Deviations in sexual development

6   Adolescence and Preparation for Marriage   61
Emotional development is unfinished at adolescence · Sexual disturbances and deviant behaviour · Models and social norms · Falling in love and its disappointments · Bases of partner choice · Premarital encounters and associations · Early marriage · The engagement

II
SEXUALITY AND SEXUAL RELATIONS

Man and Woman   77
    Differences and Similarities   77
    Male and female anatomy · Body hair · General sex characters
    Boys and Girls   80
    External sex characters · Arousal of interest in sex organs
    Adult Man and Adult Woman   82
    External sex characters
    What is Modesty?   84

The Man   87
    Male Genital Organs   87
    External Genitals   87
    Male organ, the penis · Foreskin (prepuce) · Glans penis · Phimosis
    Internal Genital Organs   91
    Prostate gland · Erectile or cavernous tissue · Cowper's glands · Ejaculation of semen · Testis and epididymis · Regulation by the pituitary · Semen and sperm cell maturation · Seminal duct · Ejaculation · Infertility in marriage · Impotence

The Woman   105
    The Female Genital Organs   105
    External Genitals   106
    Labia majora and minora · The clitoris · Hymen · Vaginal entrance · Frigidity
    Internal Genital Organs   110
    Uterus · Vagina · The ovaries · Mechanism of uptake of ova · Corpus luteum · The ova · Maturation of the ovum · Mature ovum · Fallopian tube and egg transport
    Menstruation   125
    Uterine mucosa (endometrium) · The first menstrual period

(menarche) · Cycle and menstrual calendar · Hormonal regulation of menstruation · Emotional experience of menstruation at the menarche and during the reproductive age

Sex Life 137
    The Development of Sex Life 137
    Masturbation · Petting
    Sexual Stimuli 142
    Sexual reactions · Copulatory reflexes
    Orgasm 148
    Excitation graphs · Mutual devotion · Erogenous zones in the woman · Erogenous areas in the man · Intercourse: frequency, forms, duration
    Sexuality in Later Life 156

Inheritance 159
    Germ Cell Maturation and Inheritance 159
    Chromosomes · Genes · Maturation division · Social inheritance · Asexual reproduction · Sexual reproduction · Boy or girl? · Hermaphrodites
    Mutations and Injury to Hereditary Material 169
    General mutations, radiation injury, healthy inheritance · Marriage with relatives · Effects of alcohol

Conception and Contraception 173
    Impregnation and Conception 173
    Timing of conception
    The Bases of Contraception 175
    Responsibility and sexual intercourse · Abortion and sterilization
    Methods of Family Planning 178
    Abstention from intercourse · The safe period · Basal temperature measurement · Petting · Interrupted sexual intercourse · Carezza · Other unsuitable methods
    The Apparatus of Contraception 183
    The condom or sheath · The pessary · Caps · Diaphragms · Unsuitable, unsafe and dangerous means · Chemical agents: tablets, suppositories, jellies, foaming preparations · Combinations of several methods and agents · Hormones for prevention of ovular maturation

8 Pregnancy   191
    Fertilization and the Early Stages of Embryonal Development   191
    Penetration of the ovum by spermatozoa · Union of spermatozoa and ovular nuclei · First cell division · Embedding or implantation of the embryo
    Ovarian Function and Pregnancy   195
    Maturation Stages of the Embryo   196
    Seventh to ninth day · After three weeks · From the fourth to the eighth week · The sex of the child · Development of the embryo · Relation between mother and unborn child
    Supplying the Foetus with Food   204
    Placenta · The rhesus factor
    Independence and Dependence of the Foetus   211
    False maternal claims · False claims by the father
    Uterine Muscles and Pregnancy   214
    Structure and changes in the uterine wall · Changes in uterine size
    Duration of Pregnancy and Term of Delivery   216
    Changes in Pregnancy   217
    Body changes · Emotional changes

Childbirth   223
    The Events in Labour   223
    The onset of labour · Position of the baby during labour · Opening up the birth canal · Pelvis and labour · Stage of expulsion · Episiotomy (perineal section) · Caesarian section · Labour contractions · Child's first breaths · Cutting the cord · The after-birth · Duration of labour
    The Emotional Experience of Delivery   236
    The Puerperium   238

Breast-feeding   240
    Attitude of the Mother to Breast-feeding   240
    Structure and Function of the Female Breast   240
    Glandular tissue of the breast · The nipple and areola · Development of the breasts · Breast-feeding · Weaning and breast regression   240
    Separation of the Child from the Mother   244

    Glossary   246
    Bibliography   251
    Index   253

Preface

Increasing numbers of men and women today expect to find the supreme happiness of their lives in that relationship with a member of the opposite sex known as marriage. If their expectations are disappointed, the very concept of marriage is going to suffer. But happiness in marriage is not dependent on successful sexual intercourse alone; it depends on the success of a relationship involving mind, body and soul.

For many persons this relationship is made harder because they do not know enough about each other and therefore cannot adjust to each other adequately. Understanding implies information and information acquired at the right time can prevent mistakes, provided that it is information free from anxiety. Information and understanding make for knowledge of oneself and one's partner.

This information, understanding and knowledge have both physical and spiritual elements. The earlier they are acquired, the more lasting their effect and the greater the chance that the man and woman involved will develop appropriate ways of caring for each other.

The present book is offered as a contribution to this theme, starting with the emotional development of the child and adolescent and explaining the physical and functional basis of sexuality. Throughout, the emphasis is on the body–mind relations of sexuality in both man and woman.

The book is the result of more than fifteen years' activity in medical and psychological youth and marriage counselling and the preparation of young people for marriage and family life. The illustrations have proved useful in numerous group discussions, lectures and seminars; they lay stress on essentials and are in part simplified. Thematically the text is linked to the pictures, describing organs, organ systems and their functions but it goes beyond anatomical and physiological information, deals with body–mind relationships, and takes note of many questions constantly recurring in discussion.

Thanks are due to the Evangelical Lutheran Land Church of Hanover for making available the material on which the sketches are based, and to the authors and publishers of medical books for permission to use scientific illustrations, to the painter and designer Gerhard Kapitzke for the pains he has taken to make the illustrations understandable and to bring out essentials, and finally to the present publishers. I would add my thanks to all those who have helped this book along by their suggestions and criticisms.

Hanover, July 1966
DR KARL HORST WRAGE

I

Development and Education of the Two Sexes

Man and Woman in Society

Human beings are either male or female, and they perceive, feel, think, react and act in a male or female way. Their human sexuality is not confined to the sex organs and their differences of form and function, but affects the whole man or woman, including the mental and emotional expressions of life as much as the physical ones. To be human is to be sexual.

Human life in this world therefore always involves polarity, the opposition of male and female. However, since both belong to the human species and form a group different from other living things in this world, they are oriented towards each other and enjoy a special mutual relationship. Sexual contrast and relationship determine the life of man and woman in this world, and it is in this sense that we speak of partnerships of the sexes.

Social forms
All those social forms which are contained in the concept of society arise from the association of man and woman, and in all forms of society the man–woman association known as marriage occupies a special position. It is however always incorporated in larger groupings: marriage broadens into the family, and families are united in kinships. Other and larger groups arise because the environment poses problems such as food gathering and protection from danger which are more easily solved by larger numbers.

Increased distribution of labour and specialization within a larger group make the individual members of it more and more dependent on one another, and the primary group of man and woman must also fit into the whole. The younger generation must be brought up in such a way that it may maintain and improve the conditions required for the stability of the group. The group has an interest in the physical and mental welfare of individual members and in the maintenance of marriage and family. It will take action against any threat to the interests of the group and will promote any project serving to maintain group ties. Nevertheless the special ordinances which have evolved for the partnership of man and woman, for marriage and the family, are—like all other ordinances—conditioned by time and environment. The greater the complication of society and hence of mutual dependence, the more the individual interest must be subordinated to general cooperation and coordination within the group. The success of the group is dependent on the quality of individual performance.

Group function is not confined to work alone but applies to all the groups that form within a society. In our industrialized society there are very many subgroups, each with its own interests and only in part regulated from above. These include, for example, management, political parties, trade unions, professional associations and groups with the most varied interests. Every man and woman has some relation to these. Since each group as a whole has its own regulations and is also integrated into large groups, it is clear that the behaviour of every individual man and woman is subject to a great variety of influences, which in turn depend upon the individual's activity within the group. Man and woman therefore experience life as a pluralistic entity.

Plurality of functions (roles)
The part which the individual plays within a group is referred to as his 'role'. In the course of a single day, various roles must be played simultaneously and in sequence: for example, a man may play the roles of a colleague, a subordinate, a superior, a driver, a buyer, a father, a husband, or a tenant. The man who can play his role in any given situation best will be most successful, but not everybody can adapt to all the changes in role. Roles get mixed up and the result appears to the outsider as maladaptation. The man who treats his wife as a subordinate is behaving just as inappropriately as the father who subjects himself to his children. How then can a person play the various parts correctly? Not only is it necessary to have some basic information about the role but also to be aware of acceptable attitudes. Factual, technical and intellectual knowledge alone is not enough; one must also know how to make proper use of this information.

During the course of their lives, many people find themselves suddenly forced into roles for which they are ill prepared. They feel insecure and first try out, usually with little success, some behaviour pattern familiar to them. Finally they discover the role appropriate to reality and to them, or they choose some general behaviour pattern usual in this type of situation. If they adopt the latter course they integrate into the community but lose the opportunity to give their role a personal flavour. It is true that one individual can be replaced by another in any function he has to perform, but the role he plays in discharging this function is bound to his personality and therefore not interchangeable. In fact, any role in our pluralistic society can be given a personal style.

Marriage and family in society

Marriage is only one out of many necessary roles which a man and a woman may assume during their lives. Yet marriage is a unique role because it is within marriage that the intimate interplay and intimate relationship between two persons of opposite sex find their expression. In no other role are a man and a woman so strongly attached to each other both physically and emotionally as in marriage. In all other roles the person may function well only within a part of the situation, but this is not possible in marriage. Later in this book we shall be emphasizing the high degree to which the intimate union of husband and wife, founded on mutual responsibility, care and respect is a mental and spiritual one and not merely a physical one. Suffice it to mention here that marriage does not imply a fusion of the partners but that each, the husband as well as the wife, remains an independent person.

If we attempt to represent the various human relationships graphically (fig. 1) we find it hard to delimit the area of marriage. The partial overlap of the circles 'husband' and 'wife' makes it clear that marriage is only a part of the relationships of man and woman in this world. It is however something new that transcends the individual and his relationships; it is a 'we' situation. Marriage involves the sharing of their lives by a man and his wife; though each experiences this life together differently, the result is nevertheless to unite them beyond these differences. However, this intimate union may be loosened, and the inner circles may move apart so far that they no longer intersect or even touch. But even here the common experience remains and this may lead to a renewed approach of the circles. If the couple separate, the structure breaks but what has been contributed by each partner to the common past is not lost, even if the two hate each other. For this reason the circle marked 'marriage' has been left vague except for its individual 'man' and 'wife' components, for every marriage is individual and unique. It is the outcome of this particular couple's life together.

Family is not identical with marriage, but is an additional area of living, whose content is based on common concern for the children. Yet even when the children have left home, what the husband and wife have done as father and mother and as a married couple lives on as something common and binding out of the past. Moreover the marriage remains something meaningful and functional after the communal life of parents and children has been dissolved. In Figure 1 the appropriate sex symbol has been assigned to each child to emphasize that every infant comes into the world as male or female from the beginning. The different arrangement of the symbols for children in the diagram within the family circle and their differences in size are intended to indicate that they arise out of the sexual union of husband and wife, are more or less subordinate to the mother or father during their various phases of development, finally break away from their family circle and go forth into the world, independently accepting their own responsibilities. For this reason the family circle is left open, as it always should be; it must let the world in and the children out.

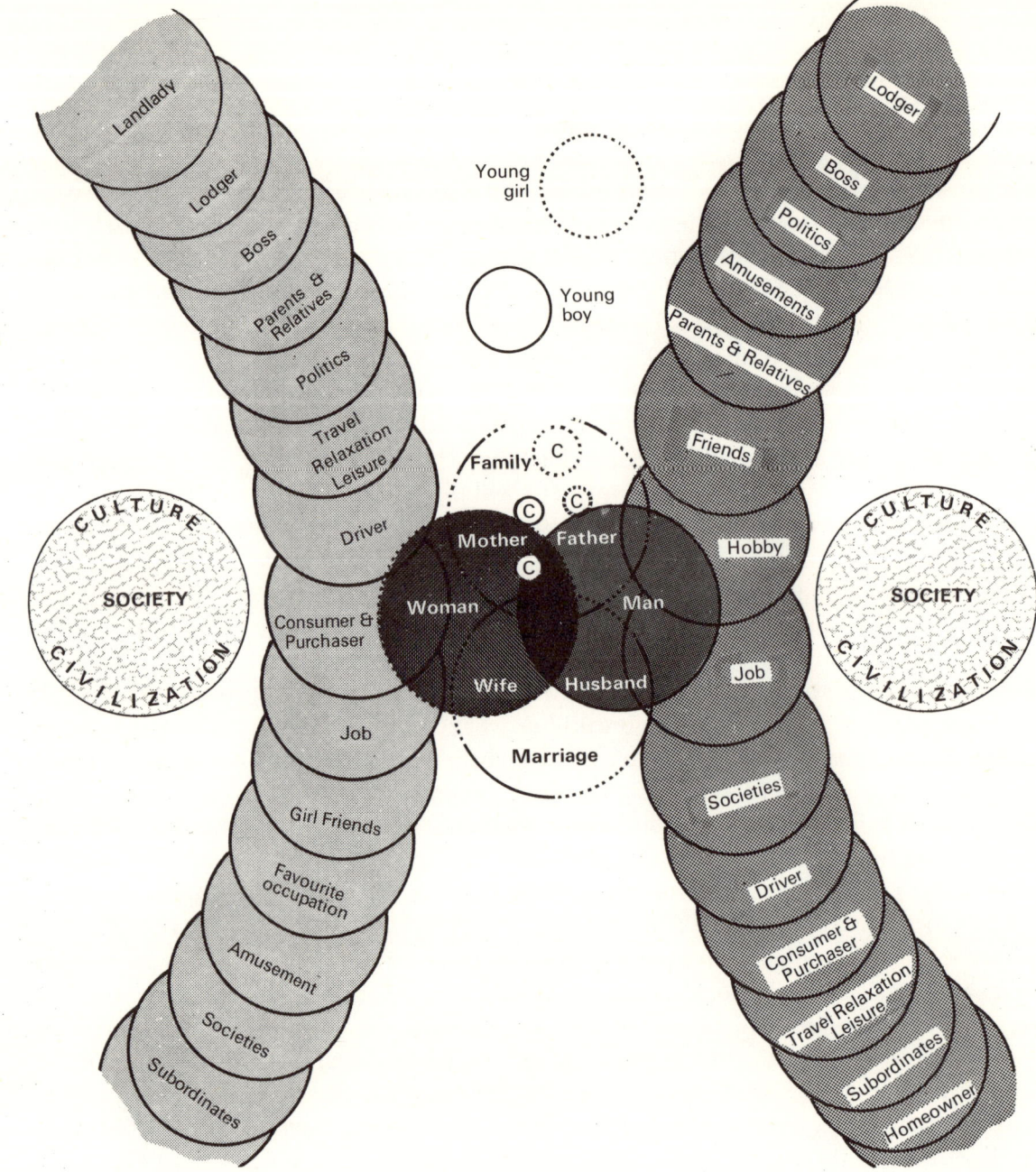

FIG. 1 *Diagram of the various circles in which a man and a woman function in our society. In marriage, in the family and in meeting the demands of the world outside marriage and the home, men and women have to assume a variety of constantly changing roles (shown in the figure as circles). (Further explanation on pp. 14–18.)*

We have intentionally left this circle without any special marking, for its nature is determined by its male–female ratio. Families with an excess of male members produce an environment different from those with an excess of females.

However, husband and wife as well as their marriage and family are constantly influenced by the society in which they live. Society helps to shape the form of marriage and has a continuing influence on family structure. Marriage and family are two basic components of society, but their structure is conditioned by history and depends on the prevailing culture and form of civilization. The influences of the many roles on the central group are depicted in the diagram as oversize telephone dials with hatched fields; although the same role concepts apply to both husband and wife, the hatchings are different to indicate that behaviour patterns differ not only between the sexes but also between individuals.

The expectations that society has of the individual are now undergoing a more rapid transformation than ever before, and this poses special educational problems and is at the root of the frequent misunderstandings between the generations. Education should prepare the young for future roles, but the demands that older generations have learned to accept of the society of their time may no longer be applicable to their sons and daughters. The uncertainty of parents, which is often responsible for inadequate guidance, has the advantage that those who are younger are not tied down but accessible for new groupings, but it also has a great advantage. Anyone who wishes to adapt to society must learn renunciation early, and this training is often neglected. For the youth of today at least, the satisfaction of one's own needs is more important than respect for mutual dependence. In our highly specialized society, the individual should learn his own limitations by his experience of dependence on others and begin to develop a sense of responsibility for the whole. Adolescents often have to learn that they are not living in the same social order as their parents and grandparents. They can therefore no longer take over the behaviour pattern of older persons as a matter of course but must be flexible. As an American sociologist has pointed out, it used to be sufficient for a young person to steer by an internal 'gyroscopic compass' implanted by parents and teachers, for the social norms long remained unchanged and the individual could use his compass for his whole life. Instead, the adolescent of today needs a good 'radar screen' with which he can continually adjust his steering and learn to determine his own position. Only then will he or she be able to live an adequate life as man or woman in a pluralistic society (Riesman, *The Lonely Crowd*).

Education, however, means accompanying an individual on the way towards an adequate existence as a mature man or woman in society. Maturity is reached when individuals on their own responsibility orient themselves with due regard to the regulations of society and its groups, take up their roles and shape themselves as individuals. Since every person born into this world is always either boy or girl, man or woman, he or she is

18 constantly involved in sexual polarity and sexual relationships. Hence all education must include sex education. In this, as in all education, the question is not only one of imparting information but also one of transmitting internal attitudes, for out of these stem behaviour patterns acceptable to society.

Sex Education in Childhood

Education and Instruction

The term 'sex education' really means education directed towards producing mature males and females, and not merely instruction about sexual anatomy and physiology. But the concepts of sex and sexuality are so firmly related in the popular mind with the sex organs and their function in coitus that sex education is generally taken to mean *only* instruction about form and function and about the wise use of the sex organs. However, the concept of sex ought to be used in relation to the whole of living and experience of maleness and femaleness. Because this book deals not only with anatomy and physiology but also with the total manifestations of sexuality, a clear distinction will be made where appropriate between sexuality as a whole and its genital side.

Just as we use the concept 'man' for male and female alike, we will use in the following pages such expressions as 'infant, child, adolescent and adult' for both sexes, even though man is either male or female at every stage of development.

Unfortunately education—especially in the area of sex—is often seen as a process similar to training fruit trees into regular shapes. The educator admits the necessity of giving information about the sex organs and their function but believes that this cannot be done without laying down moral directions, introducing ideas of punishment and arousing guilt feelings. Many parents and educators cannot recognize that sexual drives must develop and that education must imply guidance and assistance with problems of living and development.

Obstacles to sex education
What prevents the adult from approving of this free development? In the first place, a great number of personal experiences since childhood: the recollection of occasions when sexual curiosity and investigation were denounced; experiences which taught him that sex was something mysterious, not to be contaminated with explanations, or something

dirty to be avoided, or something alarming which would be encountered all too soon. The experiences that adults have had in their childhood will determine their attitudes as educators and lead—often unwittingly—to their taking up just the same attitude to their children as *their* parents took up. The emotional load from the past prevents adults from waiting to see how the child develops and causes them to impose restrictions rather than promote capabilities. Sex education becomes biased towards self-control and self-denial. Yet until a person has learned to accept himself with all his physical and mental capacities he cannot deny himself. Self-denial as a voluntary gesture presupposes a knowledge of what is being denied.

A further obstacle may lie in the fact that 'society' refuses to tolerate any behaviour pattern other than the traditional; yet society is not some amorphous mass but a collectivity of us all. Religious influence in the past has contributed to the denigration of sexuality and has associated it with guilt feelings, or else treated it as a baser part of man, and in particular the sex organs. The spiritual attraction of man and woman has been much more highly regarded than the physical. Intimacy and tenderness have received excessive emphasis in sex education while physical passion has been neglected, repressed and disavowed. The object of such education seems to have been to acquit the human race of the charge of animal behaviour. As long as human sexuality was equated with animal behaviour and separated from the intellectual and spiritual areas, which were considered more important, sexual intercourse was robbed of tenderness and became impersonal and matter-of-course. Thus isolated, and confused with genital function, sexuality was now open to attack on all sides. No wonder the result was to confound sex with inappropriate behaviour and thus produce an anxiety state from which the child must be protected for as long as possible.

The basis for such a denial of sexuality on religious grounds has vanished. Modern theologians, both Catholic and Protestant, have clearly shown that sexuality in man with all its physical enjoyment and passion is a gift of God to enjoy and to develop. The theologians have themselves freed us from an originally unchristian, centuries-old prejudice against sex and reached new conclusions because they dared to reopen the question and investigate the Bible afresh. Why have these and other new findings so far affected only a few educators and parents to the extent of correcting their own attitudes to sexual questions?

These attitudes are anchored in their consciences, are therefore deeply implanted and can be comfortably defended against any proposed changes unknown to them or never personally experienced. In consequence, parents and educators find themselves torn between the more recently acquired knowledge permitting the assertion of sexuality and the attitude of rejection originally anchored in conscience, and inevitably behave ambivalently. Their decisions are, often unconsciously, determined by these deeply rooted inner attitudes, and many will reject new knowledge as bad, false, immoral, unchristian or unnatural in order to remain true to their original attitude and avoid a deepseated internal conflict. If a time comes when such a person has to make a statement, for example in education, the fact that the statement is based on his original attitude and not on a more modern one often means that he is of no help to children and adolescents in this area. The adult's reaction in assessing the situation is characterized by prejudice and insecurity.

Since the personality gets steadily less flexible with increasing age it is not surprising that, especially as regards sex education, differences in theory and practice arise between generations. In addition, older people no longer see any necessity for studying sex; after all, their own children are grown up and it might even mean that they would have to admit that their management of the children had been imperfect. This painful process is usually avoided by claiming justification on the grounds not only of individual action but also of the prevailing ideology, laws and morals of their generation.

All this can seriously impede a modern and responsible approach to sex education. This is particularly true of ethical aspects, for, contrary to the belief of many, moral standards do not comply with any fixed law. There is an interplay between the attitude of the older generation and that of the younger, and this forms part of the basic historical problem—that progress depends on a constant interplay of tradition and renewal which must be continuously tested in the light of reality.

For these reasons, sex education often does not go beyond information; transmitting information does not require the educator to revise his own opinions. It is easy to become enthusiastic about instruction, especially if it is to be given by others—parents, school, church, medical profession and state passing the buck from one to another—or if it is to be a one-time occasion in a ceremonial setting. This disregards the most important point, the need for mental effort to rethink one's own attitudes to sex, and also neglects the essence of sex education, namely that handing out information on one occasion only is useless for moulding behaviour.

The child, and in particular the adolescent, is not in the first place interested in facts but in behaviour, observation and action. If what the educator says does not coincide with the way he acts, he simply will not be believed. It is true that knowledge is power, even in sexual matters, but knowledge brings security and self-confidence only when it can be applied. So sex education must show the child how to behave, and must always be adapted to the child's stage of development and understanding and constantly reinforced by repetition and extension. The atmosphere is more important than the words, for the atmosphere connects the information with the emotions. Knowledge associated with feelings of embarrassment or guilt is useless.

Early questions on sex
Since children very soon begin to take an interest in their own bodies and in their entourage, parents and siblings, it is not surprising that they equally early start asking questions about

sexuality. They quickly sense whether their parents find these questions embarrassing or whether they are giving honest answers. If their curiosity about the world is not satisfied they ask again, but this time perhaps using ambiguous terms to give the parents the chance to evade the questions, for they have discovered that awkward questions lead to a frightening withdrawal of love by the parents. If however the child gets a straightforward answer suited to its understanding, it will ask more, seeking to enlarge its knowledge through repetition and additional questions. It will also test out the answers by asking other trusted acquaintances—relatives, neighbours and friends. If it runs into contradictions over facts or deeds, it will return to its parents for an explanation of the contraindications only if it considers them truthful. Otherwise it will say nothing to the parents, even if such questions have not been forbidden.

In this situation such parents often think that their child is not yet ready for information, but they are dangerously wrong, for the child will simply explore the problem elsewhere. Adults are not the only source of information: he has the whole realm of fairy story and imagination as well. Quite a few children arrive in this way at the most peculiar theories of sex, which may remain in the background for a long time and temporarily satisfy their curiosity. Their concepts of sex often coincide with the mythical and magical thinking of primitive man, but there is a difference, for belief in magic was universal among the latter while the modern child's sexual beliefs must perish in the face of reality. If the child finds confirmation for his theories in his parents' evasive or unsuitable answers to his questions, he will appear satisfied until he learns from other sources facts which seem to fit in better, at the stage of insight he has reached. It is only logical that he should keep the information to himself. This is why so many children already have a comparatively clear idea of sex—however disturbed or obscene—at an age when their parents still imagine they are not interested in it. This discrepancy is an expression of the loss of confidence between parent and child, which all began with the first untrue or evasive answer to a question.

The reason for the child's attempts to explain the genitals and sex is fear of the unknown. What one understands evokes less anxiety. The most important consequence of correct instruction as tested by the parents' actual behaviour lies in the emotional area. Up-to-date, factual information helps to overcome anxiety and promote security and self-confidence as regards sex. If discussion with the child uncovers the existence of sexual fantasies and theories which have contributed so far to the child's security, they must never be laughed at or the child will feel insecure once more, since it cannot immediately take in the fresh information. It is only when the factual information has been presented repeatedly and the child has tested it and found it sound, that it can give up its myth and magic and replace this by accurate knowledge.

Incorrect approaches to education

It must be stressed that the small child first experiences sexuality through its parents and maybe in its brothers and sisters, that is to say, through human beings and not animals, let alone plants. It is therefore not only foolish but also dangerous for adults to try to teach boys or girls about human sex through the medium of animal or plant sexuality. This sort of explanation is only possible when an older child knows more about the subject. Furthermore, explanations referring to the animal and plant worlds may give the child the impression that sex is something purely physical in which the emotions are not involved, which leads back to the dangerous isolation of physical sex. If the child is taught about sex solely on the basis of animals and plants, there is no wonder that he comes away with the idea of a depersonalized sexuality related only to the genital organs. Yet this is to lower the dignity of the animal, for the latter responds correctly to its instinct, while man has no instinct. It is his lack of instinct and uncertainty about instincts which have given rise to culture and civilization. He can shape his behaviour in accord with understanding and intelligence rather than inner drives, and is not, like animals, a helpless prisoner of instinct. Hence the seriousness of the warning against beginning teaching sex from examples in the animal and plant worlds.

A third reason for rejecting this type of instruction is closely related to a widespread error in sex education. Sexuality in animals and plants is exclusively designed for reproduction, so this type of instruction would lead the subpuberal child to understand human sexuality merely as a necessity for propagating the species, albeit a pleasant necessity. This is not true, for sexuality in husband and wife serves in the first place to unite them. Sexual enjoyment and passion, tension and relaxation, intimacy and tenderness are not a reward for the act of propagation but strengthen the mutual devotion of husband and wife and their partnership and are the ultimate expression of union. Even modern parents explaining sex quite sensibly to their children usually forget to talk to them about the pleasure and joy associated with sexual activity.

This is due to a persistence of the idea that pleasure, especially sexual pleasure, is a sin, which can only be justified even in marriage because of the intention to have children (the 'pleasure bonus' of Martin Luther). Since one should not lead children into temptation, they should not be told that sex is pleasurable.

Yet all sex instruction and information is unbelievable and meaningless if it does not include a mention of these pleasures. Pleasure in sexuality and sexual intercourse has its own justification. Joy is lost through thought of purpose. It is true that the child first asks about the origin of human life and that its chief interest at first is in birth, pregnancy and propagation. But only at first, for it soon discovers pleasure in its own sexuality, and this should be accepted and not frowned upon. This is the time to tell the child that the sexual union of man and woman gives them both enjoyment and is not only designed just to produce children. It should also be explained (if the parents have answered questions honestly, the child will usually ask about this) that not every act of intercourse is intended to produce children; procreation is intended only when the parents want a child and when they can take the responsibility for its birth and upbringing. This early opportunity should be taken to stress the responsibility of husband and wife for their children and thus for parenthood.

Only factual information combined with suitable instruction about the emotional aspects of sex can overcome anxiety and either correct or dispel childish sexual fantasies and theories at an early age. At the same time suitable attitudes can be implanted and some indication of the conscious development of sexuality given long before the child reaches puberty i.e. at a time when the foundations of human behaviour are really being laid. At puberty, information about contraception can then be appropriately added to this basic framework.

Concept of one's own sex
It is essential that the child learn to think of itself either as a boy or a girl, and this is only possible when it is accepted as a boy or girl by the parents. When the parents dress up a small boy like a girl and behave towards him as if he were a girl, or treat a girl as if she were a boy, this means for the child in question: 'If you were a boy instead of a girl, or a girl instead of a boy, we would love you more.' When they do this, parents make it more difficult for the child to adopt its proper sex role, though the difficulties usually arise for the child as a young adult when most parents have long since forgotten their early remarks and behaviour.

Such an error can be seen clearly in the tragic example of the hermaphrodite (see p. 168 ff.). However even minor forms of this parental behaviour based on false expectations can lead to inadequacies of comprehension of its sex by the child and thus make it difficult to fulfil the expectations of society later.

Learning to understand yourself can also be used literally. Children of both sexes must already be aware of their sex organs in infancy, though opportunities for learning are rare since the organs are exposed only when the diaper is changed and at that time the mother is quite understandably concerned that the infant should not transfer excreta to its face or elsewhere. What is not admissible is the anxious concern hidden behind her action, namely that the child should not develop an interest in its sex organs so early. Unfortunately such an apprehension is very common and arises both from the parents' faulty attitude to sex and from the wish that the boy or girl should remain the sexless child. Failure to observe the presence of a phimosis or an undescended testicle in the boy or a malformation of the vagina in the girl (see pp. 89 and 109 ff.) is often due to this attitude. As part of this concern, the wish is expressed to have the child as a possession (own flesh and blood, see p. 211 ff.). If the mother once concedes that the child is in every sense a boy or a girl, she must acknowledge its sexuality and therefore the basis for its later choice of partner and thus its separation from her.

Care must therefore be taken that the necessary infant management is not loaded with anxiety. The child is quite rightly restrained from playing with its excreta but often in such a manner as to make it feel that not only the latter but also the sex organs are 'bad'. Not only does it find faeces and urine dirty but also later the semen and menstrual flow, for only bad material can issue from a bad organ. It is therefore not surprising when at puberty the boy finds his first seminal emission and the girl her first and subsequent menses associated with fear of all grades up to anxiety state, and feels these emissions to be bad, dirty, polluting or contaminating. Quite apart from this, the other functions of these organs, erection of the penis or mucus secretion from the glands of the labia minora, together with the accompanying sensations of pleasure, are regarded as evil and forbidden. Children of this age are often fearful of these phenomena, which they regard as signs of illness (see for secretion, p. 108; menstruation not an excretion of bad blood, p. 133). It is also not surprising that manipulation of the sex organs, first in puberty and later in adult life, is regarded as 'evil'.

From the standpoint of moral theology it is repeatedly pointed out that in spite of the removal of 'masturbation anxiety' (see p. 46) many young people still have an invincible residue of guilt feeling and dissatisfaction. This residue is only in part due to the fact that masturbation or 'self-satisfaction' (see pp. 58 and 138 ff.) can never be fully satisfying because the desired partner is not attainable and thus it remains incomplete in comparison with the goal sought by the sexual drive. The other part of the 'residue' stems from the taboo on the organs and their secretions dating from early childhood. It is this 'residue' which lets sexuality become impersonal, since one cannot and must not get personally involved with bad things. Later explanations can hardly be expected to alter implanted behaviour but are more likely to widen the gulf between the anxiety now present in the unconscious and the conscious rational acceptance of the explanation.

Sex education begins with ability to comprehend, long before verbal communication between parents and child is possible. We know for certain that the infant senses the attitudes and emotions of its mother and father and uses them as cues for its own behaviour; it is dependent on affection in its helplessness. Withdrawal of love or rejection is equated with mortal fear.

The decisive factor here is not the slap on the hand from mother because the child has played with its excreta or is about to do so; it is the basic attitude of the former which counts. To restrain oneself from slapping the infant or making disapproving noises, and instead to hand the infant a toy to distract him while he is changed is a step in the right direction but it is only the beginning. Parental attitudes to sex are more difficult to change and need some intellectual self-examination, or else they will persist in spite of apparent external change. The child will sense that there has been no real alteration in behaviour.

If the parents cannot mend their attitude, this will become apparent in the expression 'but': 'We're all for sex education *but* someone else should do it'; 'I will tell my child everything but not just now'; 'we are all for sex, but lust is another matter'; and so on.

There are other consequences of failure to understand sexuality, for an individual can modify only what he understands. If we prevent a small child from understanding sexuality, it will be much harder for him to comprehend it later. Boys and girls can do nothing about things they do not understand, and it is not enough to understand just once. We know that a child will take up a rattle, a piece of material, a ball, a piece of paper, a doll, a soft animal or some bricks again and again to play with them, often to the annoyance of its parents if it makes a noise as it tests out the object. By repetition the child must confirm its experience until the latter has been indelibly imprinted on its mind. Later the same process will take place when it tries to climb into a chair or to read and write. The time it takes to do these things varies with the individual. When the infant plays with its fingers, feet, mouth, nose or ears, an occupation its parents may regard as cute, it is really using play to confirm its possession of these parts. The fingers are emphasized in a number of nursery rhymes to show the child indirectly how important their digits are. For this reason the infant when it is changed should be allowed to feel and play with its sex organs in the bath or undressed in its cot, for playing is the child's way of learning. The infant has to learn that it possesses sex organs, and we should not teach it to associate these exclusively with excretion of faeces and urine.

Naming the sex organs

We now come to a further important point in education—what name to give to the sex organs. It is astonishing to what lengths people have gone in inventing terms to conceal from the child the significance of its genitalia. Either expressions associated with excretion predominate or those suggesting that the organ is cute and therefore harmless. These characteristic names betray the faulty attitude of the parents and their retreat from sexuality. The child will use the names it hears but each of these is associated with a meaning. One and the same word may express awe, realism or disparagement, according to the way the speaker feels at the time. In any case, an organ will be associated with the name it is given and its real and emotional content. Naming something is an essential process in relation to the object named; the name expresses the person's attitude and it also determines that attitude. Once named, the object can be singled out, classified and made available. The unnamed is always the unknown whose relation to the person cannot be clarified.

Man's dominance over the world is expressed in the Bible in Adam's giving names to all the animals and thus symbolically making them his subordinates. The fact that in marriage one partner takes the name of the other indicates their unity. The name a child is given is the key to the parent–child relationship, for it will be called by that name. Its name is the expression of its affiliation and also its duty to the group of the same name. Thus naming of the sex organs is not a matter of indifference. If the name is chosen from those denoting excretion, the organ will for all time be emotionally associated with what is 'bad' or 'of no use to the body' and this attitude will be hard to correct by rational argument later. Moreover, this kind of name omits the genital function, so that the latter is again looked on in isolation. If an unsuitable name has been used, when stirrings of desire are felt (and this can happen before puberty) they will cause confusion because the child cannot understand how an inferior organ can cause pleasant sensations; hence there is conflict, insecurity and anxiety. It is therefore essential that the boy and the girl learn appropriate names for their sex organs from the start. These must be unequivocal and plainly express the sexual character of the organ. Boys and girls must understand that they are boys and girls by virtue of their sex organs. How otherwise will they be able to comprehend that they are male and female—by the fact that the parents dress them differently?

What names are appropriate? In the critical literature on sex of recent years it has been repeatedly suggested that the technical terms such as 'penis', 'glans', 'prepuce', 'scrotum', 'vagina', 'vulva', and 'labia' which the child might learn from the start, are too unemotional, too neutral and need to be replaced by new (or newly formulated) and more homely expressions. I could mention many such popular terms, but I want to avoid all expressions and terms which may be erroneous or ambiguous as regards emotional value: I omit them also because so many of these so-called popular terms are either biased or aggressive or disparaging. All these words are only make-shifts. Either they avoid calling a spade a spade or they emphasize only one part of genital function without including their significance in orgasm (not the copulation reflex, see p. 137 ff.). We do not allude to a finger as a grasping apparatus or writing apparatus or an inducer of tenderness, nor a foot as a tool for walking; we do not find fanciful names for an aeroplane or a car when a child asks about them. I believe that behind these efforts to find new expressions for the sex organs there is the same old idea of concealing the truth about sexuality.

Familiarity with sex
Understanding and correct terminology are essential prerequisites for internal and external maturation to manhood and womanhood, but there is also a third factor. The boy or girl should be familiar with sexuality from earliest childhood. Familiarity and confidence depend in the first place on the atmosphere in the home, and the latter is an expression of the parental attitude to sex. Moreover their attitude should not be concealed but should be apparent from their behaviour. If the child is to feel easy about sex and not regard it as some secret science, the family must make it possible for anything at all to be discussed. Both mother and father should be equally approachable for discussion. The child should be able to go to either with its questions, simply choosing the person most accessible.

What it learns it should be able to present with pride as a piece of newly acquired knowledge to the other parent. The child will of course first ask that parent who seems better able to frame the answers in a manner understandable to it, but this should not lead to the other parent's withdrawal from the field or failure to declare his views, either because of convenience or lack of time or anything else. The child must always feel free to ask *either* parent about sex.

Children often ask their questions at moments when it is awkward for the parents to answer, for example on a bus or when visitors are present. But even in these circumstances the parents should take the child's question seriously (even though the bystanders may not like it or may disapprove of both question and answer), just as if it had asked about the make of a car or the function of the eye. By its question, the child has shown that it takes sex realistically. If the child knows that its parents give evasive answers, it will use public places to compel them to declare themselves, secretly hoping that other adults will support its cause. Embarrassment over their children's questions—not only in public—should lead the parents to ask themselves why these questions—and therefore the whole area of sex— are embarrassing to them. It is basically wrong to reproach the child for this. Parental embarrassment should never lead to the punishment or reproof of the child. On the contrary, the child should have its questions approved of in such terms as: 'I can understand why you asked that', followed by a remark that the matter will be discussed when they get home or when the visitors are gone. If the child has not been rendered suspicious by past experience, it will be quite content with this, but will of course expect the promise to be kept. Answers are best given directly and casually. Answers such as 'You wouldn't understand that yet' are most dangerous because such a reply simply discloses parental lack of understanding. Every question deserves a straight answer, for a child becomes a nuisance with its questions only if it has been fed on unrealistic or evasive and therefore incomprehensible replies.

One boy who asked his father about the man in the moon and got the answer 'You wouldn't understand' replied quite logically: 'So that's something else that's dirty.' The boy's reaction was correct, for he had discovered, like other children, that 'dirty' things were kept from him. If a child repeatedly finds that something is 'not worth knowing about', it will automatically put this in the category of 'bad'. If information about sex is withheld from the child, this area will also be considered 'bad' or 'dirty', something to be whispered about and learned about through devious channels. This leads to the isolation of sexuality, as does a prohibition to ask about it. In close relation is the whispering and mysterious behaviour of adults when children are present, and the threadbare excuses used to get rid of them. This seems unfair and has the effect of stimulating an unhealthy curiosity in the child.

The right place for sex education is the home. For the child, the family home is the place of safety, protection, and sanctuary from outside fears, a place which is familiar and where one need not pretend, an intimate place. Here the child learns to make its first decisive interpersonal relationship, learns to give and take, live and let live, love and be loved. Here it experiences a primitive safety in a primitive group, and learns to distinguish self from the community. It learns its place in the social group, and it learns to fulfil the wishes of the group at the expense of renouncing its own desires. Standards of conscience develop here. The child will never again be so familiar with persons and objects as those in his home. The distinction is learned between the family and other groups, and it is altogether natural that the child's knowledge of sex should in the first place be referred to his own family. Just as the child compares his own family with others, so will he compare his knowledge of sex with others, as a part of testing the reality of what he has learned in the family and in the world.

Children are interested in sharing and comparing their knowledge with others. It is therefore foolish to request them to keep to themselves any information about sex communicated to them in the family and not to discuss it with the neighbours' children. In all other areas of life, do we not encourage the child to share its knowledge and apply it because this is the only way he can hold his own in the world? Why all this secrecy? Because many parents are embarrassed to discuss the matter with the less enlightened parents in the neighbourhood. In spite of their conscious and unconscious recollections of their own childhood in which sex was taboo, they have brought themselves to give straightforward answers to their own family but it is beyond their powers to defend their action against hostility, since they fear that they may regress to the suppressive tendencies of the neighbours. Such tendencies may be demonstrated in statements: '*My* child isn't allowed to know about that—if your child talks that way, I won't let him play with ours—children of that age shouldn't know such things—you'll find out later what happens when you tell your child too much.' The reason for these fears is that the parents have accepted a change in attitude to sex education only with their intellect while deep down their feelings are unchanged. Thus forbidding their child to talk to others about what has been taught may be a protection against further involvement. This is not right because there cannot be a real transformation in their own attitude so long as they hide behind this barrier. At the very least, they should not punish their child because it shares its information with others, or complain about other peoples' children who destroy their own children's faith in the stork or similar nonsense. Such an occasion should be used to speak to one's own children openly and sincerely at last. It should be stressed that intimacies and the modesty of the individual, the marriage and the family must be respected.

Nudity in the family
Nudity belongs to the intimacy of the family. Small children parade naked before the rest of the family quite happily and without embarrassment. If they are stopped from doing this

they get the idea that nakedness is something special and something bad since it is forbidden. Their display of nudity serves the purpose of self-recognition but includes the requirement that other members of the family should also be seen naked, so that the child can make comparisons. This requirement is unfortunately often misinterpreted as shamelessness. We will discuss the question of nudity and shame in greater detail elsewhere (p. 84 ff.). It will suffice here to point out that nakedness need not be equated with immodesty, and that shame is not only related to nudity. In any case, it is not shameless behaviour when a child seeks to catch its father, mother and siblings in the nude. Small children should have access to their parents when the latter are dressing or undressing or changing their clothes, taking a shower or a bath. They have the right to know why father has a penis and mother has instead a slit between the legs, and why mother has breasts and father no breasts but a lot of hair instead. The child should receive with joy the news that as a girl it looks like mother, or as a boy resembles father and that one day when it is grown up it also can either bear or produce children and use its sex organs in the harmony of interpersonal relations. The more casually a child learns these things as a matter of fact, the more natural will be its later dialogue with its partner over sexual matters.

It is occasionally asserted that children are frightened and become withdrawn as a result of this type of parental behaviour, but this only means that the parents in spite of tolerance are still emotionally despising or rejecting sexuality and have communicated their feeling to the child, who in consequence shows ambivalence, insecurity and anxiety in its own behaviour. Or else the child has encountered parental feelings it cannot understand or as yet follow because they are strange and therefore alarming to him. We will return to this.

A child should be expected to take an interest in the sex differences of its brothers and sisters, and these differences should be explained to it in matter-of-fact terms, but it is wrong to explain the sex organs and their function *only* as they occur in children, otherwise the latter may start experimenting. Any explanation given should be applied to adults, and the transition to maturity and the adult state should be included in the explanation.

Sharing in mother's new pregnancy
The children should share in their mother's new pregnancies. She should allow them to put their hands on her abdomen as soon as foetal movements can be felt. The increase in her girth should be explained from the start, so that their observations do not become the subject of speculation and furtive sniggers in the nursery. This is the time to point out that the questioner also grew and was protected in mother's abdomen until the time was ripe for him to be born through the gap between her legs. If this explanation for the change in the maternal shape is delayed until the babyclothes are bought and the cot made ready, the older child may already have developed fears for its mother and may have already rejected the newcomer. It is also part of sex education to let older children see the baby at the breast.

The attitude of the parents towards the new pregnancy is an essential part of education
Every child regards its mother's later pregnancy with some dismay and the new infant as a rival for its mother's attention. Consciously or unconsciously, it knows that this means the loss of part of its parents' solicitude for it. If we do find a child who is really pleased over the new event, this is because either it is identifying with its parents' emotions, or it has felt lonely and wants a playmate; in a few cases the child may even feel that he has played a part in its production (see p. 46). In spite of the joy of expectation and arrival, the parents must always bear in mind that the older child up to the time of the confinement is undergoing fear that it may lose its mother. This would initiate a rivalry with the newborn which must lead to a gulf between them later. Parents should therefore take these thoughts seriously, even if the child does not express them, be quite frank about them, and give the older child the opportunity to come to them with its griefs. It is doubtful whether there should be an attempt to mention such thoughts to the child in anticipation of the event, for there is a risk of making it more anxious. At least the child should be made aware that there is sympathetic understanding for the worry and fear it suffers during its mother's pregnancy. It must be made clear that it will not be suddenly cast out from parental protection and especially from its mother's care. The child will in no way be helped by being told of the 'sudden' (unexpected) arrival of a new baby, perhaps with a hint of outside agencies such as the stork.

The most suitable interval between pregnancies is two years, since the older child tolerates loss of maternal attention badly in its first two years (see p. 36 ff.). This interval should be taken into account in family planning (p. 175 ff.). When a new pregnancy is unwelcome to the parents themselves, problems with the older children will be much greater. In such a situation, the parents should not deceive themselves into thinking that the children have failed to notice their feelings. An attitude of confidence is the only thing that will help, confidence that the parents can feed, clothe, and educate the extra child, even if they do have to make more personal, marital, social or economic sacrifices. This is the only way of enlisting the cooperation of their older children, and thus getting them to love the new child.

Thus for a variety of reasons it is important that boys and girls be involved at an early age in their mother's subsequent pregnancies. Moreover, when a small child has realized that pregnancy means a new life, stirring in the mother's abdomen, it will acquire an aversion to abortion later. Girls who have been properly prepared, i.e. without dramatization of their mother's pregnancy as a woman's burden (p. 236 ff.), will not fear their own pregnancies to come.

Modesty and nudity
Although basically nudity in the family does not offend modesty, the children should not be pushed too far in this respect. Every child after birth is so closely involved in the primi-

tive 'we' relationship of the family that it cannot at first think of itself as a separate nude object, but as development proceeds from about the second year of life on it slowly separates itself off from the original family group. It says 'I' and behaves as 'I'. (Simultaneously with this delimitation of the self, the child learns to control its organs of excretion.) During this period it may also learn to distinguish its own private area from those of others, provided of course its parents respect its privacy. If for example the parents leave it alone when it goes and sits on its chamber-pot, it will quickly learn that they also like to be left alone when they are in the toilet. If the parents or the older children leave it alone to wash or put its clothes on, as soon as it is able, it will in turn leave the other members of the family alone. If father, mother, or brothers or sisters put on a dressing-gown when they go from the bathroom to the bedroom, the younger child will soon want to copy them; in fact it will probably demand a dressing-gown to show how grown-up it is, even though it already has a secret desire to see its parents naked. The behaviour of the parents will often lead to imitation without the need for admonition. Thus, a natural modesty develops without prohibition of nudity as the child's private world separates off, although the knowledge of how adults look when unclothed will persist. The child is also well aware that father and mother, husband and wife, see each other in the nude.

As we have seen, this type of education is possible only when the family takes nudity as a matter of course. This type of nudity is not immodest, for it is not an exposure of one's intimate area to strangers (see p. 84 ff.). Furthermore it has nothing to do with the cult of nudism and similar cults which over-emphasize exposure of the body. The philosophy of the nudist and his desire to bring the body in contact with natural elements is controversial; the form it takes of bringing members of different families together in the nude deserves critical study. There is no doubt that children from a certain age on do have genital-erotic wishes (p. 46 ff.); these cannot be overlooked and they do not fit into the pattern of nudism. Within the family, these perfectly normal wishes can be recognized as a part of development but must not be fulfilled, since daughter cannot marry father or brother, while son cannot marry mother or sister, nor can they form erotic attachments. They must look outside the family for their choice of partner, and their wishes so directed outside the family will certainly not be intellectual but contain a genital or erotic component. In the nudist movement, however, such desires are supposed to be suppressed. Young people encounter problems later in life if in nudist camps they have been allowed to look but not to touch and have been obliged to conceal their sexual excitement. As might have been predicted, this causes a profound conflict, for the mores of the camp demand that emotion be neutralized, that the erotic be separated from the genital, and that sex be isolated (though this time from another angle). Where the rules of the nudist camp do not hold and the erotic is not separated from the genital, as in certain private clubs for bathing in the nude, the danger of promiscuity is great. This will be discussed later (see p. 62).

Children in the parents' bedroom

To have the child sleeping in the parental bedroom is to impose a strain beyond the natural nudity in the family and the limits of what the child is allowed to see. In many countries, however, housing is hostile to the family, i.e. too small, so that some other way out of the difficulty must be found. This may require a rearrangement of the sleeping quarters so that one or more children use a living room for sleeping apart, undisturbed by the parents, whose different sleeping habits and rhythm can be a nuisance to the children. This also belongs in 'responsible parenthood' (p. 176 ff.).

Why shouldn't infant and toddlers sleep with the parents? Isn't it better on many grounds for the mother to sleep close to the smallest child? Is there not a risk that the child in its sleep will get its face into the pillow and suffocate without anyone's noticing?

Certainly the baby could get into such a position that it suffocated in its pillow, but then it should never sleep with a pillow. It is better for the vertebral column and its posture if it only has a mattress. The newborn will not toss about, and the older infant should sleep under a properly designed cover so that it cannot suffocate itself under it. It is quite wrong to have pillows for infants. Provided this error is avoided, there is no need to worry any more about suffocating; in any case if the child were in its cot during the day and the mother in the kitchen, she could not hear the child moving about. The particular fear of darkness has other causes; it is a projection on the child of the mother's own fears at nightfall. She fears the takeover by her emotions at night (therefore she imposes some duty on herself) and this is associated with fear of sexual intercourse (which is impeded by the presence of the child, since she must be constantly on the alert for the latter). A spurious claim to 'possession' of the child is often involved (see p. 211 ff.) and used to reinforce the mother's worries.

The breast-feeding mother is still linked with her child though there are two closed doors between them, but it is incorrect to regard this close linkage as due to mother instinct. It is a change in direction of attention governed by hormones (see breast-feeding, p. 242 ff.) reinforced by the primitive emotional 'we' relationship and by a lowered threshold for stimuli emanating from the child (p. 142) but not from elsewhere. It is a common observation, for instance, that a collision between a couple of cars outside the house will not wake the mother while the slightest whimper from the baby in another room will do so; on the other hand, the husband will jump out of bed on hearing the collision but will never notice his wife's departure to see to the baby or her return to bed.

Naturally the mother would be a lot more comfortable if she did not have to get up for the child, but that could be the beginning of spoiling it; such behaviour would not help it to learn to do without its mother and greatly increases its dependence on her. Mothers of this sort are disturbed and annoyed later on when the child is always tied to their apron strings, will not leave the house to play with other children, and so on. To prevent this behaviour, the child must learn early to expect to be alone at times. It will learn this more readily if its mother shows that she is there when it really needs her. A child that has learned this lesson early will soon play by itself and will achieve independence and satisfaction earlier than others. Hence the mother's indolence could have late consequences which are even less agreeable than getting up at night when the baby is tiny.

There is another reason why the baby should not sleep in its parents' bedroom; it should not be a witness to its parents' sex life. This applies not only to the observations an older child may make but also to the baby. Because of the close and primitive 'we' relationship between child and mother, the baby will perceive the change in focus of attention when the mother has intercourse, and of course more clearly when it is nearby. This experience is alarming, and the child becomes anxious because it fears the loss of its mother. It is often awake but is so paralysed by anxiety and fear that it neither moves nor cries. The parents often think that the child is asleep and are annoyed when they accidentally notice that it is awake and still. Other children become disturbed and may scare their parents by yelling, though the yelling often begins only when intercourse ceases, for the child's crying is a subsequent working through of the experience that frightened it. Accounts of dreams of somewhat older children who used to sleep with their parents but no longer do so have demonstrated that they experienced parental sexual intercourse as dangerous for the mother. For example they may have dreamed that mother was run over by a lorry in the total absence of any such danger. Another couple observed that whenever they had intercourse their four-year-old son in the next room always put on his bedside lamp for long periods. When his father looked into his room later, the child was asleep again and did not waken even when his lamp was put out after intercourse had ended. The child cannot follow the powerful interpersonal tensions and emotional explosion of orgasm in its parents, because this emotional area is still closed to it. As a result its participation in the experience due to its intense emotional tie with the mother must remain incomprehensible to it and therefore alarming. In most cases sexuality and sex education are forbidden ground to it and it is experiencing something prohibited. If the child is even older and has not been correctly informed about sex, its curiosity and the attachment to the parent of opposite sex which is a part of natural development (p. 46 ff.) may lead to persistent damage through observation of intercourse. The damaging influence may become apparent only later in the person's sex life and is hard to comprehend and remove, since these early experiences have disappeared from consciousness and are firmly anchored in the unconscious, from which they exercise their effects on behaviour and attitudes in the sexual sphere.

Because in our culture sexual intercourse is exclusively related to the private life of one man and his wife, neither infants nor older children, either asleep or awake, should be witnesses of the act. The presence of the child represents an intrusion into privacy which it cannot understand, however well informed it may be and however healthy its attitude to sex. Where it is impossible to separate parents and children at night, the parents should assume their responsibilities by reserving their intercourse for the living-room.

Society, and in particular those parts of it responsible for housing, should be aware of the responsibility for constructing dwellings suitable for families, and not only for the reasons set out above. Engaged couples and newlyweds should give some thought to these matters and plan accordingly; their assumption of responsibility begins at the latest with the first child.

Consequences of erroneous sex education in childhood
We have shown that understanding, correct terminology and familiarity with sex are indispensable for healthy development to adult maturity. If this education is neglected and therefore sexuality, in which every child obviously has an interest, is excluded from the total area of human experience, the result can only be a fear of sex. This fear comes to the surface at the latest during the maturation of the child. It is absolutely essential that this anxiety (which, however, scarcely a boy or girl of the relevant age can admit to) be overcome, for everyone wants to live without anxiety. There are only two ways of overcoming this consciously unconfessed sexual anxiety. Either the individual must strive to suppress his sexual drives entirely or he must ignore his anxiety with the thought that sexuality is just something natural in the animal kingdom. In both cases, sexuality is isolated from its context. In the first instance, the result is prudery, in the second lack of restraint. Even in the best informed child one of these two attitudes can develop unless appropriate types of behaviour are taught and unless sex is represented in its totality with its physical, sensual, intellectual and spiritual parts, something designed as a creative thing and consciously used for this purpose.

Bases of Sex Education

Shaping of conscience
The child's assumption of behavioural attitudes and patterns modelled on those of parents or at a later age those of educators, or its identification with these persons, is a complicated mental process which cannot be entered into here. We will limit ourselves to a few basic points. Every child, like every adult, wants to be happy. Happiness depends on a very wide variety of human wishes—often secret. There will always be argument about what 'happiness' really is, even in cases where all one's wishes appear to have been granted. This is as true of adults as of children. The adult is in a position to fulfil many of his wishes himself, whereas the child has to a large extent to rely on his parents for this fulfilment. It very soon has the painful experience of discovering that not all of its wishes are going to come true.

In consequence it feels that its parents, and in the early months of life this means mostly its mother, do not love it, for it reasons that withdrawal of love by mother is responsible for its feeling of unhappiness. So it tries even harder to get its way. If it does not succeed in spite of all efforts the only thing left to regain happiness is to renounce the wish, for only thus can it win back its mother's love. By adopting this course it conforms to the demands of the world as represented by the parents or mother, in order to bask in her love again. Naturally there are other wishes of which the world does approve and which it therefore does not need to abandon. As a child comes to terms with the environment in this way it acquires internal standards of values or in other words it develops a conscience.

This internal modification of wishes is first activated through the voices of its mother and father. Their behaviour and their attitude to their child's wishes are therefore decisive in shaping its conscience, the elasticity or rigidity of which is directly dependent on parental attitudes. It is only later that the child will gradually assume a wider set of values; even then it will mostly choose those acceptable to its parents. In other cases, there are conflicts of conscience, though the values imprinted by the parents will be the real standards for what is permissible. Knowing what ought to be done, and knowing also that one is in conflict with this, leads to a 'bad conscience'; knowing that what ought to be done coincides with one's wishes leads to a 'good conscience'.

Four areas of communal life are especially important: contact, possession, status and love. All wishes leading in these directions underlie the processes of identification described above, and therefore although they are innate they can be influenced by education. They are, of course, never isolated but always interrelated. For descriptive purposes, however, it will be convenient to deal with them separately.

Striving for contact.
It is well known that human beings are to an extraordinary degree dependent on their relations with others. An essential agent in this is the exchange of words through conversation or dialogue with other individuals. But conversation is not the only expression of this need for contact, for every relationship which begins with a dialogue continues with a desire for tangible evidence of physical presence. The need for belonging is thus reinforced by a feeling of security. This tangible evidence of physical presence is expressed in many ways: shaking hands, embracing one's loved ones, relatives, friends and acquaintances, or even conveying by a look a sense of security, protection or trust. Trust increases the self-confidence of the person trusted and this in turn enables the latter to trust his partner without fear. Through a healthy self-esteem achieved by the trust of another person, the individual's capacity for devotion to another will grow, and by extension his capacity for devotion to a cause. Self-esteem is the only thing which makes it possible to face the world without fear.

Every child is born with a positive attitude towards the world. It therefore responds spontaneously to an environmental stimulus, seeking to become familiar with the latter, to establish contact with it and to hold on to it. But already in early childhood this desire for contact becomes inhibited by the discovery that wishes cannot always be fulfilled but may at times have to be foregone. A further limitation arises through the development of the critical sense, so that the child begins to feel the need to try things out. These limitations play a part in the growth of the healthy child, in that they develop its capacity for putting a distance between itself and its own wishes and needs as well as the attractions of the outside world. Both the capacity for familiarity with the world and the capacity to stand aloof from the world make it possible for human beings to behave appropriately towards persons and things. These capacities and their development are particularly important for the shaping of subsequent relations between man and woman.

The crucial expression of desire for contact and relationship takes place in the first months of life. The child gets its first impressions of contact when its skin touches its mother's skin. Words of affection and tenderness and the mother's bearing and feelings are answers to its need for a personal relationship, without which it will languish physically and mentally. To feel oneself loved confers self-esteem even if, and indeed precisely when, one is obliged to renounce one's wishes either temporarily or entirely. The manifold wants of a small child for environmental contact must be channelled by the parents. An excess of these must inevitably lead to superficiality of contact and also to a shrinking away from offers of contact. Too little on the other hand causes an inability to make relationships. If there are not enough stimuli to development the child will lose its delight in its environment. Since every possible type of behaviour, if only in outline, is practised in childhood, and since learned behaviour patterns are later continually repeated because they are familiar, the natural and continuing affection of its mother are of vital significance for the child's later abilities. There are therefore serious consequences if early in life contact is broken because the mother is away or because she is unable to make meaningful contacts. Apart from severe mental and emotional illnesses, breaks in contact lead to poverty of relationships, anxiety about them, emotional insecurity and lack of confidence, anxiety in the presence of others, and inability to surrender to others. Another consequence may be an inability to keep one's distance.

People who have suffered from this poverty of contact and have always had an unsatisfied need for this from infancy often seek a rapid succession of superficial sexual relations in the hope of finding in these incomplete episodes the human contact they desire. They cannot however maintain a lasting relation. All these superficial affairs simply delude them that they are not lonely. Not infrequently these people expect from their partner unconditional affection and unconditional trust, but adults cannot comply with these extravagant expectations, so that disappointments arise which the disturbed person cannot work through because he has learned neither to be intimate nor to remain apart. As a result he withdraws further from the world and his inability to make friends gets worse. Since his 'loving' relationships do not involve the whole person, they become purely physical. The ability to give oneself is often disturbed because the patient is just not aware of it, so that disorders of orgasm and potency frequently follow on these disturbances of contact. It will be obvious that such disorders of sexual relationships cannot be cured by drugs or by an act of will. The patient still needs to mature mentally and emotionally, and this means psychotherapy.

These examples show how important for a meaningful sex education the presence of the mother and her emotional and physical affection are during the first months of life. Grandmothers and crèches, although they look after the child quite well in the sense of feeding, clothing and caring for it, are in no position to replace emotional contacts with the mother. If human society lays any value on preventing poverty of emotional life among its members, it must in spite of industrial full employment see to it that mothers are available to their children. It must also teach these mothers and fathers how to develop relationships with their children in a sensible manner. The decisive part of this learning lies in the first months of the child's life, up to about the end of the first year, though contact and relationship are still needed later for the development of the child.

Modern sexual permissiveness and instability of relationships, the Don Juan philosophy of the men and sexual promiscuity of the women, their failure to govern their own sex drives, to which they must childishly give way at once without constructing a relationship based on feeling (or their contempt for the latter), are clearly results of this poverty of contact. They cannot be overcome either by explanations or discipline, but only through forming correct attitudes in early childhood. This is a social problem which can be solved in the future only by sensible education, which will require the collaboration of all parents and educators.

Striving for possession
The human desire for possession is already demonstrable in earliest infancy, the first sign being the wish for food. The fulfilment of this wish is associated with evident pleasurable satisfaction, while its refusal evokes the strongest feelings of displeasure. Long after the child has been weaned from its mother's breast, it still tests its possessions by putting everything in its mouth (see p. 244 ff.). For a relatively long time the mouth is the preferred part of the body in the striving for possession. The feeling of satiety is not limited to the organs which serve for intake and digestion of food but is in close relation to the acquisition of needs, affection and recognition. Soon however it is not the mouth but the hands which are the grasping and grabbing organs. They play an important part from the start. With further development, sensory organs are finally involved in taking the environment into custody. The nose strives to inhale the whole world, the eyes want to encompass the whole world in

the gaze, the ears seek to hear all the noises present; finally, the understanding wants to penetrate the secret of the world and conquer it with knowledge. An enormous hunger for the world distinguishes the healthy strivings of man for possession. Basically this is a primitive desire to have things, spreading far and wide into the moral area of positive response to life and joy therein. To this need to possess things belong the exploration of the world as well as the collection of goods, requests, comprehension, desire and pleasure at receiving gifts.

Education of any sort must teach the child to adapt his desires to his needs. To this belongs the ability to give things up spontaneously, renouncing one thing for something else of more importance or value. Every endeavour, including that for more possessions, must be directed in this way because the possessions and freedom of one person end where those of another begin. This boundary can be crossed only by mutual agreement.

If the child grows up in an environment in which instead of cooperation it encounters rejection and refusal of its wishes, it will find its early striving for possessions inhibited. According to the category of the refusal, this child will seldom or never experience pleasure from obtaining things and will wait to be 'fed' by the world and the people in its environment, because its parents have given it what it did not ask for. However the world outside the home will give it nothing it has not wrested from the environment. On the contrary the world constantly demands things from the individual. A person who cannot grab for himself will fear the demanding world. From such attitudes, docility, excessive modesty, resignation and envy develop as well as the idea that it is actually reprehensible to try to possess the world.

Encounters with possessions are not limited to acquiring things but include keeping them. A child who is not allowed to learn how to keep things in an appropriate manner will have difficulty in learning how to look after itself or its belongings.

Another aspect of the life of property should be mentioned—the desire to give presents. Quite a small child will give things away or share its experiences. The desire to give spreads widely in life up to the limits of personal devotion or sacrifice, but a person can give freely and joyfully only when he can equally freely acquire and keep things.

Giving and taking is of the utmost significance in the relations of the sexes and therefore in sex education. Errors in this area may make it difficult for an individual to open his heart to his partner and share confidences; it will also be difficult to participate in the joys and sorrows of another. There may be problems in understanding one's own sexuality and that of the opposite sex. Dialogue between partners can suffer greatly if one partner never says what he is thinking but expects that the other will know without being told. Inability to request can lead to as severe sexual and marital disorders as inability to give. Frigidity is due to inability to give oneself; impotence is due to an unconscious aversion from giving one's semen. False attitudes in daily conjugal life bring wearisome arguments over trifles and a variety of tensions in marriage, because every intimate relationship requires surrender, possession and keeping of what has been obtained. Finally, all such disorders if repeated continually conjure up the spectre of separation and lead to both mental and physical illness.

Striving for status
The desire for status is also present early in life. It may however be overlooked if one does not notice that the infant is always drawing attention to itself (by crying for example) whenever it is without its parents or its mother for a while. This technique of drawing attention to itself is a simple sign that it is seeking status. Mature forms of status-seeking are detectable only very much later. It is important to note this development, for the personal relations between husband and wife are involved. Personal status depends on a number of things—rank and self-assertion, natural authority and healthy pride, worth and sense of one's own freedom, and ability both to give and take criticism.

Every living being seeks to enlarge its area. Even the smallest child would like to enlarge its tiny world by action, but for this it needs to move around. Movement is a fundamental characteristic of living things. The older the child, the greater its mobility and the greater also the dangers of the environment. Anxious behaviour on the part of the parents may limit the child's movements and thus limit its delight in movement and make it dependent through fear. On the other hand, too early encouragement of movement may produce later a person who demands too much of himself, is therefore frequently disappointed and thus feels inferior.

Enlargement of its horizons is associated with activities which help the child to realize itself, though the adult may see these activities only as a game. It is important to tolerate these games and to encourage them, since they form the basis of creative imagination. The child derives real pleasure from them only when its actions are taken seriously and approved. Thus the capacity for collaboration with others is exercised. This capacity is of significance not only for marriage but also for other forms of communal life. A few examples of disturbances caused by lack of this ability are doubts and fears in matters of cooperation, abhorrence of human ties, and delay in making decisions (for example in fixing the wedding).

In an early phase of its development, the child learns to speak, to think and to construct a conceptual world. As with all other forms of activity, testing is a prominent feature. Parents are pleased when their offspring make bits of words out of 'nonsense' combinations of vowels and consonants to express ideas; later with practice, children learn to put the correct sounds together to make sense. By showing their approval of the initial dissection of words and terms into their acoustic components the parents recognize the child's attempts and enable him to learn to speak correctly. What is true of speech is also true of the child's method of learning to handle things, by first taking them apart. It experiences delight in its own strength when it pulls things to pieces, but all too often the child is thwarted during this stage of development because adults cannot tolerate watching it at work in the purely destructive phase. They do not stop to think that every constructive activity, whether material or mental, needs material for construction. The child can obtain this material only by taking something to pieces. When the components are there, it can build them up into the old structure or something new. It is therefore absolutely essential to let the child destroy things so that it can learn to construct later. Ability to dissect or take things apart is also a prerequisite for ability to criticize. Encouraging, helpful, positive criticism is the 'leaven of marriage', for there is no ideal partner and no ideal marriage except in quiz programmes and the imagination. Every partner has strong and weak sides; the thing to do is to give due acknowledgment to the strong side and either accept the weak or correct it by encouraging criticism. This is possible only if one can without envy recognize the strength of the other partner, and this in turn is possible only when one is sure of oneself. Otherwise the criticism becomes biting, hurtful and humiliating and leads to rebellion in the other partner, whose rejection of the criticism is a further obstacle to his development.

Ability to criticize constructively is absolutely essential for the real exercise of authority, but nobody can be an authority in every field. It is therefore necessary in a partnership relation for the different authorities to delimit their zones of authority in free discussion and through experience.

Development of *will* in the child is closely linked with the awareness of its own value as it conquers the world in play and as its faculty for critical attitudes grows. The child again starts by testing, first going from one extreme to the other to see how far, how long, to what limits and against whom it can impose its will. If the child has been loved by its parents for its helplessness and clumsiness and maybe spoiled on that account, they are often surprised to find that it has developed a will of its own which does not suit those around it. The child's defiance is its own 'no' to the environment and also a protest against the 'no' of the environment; it is a necessary stage on the way to independence, and this phase starts about the third year.

The child acquires strength to develop a will of its own through its ability to direct its movements more surely towards a goal, through its independence and through its increasing awareness of itself as a person. In other words, it recognizes that it is somebody separate from the rest of the world. Symbolically, children of this age see themselves unconsciously as the centre of a circle. The larger this circle the greater the claim to make their own decisions and get what they want. This is a difficult time for the parents, since the child wants to subject everything to its own will and take in more territory all the time. It becomes obstinate; in other words, it develops its own inclinations. Only through the phases of defiance and obstinacy does a person win through to becoming an individual. It is entirely wrong to thwart this development by attempting to bend the child's will to that of the more powerful parent. The old Prussian principle of education produced subordinates who all too readily degenerated into uncritical hangers-on. If the development of the will is hindered there is a danger that the child will become incapable of forming its own opinions or taking its own decisions. These persons become straws in the wind of other people's opinions, pliable and docile. It is however just as dangerous to give way to all the child's demands for power, and retreat before every expression of the child's will. The child will get the idea that it can do what it likes, for it encounters no opposition and does not know where to stop and take its bearings. It is, in fact, unprotected and neglected. The child must therefore be taught to respect certain limits, if only to protect it from its own exuberance. It must learn how to assess reality correctly or it will go under later.

As in all education, one must approve in principle the child's wish to shape and try out its own will, even if in the better judgement of adults the realization of the wish cannot be permitted. At the same time the child must come to realize that between all and nothing, between either and or, there are a whole range of possible decisions which permit freedom of choice.

Development of these faculties is of great significance for relations between partners. The faculty for choosing a suitable partner depends to quite an extent on the capacity for assessing correctly the real facts of conjugal life. Give and take in marriage, even in the most humdrum matters, always requires mutuality between the partners, each recognizing the rules and limits of action.

Self-assertion is linked with aggression even in the earliest stages of development and there is growing pleasure in combat; strengths are assessed and compared and the infant both attacks and defends. Siblings and children of like age will fight over the distribution of power, love and influence and over ideas and opinions. After the fight comes a short period of isolation and then, with growing reliance on its own powers, the child develops a capacity for collaboration. The wish to unite one's will with someone else's to improve achievement develops best if parents have not interfered in the previous stage of hostility, since only differentiation from others permits the child to appreciate its own powers. Mutuality, at first between parents and child, is associated with the recognition of the help that parental authority can bring. If the parents are exercising a false authority, however, there can be no real mutuality and the child will continue to protest. If it realizes that its parents possess real authority, it will come to understand that rules are necessary and that these enable the individual personality to come into its own. That rules can be helpful is first observed when the child begins to appreciate that for some tasks the combined powers of a number of persons are needed. The value of an orderly life as a whole is only later understood when the child can fit its own plans and intentions into the system. Thus self-assertion grows into a feeling of personal worth and finally into a capacity for adaptability. Modern neglect of order must certainly be linked with the experience that so few parents now use their authority in a helpful way to do things together with the child instead of forcing the latter to make all its decisions alone at too early an age. Without some submission to rules, there can be no respect for others nor can one play one's proper part in society.

Self-confidence is a logical consequence of this development, which makes it possible to meet the world's demands in suitable terms, to conquer the world of knowledge, to overcome problems through planning, to enjoy what the world offers and to obtain status and recognition. The individual becomes sociable and acquires the qualities needed for a successful and therefore happy sex relationship. If however the individual's desire to assert himself has been repressed and he has not been allowed to seek status, he will give up the struggle later, feel inferior, and hide his excessive greed for recognition at any price beneath a mask of submission. On the other hand, he may become arrogant and distort his unfortunate search for status into an overwhelming ambition. Giving no quarter to anyone, he will seek to force his claims upon the world. Because he has never been given a sense of status or of security, of healthy pride and self-respect, he will find a subordinate position intolerable and demand a better one. We all know of unhappy couples in an eternal struggle for power, with a sexual life usually in ruins. In normal marriage there should be collaboration but the leadership should change hands according to the situation, one partner being temporarily dominant while the other cheerfully accepts this.

The real partnership of modern marriage can only be achieved if the personalities of the partners have not been hampered in their development. It is all too clear that relationships of husband and wife are very definitely determined by influences entirely outside sexuality.

Striving for love and tenderness
The desire of the individual for love is a basic need with many strata; relief of sexual tension is only one of the goals. This drive includes a longing for devotion and tenderness, a search for psychosomatic harmony, as well as sexual drive in the narrowest sense. An adequate love relationship, however, always depends on the correct organization of the pursuit of contact, possession and status. Devotion must be preceded by trust, inclination and security, and these emotional factors can develop only if they have been cultivated in early childhood by suitable parental attitudes. Moreover, the capacity for devotion depends upon the ability to make contacts and to give of oneself, and these faculties can grow adequately only in an environment of security and confidence (see pp. 37 and 39 ff.).

The need for safety. This is usually adequately satisfied by the mother. Her presence, and indeed the home as a whole, become sanctuaries of peace and contemplation even when the older child starts going its own way. It is important for the child to retain this feeling even after it has left home. If he feels that protection has been withdrawn because he is becoming independent he will experience this as something more significant than the challenge of life outside and he may abandon enterprise in favour of safety. Later on, such a person will be more and more concerned with safety and therefore may make unreasonable demands on his wife for love; she should however never be expected to take the place of his mother.

The child must also learn at an appropriate age that security involves personal effort. It is not uncommon to find that men to whom this idea is foreign have a strong desire for security in later life but no capacity for getting it. They introduce all the latest labour-saving devices in their home, shower expensive gifts on their wife and furnish the home extravagantly but the atmosphere remains cold because they themselves are emotionally cold. These people have often not learned to share their feelings, and in fact they have frequently been forbidden as children to show their emotions. Although they expect a lot of affection they are themselves incapable of it. A hardening regime in childhood in particular will lead to emotional coldness and seriously disturb the capacity for devotion and affection.

But there are limits, and the child must gradually learn that it can keep its feelings to itself and does not have to communicate everything it thinks and feels, otherwise it will grow up a gossip and a chatterer. Its poor spouse will then be overwhelmed with a flood of immature thoughts, feelings and opinions and will be expected as a mother or father substitute to comment on its mental life. Inability to achieve the right balance between intimacy and excessive aloofness may also impel a person to demand of the spouse that she recount even her most trivial thoughts, so that she gradually loses her independence.

Striving for affection starts with physical contact and gradually widens to include caresses, and attention and fondness in general. It is early observed that children of both sexes want a soft doll or a teddy on which they can bestow affection through contact without protests from the doll! This shows more clearly than in the mother-child relation that the search for affection implies a two-way traffic—receiving and giving. We know however that this capacity can develop only if the child has been shown tenderness and affection in its first contacts with mother and father.

Excess of affectionate contact in childhood is equally disadvantageous for development, since life's problems are not to be solved through loving contacts but by suitable action and by dissociation from persons and things.

Whereas devotion and affection were formerly the province of the mother alone, the greater leisure now available to fathers has led to their more frequent contact with their children. If in addition they have been successful in life they can endow their offspring with even more confidence and security than the mother could formerly, from her usually limited domain of the home. It is probable that future generations will be more self-confident and therefore increasingly able to demonstrate their affection and devotion. The child's observation of the relationships of mother and father at home and their daily exchanges of affection are more important for it than any amount of talk. Here again in a modern industrialized society with greater leisure, conditions are more favourable than they used to be.

The need for harmony of body and mind is not only related to grace and beauty but also to harmony with one's partner and the world. One of the first satisfactions of this nature which the child experiences is its rhythmical movement in time with the mother's motion as she rocks it or sings to it or carries it around. The desire for harmony however soon comes in conflict with the child's own will, so often in opposition. If the child comes to look upon familial harmony as more important than its own primitive needs it may grow up with the illusion that complete understanding between it and its marital partner is essential. This expectation is mostly closely coupled with an inability to tolerate disagreements and overcome them in a sensible manner.

Striving for physical sexual satisfaction and erotic sexual relationships
Both of these are primary needs in terms of sexual drive and are both demonstrable in small children.

It is a prerequisite for proper satisfaction of sexual needs, quite apart from knowledge of sexuality, that boys and girls be aware of their particular sex characteristics. In this respect there is a temporary phase of competition between boy and girl over function. The boy learns to use his penis on urination to make bigger and bigger arcs and thus employs it actively, while the girl often feels that in comparison she has been short-changed. It is true that she occasionally becomes aware of her clitoris and wonders whether it will grow but she usually realises that it will never rival a penis in size. During this phase of development it is important to call the girl's attention to the merits of the feminine role (though this role is yet to come) and to accept her femininity as well as the boy's masculinity. If this is not done she may later in adult life get stuck at the stage of aggressive competitor with males and thus be rendered incapable of partnership with a husband.

In this developmental stage children like to display their sex organs to each other or to adults. Boys and girls want to know exactly what the other looks like, and at this age there is no reason to stop them, though they need some direction (see p. 29 ff.). What is forbidden at this age will be repeated at school outside the parents' reach and may then meet with disapproval from others. But even this should not be dramatized by adults but on the contrary used as an occasion for helpful leadership. If at an early stage of development the child is forbidden to look at and display the sex organs, this may start him on the road to later perversions, in which sexual stimulation and enjoyment can be obtained only from looking at (voyeurism) or displaying (exhibitionism) the genitals.

Parallel with this development goes the discovery that touching and playing with one's genitals leads to pleasurable feelings and enjoyment and in the male to the visible changes of erection. This situation is quite normal and should not cause any worry. It serves to make the child aware of its own possibilities for physical satisfaction. To react with dire threats, prohibitions or blows may lead to later sexual disorders, or to a secret counter-reaction of greater activity by the child (see p. 58 and p. 138). Excessive autosexual activity in early childhood is always a sign that the child is relatively inaccessible to human contacts and does not enjoy playing with others. In these cases, playing with the genitals should not be punished or prevented but a serious attempt should be made to determine and remove the underlying cause for the disorder.

This pleasurable activity is still generally known as 'masturbation' or by the misnomer 'onanism' (unfortunately even in scientific circles). The latter term carries a deplorable connotation of sin, for it comes from a Biblical text, though the idea behind the use of the term is entirely erroneous. In Genesis 38 we read that Onan refused to impregnate his dead brother's widow and instead 'spilled his seed upon the ground'. It was later concluded from the fact that Onan was punished for this that any stimulation of the sex organs without the design of procreation was sinful. What the protagonists of this idea overlooked, however, was that a Levitical marriage was involved in Onan's story and that such a marriage had some unusual rules prescribed by Jewish law and even noted in the New Testament (cf. the question put to Jesus by the Sadducees). In Levite law a barren marriage could not be remedied after the husband's death either by recognition of illegitimate children or by adoption. The purpose of Levitical law in such cases was to ensure that the dead man's name and possessions stayed in the possession of the clan, and Onan was therefore expected to comply with the duty laid on him by law and give the widow children to which she had a right in law. Thus Onan's action flouted the law, refused the widow her rights and was hurtful to the whole family. He was certainly not punished simply for interrupting sexual intercourse (p. 181 ff.). It is thus quite clear that the name 'onanism' is wrong and that masturbation can no longer be regarded as a sin. We will return to this question (p. 138).

Relationships with persons of the same and the opposite sex, the search for erotic and sexual ties, are first contracted between the child and its parents. In early childhood the parents' marriage is taken as a matter of course by the child but later there is an active attempt to manipulate it because of the unconscious drive towards a close relationship with the parent of the opposite sex. The boy wants to have mother for himself alone and the girl wants to take over her father; both show a tendency to seek close physical contact with the opposite parent. Not uncommonly the boy has the unconscious wish to marry his mother and replace his father, and occasionally he will say so. Similarly the girl is attracted to her father, comes into unconscious rivalry with her mother and makes up to father. There may even be an unconscious wish for sexual relations with the father. These strivings are elementary in a child of 5 to 6 years old, and have found their expression in early human history in myths and sagas. Anyone who has noted this will be able to observe the phenomenon in uninhibited children in a great number of variations. Boys seek to imitate their father in behaviour towards the mother and show that they are men; they may be especially attentive, helpful and tender. The girl imitates her mother and seeks to draw father's attention to the fact that she also is a woman. This brings the children in competition with their parent of the same sex and their siblings, whom they regard as serious rivals, trying to cut them out at any price. Boys and girls also find their parent of the same sex more powerful and feel that their desires are threatened by the latter; hence they seek to avoid this threat by once more identifying with the parent of the same sex, the son with the father and the daughter with the mother.

Children cannot disturb an intact marriage and are therefore disappointed and obliged to overcome their sexual and erotic wishes within the family by a return to identification. They have learned in this phase of development (up to about 6 years old) that they must look for their sexual goal outside the home, so they now seek it in older persons of the opposite sex though their veneration often goes unnoticed. Then follows an inclination to children of the same age with whom ineffective but sexually tinged relations are attempted.

These childhood wishes may have serious consequences for a disturbed marriage. If for example the mother is not getting enough affection from her husband she may all too readily respond to her son's sexual wishes by creating a fairly powerful bond between them. The resulting 'mother's boy' is not usually too much harmed, but it becomes tragic if a bond of this kind cannot be broken to enable him to choose a partner. Either the young man is then incapable of attachment to a girl of his own age, or he simply looks for a mother substitute in his future wife. It is not uncommon for marriages of this sort to be upset by the man's impotence because he has unconsciously transferred the social barriers against incest from his mother to his bride. Moreover in such a mother-son relationship there will be constant competition with the father, since there is no possibility of identification with him. In consequence the mother's boy has difficulty in working with other men and tends to be either a solitary person or an unpleasant thruster.

If however from the start the mother rejects every affectionate and erotic approach of her son, as she has done with her husband, both father and son will end up by taking a defensive position against women. The boy will later prefer homosexual relations, even when he should be thinking of marriage.

Just as significant are the results of an incorrect attitude of father towards daughter; indeed most fathers respond all too well to their daughter's blandishments, perhaps because the ageing male is flattered by her attentions. He considers that a response to these is less dangerous than one to the adoration of a girl unrelated to him. It is remarkable that the expression 'father's girl' is virtually unknown although every young girl wants a husband who—like her father—is superior to her, can guide her, can be leaned upon, and can be looked up to, rather than a true partner. This view of errors in paternal behaviour and their consequences is supported by the finding that in our culture girls obviously still cannot regard their femininity as of equal value with masculinity; they still think they have been short-changed and therefore seek the support of a male, which of course they can get only from someone stronger than themselves. A strong bond between father and daughter can later upset the girl's marriage by interfering with her sex life even to the extent of causing frigidity, if the social ban on sexual relations between father and daughter has been transferred subconsciously to the husband as a father-substitute. If however the father totally rejects his daughter's sexual advances, as he has done with his wife, mother and daughter may combine to gang up against the male sex. Thus the natural rivalry of women and their traditional wooing of the male may be completely reversed.

It is obvious that the development of ability to love may be hampered and indeed destroyed in many ways through errors of behaviour of the parents. One of the greatest misunderstandings as regards love will be the individual's later confusion between loving and being loved. A person often believes himself to be greatly in love when his real wish is to be loved, though he can only be loved to the extent that he is himself capable of love. All expectations beyond this will be doomed to disappointment. Hence the first six years of life are of the greatest importance for the sex education of both sexes; what is not learned then will never be learned. Fortunately, nowadays there are means available to help a personality to mature when the causes of the trouble are correctly assessed. These aids include the counselling of both children and adults as well as the actual treatment of the maladjusted.

Answering Children's Questions

The first questions

The first questions about sexuality will come when the child is about 2 to 2½ years old. These questions, like all others at that age, are factual and should be answered factually and straightforwardly in accordance with the child's understanding. This will be easier if the parents have talked to each other freely about these things. Experience has repeatedly confirmed that if parents are to give a child the correct answer at the right time (determined of course by the child) they must have previously talked about these matters more than once among themselves. It is not enough to read up answers, because when the moment comes the parent's inhibitions may prove stronger than his book knowledge.

For example, a teacher discussed the origin of babies with a class of girls, all of whom listened intently and then promised they would tell their own children the truth. When however they went over to acting parts in a play, one actress who was asked about babies said promptly that the stork was responsible. After initial laughter the class were brought to see how strong the tendency is to repeat what one has heard in early childhood. This is also true of adults, parents and teachers unless the latter take care continually to bring their new knowledge in line with changes in behaviour (p. 20 ff.).

The first question related to sex will be: 'Where did I come from?' or 'Where do babies come from?' This question may be stimulated by the arrival of a new baby in the family or among the neighbours, or by seeing a baby in a pram, or from casual remarks made by adults. Thus, one 2½-year-old boy discovered a briefcase and asked about it; he was told that his mother had used it when she used to work. Since he had no idea that his mother had ever worked he asked: 'And where was I then?' In such a case a correct answer would have been 'You were still in mummy's tummy', or with a variation in the question: 'Babies come out of mummy's tummy'.

In the first place, this answer is true and need never be contradicted. Secondly, for small children the abdomen is the centre of life. All small children refer their physical and mental pain to the abdomen, and at this age it is indeed the centre as far as anatomical proportions are concerned, while this is the age at which a child tries to possess an object by swallowing it. The answer: 'You were under mummy's heart' is only *apparently* a factual answer since it avoids the facts by displacing pregnancy to a higher plane above the diaphragm. Adults who give this answer want to emphasize the close association between mother and child but they overlook the child's belief that the abdomen and not the heart is the focal point. Using the fable of the stork is quite wrong, for it represents the parents' retreat from sexuality as much as do other popular explanations, but it does contain sexual symbolism, with the stork's beak as the penis, the pond as the ovary, uterus and amniotic fluid, the chimney as the vagina. However the child in our age and culture is inaccessible to symbolism, and we do not speak in symbolic terms about anything else.

It is equally reprehensible to describe God and Heaven as the origin of babies. Such an answer evades the real issue in the child's question, and it is dangerous for the parents to refer to 'the loving God' just because they do not want to give the child the good news about the use of His instrument of sex. This is not to say that biological facts should be divorced from religious beliefs but the spiritual truth of the origin of the child from God's hands must not be made a handy substitute for a straight answer to a straight question. True religious belief ought to be a direct stimulus to give to the child the correct facts in a clear and open manner, so as to awaken in it reverence and joy over what God has allowed to happen.

The negative answer 'You weren't born then' is evasive and puzzles the child, for it cannot understand 'not being' quite apart from the fact that the word 'born' means nothing to it unless it knows about the birth process.

The child's second question is usually the direct consequence of a correct answer to the first: 'How do babies get into their mummy's tummy—how did I get into it?' The question has several causes. First of all, the abdomen is a part of the body into which something goes (food) and from which something else comes out again (faeces). The child is therefore asking in logical sequence, though it also cannot understand how an object as big as itself could find room in mother's abdomen. There is also a wish to return to the protection of mother's interior, while there may also be an unconscious fear of being 'eaten' by mother. (Children of this age love to hear stories about people being eaten, e.g. Red Riding Hood. Thus they work through their fear of being eaten and their joy in being alive.)

Hence the answer to the second question must be the truth; it must satisfy the wish for security and relieve the fear of being eaten. It must also be borne in mind that the child has *not* asked about sexual intercourse. Many parents assume that it has, and are consequently embarrassed about answering. The answer should run: 'You were in mummy's tummy ever since you were a small egg' (p. 116).

The child's third question, which may follow at once, is 'How did I get out of your tummy?' The answer should be something like this: 'After you had grown from being a little egg into such a size that you hadn't enough room inside mummy you were born through the hole between mummy's legs'.

With increasing knowledge of the physical difference between man and woman (see pp. 24, 26, 27), the child will ask where father comes into the picture, but this question often comes a very long time after the other three. When it does come, the question is also related to emotional attitudes towards mother and father (p. 46 ff.). Since it often does not know how to frame its question, for it probably does not know what it is aiming at, the child may wrap the question up, for example by saying: 'What grows inside daddy?' or 'Is daddy only here to earn money?' or 'Am I related to daddy?' or 'Can't another daddy earn money for us?' In answering these questions the chance should be taken to repeat and add to what the child has been told previously. A dialogue between father or mother and a 5- or 6-year-old might run like this: 'You know that babies grow in mummy's tummy. But to make the egg into a baby daddy has to add a seed to it. The seeds are in daddy's testicles and come out through his penis. If two people love each other, and want to live together and marry, and then want babies, they lie close together. Then the husband puts his penis into a passage between his wife's legs and his wife takes his seed in. When seed finds the egg, the egg begins to grow inside mummy's tummy'. 'Is that what happened with me?' 'Yes, it always happens that way if the egg is to grow'.

As a result of its own observations in the neighbourhood, the child may then ask about the situation when a mother is unmarried, and of course this point will arise if the child is personally affected. It is a hard thing for the unmarried mother to have to explain indirectly or directly that she did not have the security of the marriage she is recommending to her child when she took a lover, but for honesty's sake she must admit this. When she does, if it is at all possible she must also tell the child that at the time she became pregnant she and the man really were fond of each other. This is important, for these children need to be assured that at the beginning of their lives love was present. Then in spite of the absence of a father they can create for themselves a positive father image. For a widow all this is naturally much easier.

Step-parents or adoptive parents also have difficulties when the child asks about its origin, but this must be cleared up before the child goes to school. If not, the lie involved will exercise a corrosive influence on confidence and trust and become a significant source of disturbance in the family. Not only that but the child will have the additional pain of learning the truth about its origin from classmates or other adults.

All the facts mentioned above ought to be imparted to the child before it goes to school. It can then, together with the capacity for social life it has acquired (p. 42), solve the problems of detachment from the parent of opposite sex and identification with the other parent (p. 46) and apply its school work to its plans for gaining experience and conquering the world.

Questions before and at puberty
As a result of reflections or conversations with its schoolfellows the child will at the age of about 8 or 9 years start repeating its questions about the origin of babies and about procreation in general. This wish to know more is often clearly detectable, and this runs parallel to the discoveries about its body the child makes before puberty, when the boy observes his first erections and the girl finds out that it is pleasurable to touch her external genitals. In conversations with children, the parents should prepare them for puberty by pointing out that sexual intercourse is an integral part of marriage and is not related to the intention to have babies. After repeating previous information, the male parent may say something like this to his son: 'You've noticed that when your penis gets bigger and stiffer it feels very nice. When you have grown up, it will feel even nicer. Women also get these nice feelings'. For a girl one might say: 'When you're older, you'll find that as a woman you get nice feelings. Men have them too'. For both: 'Wives like to feel a penis inside their vagina, and husbands like to put their penis inside their wife. Because it is so nice, parents do this often and not only when they want a child. It is a very important part of being married. But because they may start a baby any time they do this, they must think carefully before marrying, for it's important to stay together for always, so that there will always be a mother and a father to look after the children'.

There may be opportunities with children of this age to exert an influence on factors involved in later choice of partner. Both boys and girls often express their thoughts about girls or boys they like and might perhaps marry. For example, one boy of $9\frac{1}{2}$ asked if his family was related to another one. After he had been told that they were not, his mother asked why he wanted to know and he answered that if they were not related he would be able to marry the other family's daughter. Mother then asked why he was interested in this girl and there was a long conversation about choosing partners, with lively participation from the boy. If we remember that it is very difficult to have conversations of this sort with 16-year-olds because they have entered puberty and are therefore not disposed to take any notice of their elders about things they have already decided on, the extraordinary importance of such earlier discussions becomes obvious. In addition, if adolescents have been prepared in this way and have freely discussed the topic at home, they will later be willing to engage in further discussions spontaneously and without emotion, although any decisions must of course be their own independent ones.

Unfortunately many parents inhibit such questions and discussions from the start by telling the children that when father and mother love each other they have a child. Information of this sort narrows down marital love to procreation, and in consequence the children will draw the conclusion that their parents no longer love each other because no more children appear. Moreover, when the concept of love and conjugal life has been so narrowed down to the sex act the adolescent will conclude that love must and can only be expressed in intercourse, that a child will follow and that then people get married. This idea is still widespread but it has a somewhat limiting effect on choosing a partner.

In talking to children about the significance of sexual intercourse in marriage, it is also necessary to point out the possibility of preventing pregnancy and that this possibility is utilized, thus introducing the idea of responsible parenthood (p. 175 ff.). How far the child is informed over means and techniques of contraception can be left to the individual situation, but the information must be given. It can be discussed in greater detail when the child has made some discoveries for himself or had his attention drawn to the matter by third parties. This happens not infrequently by the age of 8 or 9, and children will come with their questions to their parents only if the subject has already been mentioned at home.

It is a good thing for parents to illustrate their explanations with some simple sketches or with pictures such as are to be found later in this book. The child should also be told where to find more pictures and text about the subject, thus avoiding the need for it to search in pornographic literature or make secret raids on the family bookshelves. It is clear that the first answers will need to be expanded and their content repeated as the child develops.

Before they reach puberty, i.e. at the latest by the ninth or tenth year, boys and girls must be informed of the structure and function of the sexual organs of both sexes, know the essential about marriage and the family, and be aware in principle of the primary part played by mature sexuality in the relations between husband and wife not only in production of children: a responsible approach to choice of partner, marriage and parenthood must have been created.

Influences outside the home
As he grows older the child is also influenced by factors outside the home, by conversations and activities with other children and with adults. In both instances the child who has been well prepared by parents and well informed about sexuality has the best defence against evil influences. However every child, just as it should be informed by degrees about normal sexuality, should also be warned about the dangers of abuse and sexual violence inflicted by

perverts. The latter seldom start talking about sexuality with children but awaken their curiosity and desires for other pleasures first and thus seduce the child into going with them or doing things with them. It is important in this connection for the child to be sceptical and not gullible (p. 43 ff.), and also to know that he can confide to his parents all his wishes, experiences, discoveries and observations and not be obliged to keep silent for fear of punishment. All members of society must, however, bear in mind that children are particularly easily seduced because of their constant search for new experiences, and therefore are in need of protection. We also know that the type of child who has been prohibited from learning about sex in the ordinary way will turn his vague curiosity and his desire for novelty in other directions, and is therefore a ready prey. It is not surprising that seducers and criminals almost subconsciously choose these children as their victims. Hence apart from the protection which society must extend to its young, a sensible sex education, carried out early enough, offers some security in this respect.

The child starting in nursery school will come under other influences, and the staff should be informed of the state of its sexual knowledge so that they can cooperate with the parents in dealing with its questions, as expressed verbally or in play. Experience has shown that heads of nursery schools perform a service by reminding their charges' parents from time to time of their responsibilities for sex education, by communicating their own observations to the parents and by offering help, for example with books, in this respect.

This is equally true of primary school. In the first four years of primary school, the most important task the teacher has as regards sex education is to keep reminding the parents, collectively or alone, of their responsibility and to offer help with it. Both male and female teachers, by reason of their training, the guidelines laid down by government and school administration, and the support of the parents, should be able to introduce suitable discussion into the curriculum, taking constructive, educational and systematic action. I have already pointed out that this is not so much a matter of explanation as of continuing guidance along the road to maturity, and that this is part of general education rather than of biology.

After the first four school years this education should continue, but it must be stressed that the work done by the school can never replace the parental influence; it can only support it. However, sex education belongs to the inalienable tasks of any school that takes its job of preparing people for life seriously. The better the school does this, the sooner will the future parents be in a position to bring up their children properly.

Puberty and Adolescence

Development and Education before and at Puberty

Puberty begins with the appearance of physical maturity and ends with the full anatomical and physiological development of the sex organs and the so-called secondary sex characters. It is impossible to state exactly the age at which this happens, for the processes are subject to very considerable individual variations. On the average the first menstrual period (menarche) in girls appears between the twelfth and thirteenth years, though girls are not uncommonly menstruating by the age of 10 or even 9. The first seminal emission or ejaculation in boys appears at about the fourteenth year, but there may be emissions at night by the age of 11 or 12. By about the seventeenth to eighteenth year the genitals in both sexes have reached their final size and functional potency (shown by production of predominantly normal mature spermatozoa or sperm cells in the young man and by regular menstruation in the girl), while the secondary sex characters (hair growth, voice, breasts, typical build) are fully developed.

Emotional tensions in puberty
Parallel with this physical maturity caused by hormones there is a process of transformation in the mental and emotional areas which is even more remarkable, and this process is already heralded in the so-called pre-puberty period. This period before maturation generally begins between the eighth and tenth years and lasts until the first signs of genital function, at about 12 to 14.

Pre-puberty is characterized by increased mental activity, increase in strength and a very marked self-will. This self-will is an attempt to separate off one's own sexual role from that of the opposite sex and to identify the role with those of one's peers. Of necessity therefore the members of the two sexes isolate themselves, cannot bear each other and are extremely rude to each other. The ideals of independence and self-will are excessively displayed in a second 'negative phase' and at the same time the subjects become more irritable (especially girls, who often have emotional storms), or obstinate as well as impatient (especially boys). Simultaneously there is a second change in bodily configuration with disproportionate growth of the limbs, ushering in the beginning of the maturation process.

The emotional phase of development before puberty marks the end of childhood, and leads to a second phase of coming to terms with adults. The tendency to take the initiative and bring one's own forces into play is in internal conflict with a simultaneous longing for loving protection, safety and security in the home. There are inevitable internal and external conflicts with parents and other persons in authority. It is therefore important that teachers recognize all these changes as a normal part of development and do not give them exaggerated importance. The child about to become an adult must get a chance to work through his commendable struggle for independence. At the same time he must be able to feel that the parental protection will not necessarily be withdrawn just because he wants to be independent. But an adolescent should not only be allowed his head; in spite of his revolt he should be integrated into the community of the family, given some serious commissions, and shown that the family takes a sympathetic interest in his problems. This is the only way to incorporate his mental and emotional powers into a new form of sociability.

With the onset of puberty the subject retreats within himself, for the first stirrings of sex upset all the familiar forms of relationship with his environment; it takes a few years before he succeeds in getting his internal and external bearings and reaches stability. With good handling there will develop out of the negativism a goal-centred and differentiated appreciation of will and thus reintegration into the world. During this transition, at first involving all areas of experience, there will be ambiguities, uncertainties, and sudden swings from one extreme to the other. They are experimental, while the subject is seeking a way between opposing tendencies.

Puberty (together with pre-puberty) has been described as 'the melting pot of the personality'. This is the time when all the basic needs of the person (now stronger and more independent) and all previous attitudes and behaviour patterns are once more put in the melting pot for clarification and purification. Unresolved conflicts from the earlier years break out with renewed ferocity. If the child's wishes for relationship, possession, status and love meet with the same rejecting attitudes from parents and other mentors, the negative traits in construction of his personality will become more firmly fixed. These will lead to dramatic conflicts in the dynamic years of puberty and finally to firmly established deviate behaviour attitudes in relation to his fellow men and the world. Yet pre-puberty and puberty present a wonderful chance to create a great gulf between childish behaviour patterns and adult personality and to correct the errors of childhood by giving sympathetic leadership to the adolescent. This will happen only if the adolescent can contract a firm relationship with an adult (parent or mentor) prepared to show understanding, love and frankness and to give the time to it.

Crises involve all areas of development. They are normal and need not give rise to anxiety if one recalls that all these experiments in the areas of relation, possession, status and love are based on powerful drives. Attitudes considered valid in childhood are now rejected and the insecurity and ambiguity characteristic of puberty worked through.

At the same time the young person is trying by taking someone as a model to steer a way between intellect and impulse, between what should be done and what he wants to do, until he has formed his own new system of values. He can then manage his responsibilities, armed with his own powers. Adolescents who do not go through these obvious crises should be suspected of developmental disturbances just as much as those whose crises have ended in insuperable and continuing conflicts with the world. Both types of disturbance require expert help which will mainly consist in a change of environment. It is quite wrong to believe that these disturbances will be grown out of in time. Puberty, like early childhood, is an optimal time for corrective education.

Sexuality in puberty is one of the areas of crisis, and this is particularly so in the average adolescent because this area is still to a large extent taboo in society. One further problem is that although physical and sexual maturity come early, sexual activity is approved of only after marriage. And statistics show that on an average European men marry for the first time at almost 25 years of age, and women at almost 24 years. Thus there is a period of almost 15 years in which sexual drive must find an outlet other than intercourse. Because society is aware of this (and also the educators) there is an unfortunate delay in explanation and information about this drive, in the belief that this atmosphere of ignorance and prohibition will make it easier for the adolescent to suppress his sexuality. This is entirely wrong, for only when it is fully understood can the adolescent, with growing sense of responsibility (p. 25) and with personal insight, deal with it in a sensible manner. This assumption of responsibility in sexuality is also true of other basic drives. The powerful drives towards contact, possession, and status, which the adolescent would like to satisfy immediately, must be under conscious control. They can be satisfied only through work and achievement inside society and not through sycophancy, theft, or fraud. The wish to satisfy sexual urges immediately is thus only a pubertal attitude and not that of a mature man or woman.

Informed education

In pre-puberty and puberty, factual education is therefore the watchword. It even has priority over transmission of attitudes and behaviour patterns, because the adolescent will himself learn to take decisions and find out his personal limitations. But he can do this only if he has enough factual information available.

However in pre-puberty or puberty any attempt to convey fresh information as advice may run into difficulties because of the common adolescent protest against adult superiority.

In imparting information there must be understanding of the young person's problems and he must be taken seriously at every stage of development. One must remember how easily adolescents are offended and that they have sexual and erotic wishes which at first are undirected, then during puberty charged with imagery and only later goal-directed but even so often unreal. If the information can be added to earlier education as a continuation of the latter, so much the better. It is not enough to give adolescents books to read. This can help only if preceded by sympathetic dialogue, repeated from time to time and from various angles.

Boys and girls need some preparation for the appearance of ejaculation and menstruation, usually at about 10 years but at the latest when a spurt forward in growth heralds the imminent onset of genital function. This preparation must include detailed information on the anatomical structure and function of the sexual organs in both male and female, so that the child's own maturation can be seen in relation to that of the other sex. The fact that when the boy first experiences an ejaculation he has a hitherto unknown sensation of pleasure, in contrast to the girl, who regards her menstruation as 'being unwell', must be taken into consideration. It is important to note this distinction and to state why, for at this age of critical study of the world the young person expects statements about processes or behaviour patterns to be justified, and any educational effort not backed up by evidence will be rejected.

Physical maturation
The boy experiences seminal emission as biologically necessary and agreeable, since the process serves to maintain human life on earth by fertilizing the ovum. All physical processes and conditions which serve to maintain life, such as eating or drinking, warmth and harmony, are experienced as pleasant, while all events threatening life, such as hunger or thirst, cold and quarrelling, are experienced as unpleasant or injurious. Hence, the menstrual flow must be experienced as unpleasant for it is the visible sign that an ovum, that is, a possible life, has died off for lack of fertilization.

Boys and girls alike must be taught the details of sperm and ovular maturation and of procreation, fertilization and birth, which they are well able to understand at this age. They must also be taught about the significance of choice of partner and must recognize that sexuality needs to be integrated into the whole relationship between husband and wife. Only if the parents discuss these questions openly, confidently, honestly and seriously can the adolescent develop a healthy attitude to sex and also a genuine feeling of modesty. We will deal with the preparation of the girl for menstruation in the section on the menarche and menstruation (see pp. 133 and 135). However it is also important to teach boys to realize and recognize the emotional lability of girls during menstruation. Here the boy can begin to learn to be considerate of feminine feelings.

It is important for the boy to have his new feeling of pleasure endorsed. He should be happy to have adult male feelings, just as the girl should be happy to be classed with adult women now.

In opposition to educational principles still being enunciated, it cannot be sufficiently stressed that a child is bound to take an interest in what gives him pleasure. It is therefore entirely wrong to minimize the ejaculatory pleasure of the boy or the menstrual malaise of the girl. Neither can take up their proper role unless they are allowed and able to be positive about their genitality. It is equally important for them to know about their different areas of experience. This is the only way to avoid errors of expectation or action due to ignorance of the opposite sex. Girls must learn later that every time they approach a boy erotically they stimulate him sexually and that the approach is regarded by him as a challenge to sexual activity. Young men ought to be told that the girl who has begun to menstruate experiences a double and often contradictory reaction to his approach in that she wants to respond erotically but not sexually. She realizes better than him that her sexual surrender includes the possibility of pregnancy and therefore feels fundamentally responsible for playing the parts of both sexual partner and mother. Failure to bear these differences in mind leads to misunderstanding and also to disappointment and misinterpretation of behaviour which all too often can end in an unwitting mental rape of the partner and unfortunately early and premature sexual relations. Both boy and girl are being challenged beyond their state of real maturity. The information given at this age about responsible parenthood and contraception will not be used as a licence for early intercourse if it is correctly integrated into education.

Both boys and girls indulge in masturbation, pleasurable play with their own sexual organs, often before puberty but usually at the time of genital development. In the male this is followed by pleasurable ejaculation and in the female by a feeling of sexual pleasure similar to orgasm. Masturbation is a normal accompaniment of development and is now almost the rule in both sexes. It is at first purely referred to the organ and during puberty is increasingly accompanied by sexual and erotic images (nocturnal dreams). Frequency of masturbation varies greatly, from once a day to once a month. It does not lead to physical or mental injury; any harm done is due to punishment of the practice and the feelings of guilt or inferiority aroused by punishment. It is abnormal only when practised with far greater frequency than usual, but even then it is merely a sign of other disturbances, usually of contact. Masturbation is a stage in healthy development which is spontaneously abandoned in later years. (Masturbation as a stage in maturation is discussed on p. 138 ff.; see also pp. 25, 45 ff. and 72.)

Development of sexual drive
Awakening and development of sexual drive run parallel to physical maturation. At first,

both girls and boys experience their genital tensions as related to themselves alone, so that they feel an undirected drive and indefinable longings. These lead to enthusiastic adoration of and passionate rapture for older persons of the same and the opposite sex, often far away and unattainable; they also lead to tensions with the parents accompanied by sexual fantasies related to the latter. In addition, in continuation of the prepubertal aversion to the opposite sex, there are feelings of love directed at partners of the same sex. These should be regarded as completely normal provided the partner is of similar age, even if the relationship involves individual or group masturbation, usually undetected by parents and educators. On the other hand any love relationship to older persons of the same sex must be viewed with suspicion (see p. 60).

Only gradually do partners of the same age group but opposite sex appear in the imagination and in reality. However, the latter are not desired sexually but only idolized and treated with excessive emotion. If sexual wishes are totally repressed at this stage there is a risk that development may be arrested here. The result in the male may be that he desires his wife only mentally and emotionally, separating off the despised but persistent need for relief of sexual tension which he satisfies either by masturbation or by intercourse with prostitutes; in the female, the wife's desire for the man may be arrested at the stage of tenderness while sexuality is repressed. If we briefly recall what has been said earlier about the sexual and erotic developmental stages in earlier childhood (p. 46 ff.), we will see marked analogies and effects. It is only gradually that a boy or a girl succeeds in concentrating the different needs and sexual wishes on one partner. In the beginning there are approaches highly coloured with aggression, the latter serving for self-protection and expressing the insecurity which is still making it impossible to surrender oneself. Boys like to romp, wrestle and argue with girls, and these incidents always have an undertone of sex and eroticism, as can be seen by observation or by the later discussions among companions of the same sex. Girls begin to behave coquettishly but when a boy responds they retreat at once into flippancy and haughtiness. This is the prelude to flirtation, which is usually indulged in by groups. Groups of boys or girls often express a quite honestly entertained resolve never to marry, but gradually the front gives way and the first timid attempts are made by individuals to approach individuals of the other sex directly, and to make harmless appointments to go out together. Rivalry among groups of the same sex then sets in and the groups dissolve. At this time there is often a change in appearance, and in an effort to please the partner the individual often resorts at first to the parental fashion in dress, only much later developing his or her own style, a transition aided by a sensible attitude of the parents.

These first delicate approaches may quickly break up and be followed once more by a period of isolation from the opposite sex until a renewed personal approach is made. In this respect differences between the more intellectually and the more practically oriented are seen, for the intellectual lets a long period elapse between his very first love and his next experience while he develops his mind, whereas the practical person rapidly deepens his relationships. This holds good for both sexes.

With the step towards pairing off of the sexes the ties with home are usually first perceptibly loosened, and there is an end to conflicts due to pubertal insecurity and excessive wilfulness, provided the parents accept the situation and neither ridicule these flirtations nor attach excessive importance to them. The rivalries between father and son for the mother and between mother and daughter for the father are now transformed into real rivalries between peers and become superfluous. If the parents try to show the child that his first inclinations represent only an incomplete form of love, the latter may be led to protest (even to the extent of marrying for spite) or to withdraw into himself through lack of confidence. Undue emphasis on these first relationships because the parents would like them to be serious puts too much strain on the child, who needs some variety in his first contacts in order to develop his own style relating to the opposite sex. He cannot therefore entertain steadier relationships as yet.

At the end of puberty the possibility should exist of letting genital needs grow into tender inclinations, with formation of the first heterosexual friendships. These friendships are at first not genitally directed; in fact, sex is still kept out of them. Moreover, with the beginning of heterosexual friendships the activity of the sex organs loses its significance; for this reason, masturbation usually ceases with the end of puberty.

Deviations in sexual development
Deviations in sexual development in the widest sense occur when the above capacity is unattained. At the present day, delays in maturation are not infrequent, but what is more important is arrest at a stage in which sexual drives diverge widely from wishes for tenderness and interpersonal mental and emotional harmony. If the desire for release of sexual tension becomes obsessional, this is usually a substitute satisfaction for other unfulfilled areas of experience; and the youngster may harbour, usually unconsciously, the dangerous illusion that he can solve his problems by sexual satisfaction (either by masturbation or by early heterosexual contacts). If rivalry is unsuccessful (either in early childhood, see p. 47, or in puberty in relation to people of the same age) the unattainable partner of opposite sex will be devalued at the same time. But this leads also to a loss of self-esteem and a feeling of inferiority in relation to friends of like age; and the individual strives to become at least a man among men or a woman among women. Here lies the environmental basis of homosexuality in man or woman, in addition to the congenitally determined deviations.

If there is total failure to establish love relationships, sexual drives may be directed to substitutes. When for example the child at puberty already shows deviant inclinations towards smaller children (paedophilia) or animals (zoophilic inclinations), often following prepubertal eccentricity or an outsider attitude, the possibility of congenitally determined deviation must always be borne in mind. There may be deviations in sexual needs with substitute satisfactions for sexual activity as the goal. These are mostly due to severe mental disturbances in which either a part of the normal sexual sphere or parts which have played a special role in sexual development are valued for themselves alone and can alone lead to release of sexual tension. These substitutes include cruelty (sadism), infliction of pain on self (masochism), exhibitionism or the deviations in which only certain parts of the sexual partner such as parts of the body or items of clothing can induce orgasm (fetishism). Even these disturbances are foreshadowed in puberty and recognizable by the skilled observer. They require intensive treatment. One other form of deviation consists in wearing clothing of the opposite sex (transvestism).

Adolescence and Preparation for Marriage

Emotional development is unfinished at adolescence

Adolescence begins at about the seventeenth year, and by about 20 to 21 years physical development both in height and breadth is finished. But in our culture of today mental and emotional development does not cease until about 22 to 24 years for girls and 23 to 26 years for men. This leads to difficulties both for the adolescent and for society. Young persons of this age group find themselves in full possession of physical powers and intelligence (mostly determined by inheritance and developed as a result of external influence), must often work hard at their professions, perform well, and earn well (often more than their parents) and can scarcely credit that their process of maturation is still unfinished. They measure their value frequently on the basis of the money they earn through physical or mental labour. Paradoxically, to be aware that one is not mentally and emotionally mature, one would need to possess the still absent maturity. Students also feel that by reason of their knowledge and their special studies together with their energy and ideals they are far superior to others. A certificate or degree conferred by school or university however does not testify to maturity but only to intellectual performance, just as the apprentice's certificate testifies to his skill in his craft. Society, which must introduce most adolescents to employment and social institutions, is in a dilemma because on the one hand it must acknowledge their achievements (so-called legal majority at 21 years) and on the other hand knows that they are not yet 'mature' in the sense defined by Schwidder as 'full and unimpeded capacity for freedom of decision and of action according to personal standards of order and value'. Experts now agree that this capacity is first reached in women at 22 to 24 years and in men at 23 to 26 years. 'It is only at this age that emotional development, capacity for love and acquisition of experience in inter-personal relations have proceeded so far that clear decisions free from illusion as regards choice of partner can be made' (Schwidder). Thus persons are mature enough for marriage only at about 24 to 25 years, when adolescence ends.

With the onset of adolescence begins the 'early childhood of adult life'. In comparison with puberty of course, emotional reactions and moods are more balanced, but the subject is in general still not very critical of either the world or himself. His plans and ideas still lack the test of reality and his enthusiastic espousal of high-flown ideals applies both to the world and to his aspirations for a sexual partnership; many years must go by before experience adjusts itself to reality. For this 'a system of guidelines and values for the direction of personal behaviour' (Schwidder) must be found. This is the main problem of adolescence.

Sexual disturbances and deviant behaviour
Inadequacy of contact in its widest sense leads to isolation, loneliness and poverty of experience and prevents or renders difficult the acquisition of real and practical knowledge. Disturbances in attitudes to possession manifest themselves either as failing initiative or acquisitiveness, or by the failure of the subject to handle money properly or else by his overvaluation of the commodity. There may also be disturbance of ability to acquire knowledge. Disorders in the area of status lead either to inappropriate thrustfulness (excessive aggression) or failure to stand up to others (pliability). The associated disturbance of the critical capacity makes it hard to gain one's own point; this is also commonly overshadowed by the excessive need for self-assertion. Disorders of sexuality are revealed not only by withdrawal from the opposite sex but also by perversion (see p. 61). Sometimes 'hyperactive' solutions may be sought which affect only parts of sexuality and doom to destruction any wholehearted partnership.

It is not uncommon in male adolescents to find unbridled sexual licence, whose origin lies less in heightened sexual needs than in disorders of contact, possession and status, which the subject tries to overcome in this way. The traditional recounting of sexual adventures at work and in school is a sign of this, for it is seldom the younger adolescent who takes part but rather the older man who ought to have reached maturity but shows by his talk that he has not. These discussions represent a considerable danger to younger boys still looking for their own value systems and led to believe by the others that sexual success is in itself valuable. This is yet another example of the significance of emotional impoverishment (see p. 37). It also demonstrates an attitude in which sexual intercourse is measured by material standards of performance and so introduced into the realm of competition and prestige. This isolates it even more from the human experience as a whole, and often makes sex a consumer good that cannot be dispensed with. Such an attitude usually leads to a frequent change of partner (promiscuity).

Sexual licence in young men, the Don Juan complex or more properly a manifestation of disturbance of contact, and its counterpart in women, must always be looked on as a sexual deviation, even though half the male population often or regularly have intercourse with a variety of partners before marriage. It should be noted that in contrast about a quarter of women have had premarital intercourse only with the future husband while another quarter have not had premarital intercourse at all. This does not mean that women and girls do not also indulge in sexual boasting, but because of their awareness of the relation between intercourse and pregnancy they are somewhat shyer of indulging sexual wishes without the protection of marriage. Whether this shyness will recede now that efficient contraceptive methods are becoming widespread remains questionable.

These disorders should be distinguished from signs of deviant behaviour, seen in young men as homosexuality. Such signs are commoner in girls, and are caused by a poverty of emotional contact which leads to an unfulfillable longing together with fear of entering into a permanent contract. These disorders may be expressed in idle wanderings but may also readily lead to changing sexual partnerships and to prostitution. Where there is such a tendency to deviant behaviour the combination of an attractive appearance with a low intelligence favours the slide into prostitution. It is very rare for excessive sexual drive to lead to promiscuity or prostitution; most prostitutes are in fact completely lacking in sexual feeling.

In cases where the search for firm guidelines and standards as a key to personal contact, possession and status has not been successful and has led to the above disorders, effectiveness and creativity may also be considerably impaired. Moreover, at times of crisis in human relations, at work or in sexual relations the internal conflicts arising may be so great as to cause physical or mental disorders. Treatment of these disorders can be successful only if it takes into account the psychosomatic relations and the underlying developmental disorders. An attempt must always be made to overcome these last as rapidly as possible; if these developmental errors are first encountered at the time of choice of profession or partner it is much more difficult to correct them, for already the consequences of earlier faulty decisions complicate the matter.

Models and social norms
The best aid to sound development in adolescence is the continuation of sensible sex education begun in childhood. As we have seen, this education depends to a large extent on models (more than prescriptions) with which the young individual can identify himself. In our time of reorientation of society on general democratic and partnership lines (instead of traditional and authoritarian and patriarchal ones) models are no longer reliable and may themselves be victims of insecurity, so that identification is harder. For these reasons the actual behaviour of adolescents may often seem in contradiction to their stated goals. They are plunged into insecurity by the very source from which they expect valuable standards to

guide their inner exuberance. Since also no definite ways to their goals can be pointed out, they are faced by the problem not only of finding their own goals but also of mapping out the course to the latter. Because this happens at a time in life when ideals and self-will are coupled with enormous ability to make their way, there are bound to be great deviations from the rigid and apparently invalid views of their parents.

The essential adolescent search for independent measures of order and value is never conducted in isolation but always in relation to the prevailing society. Standards are also dependent on attitudes acquired since early childhood, which are taken over as norms of behaviour. There is, however, no doubt that the individual of today increasingly regards norms as relative, and that their absolute validity has been shaken and is questioned everywhere. In ignorance of sociological relationships it is often proclaimed that, as a result of the loss of definite standards all round, these regulations devised by society in relation to sexual life are also invalid and should be dropped in favour of an unlimited and completely voluntary form of sexual behaviour. This idea is however not in accordance with the fact that maintenance of order is essential for the continued existence of a group. Since, unlike all other living things, man is lacking in instinct, and is therefore uncertain in his attitudes to nature, he must try to regulate his relationships by intelligence. The result of this intelligent arrangement of the general and human environment is his culture which lays down the rules that make social living possible. The norms of society are therefore as necessary for the individual as for the total cultural circle.

These norms are associated with a particular culture. Although we know that in another culture other norms are used effectively we cannot just transplant these spontaneously. Because sexual mores depend on the total culture it is impossible to designate one or the other as 'natural'. If we compare cultures and look at what they have achieved in terms not only of progress but also of regard for the intrinsic value and personality of the individual, we find an almost direct relationship between renunciation of sexual licence and height of culture. It is impossible on the long haul to enjoy the advantages of a high cultural level and at the same time unrestrained sexuality.

In our form of culture, man and woman as individuals and in the group are so closely related to each other that a general dependence of everyone on everyone exists (see pp. 13–18). Hence our culture demands of all that they take care of one another. This demand also sets the standard for sexual behaviour, for the personal encounter in sexual relations is more than release of sexual tension on a love object (see p. 70) and becomes complete within human limits only over the long term. Thus it needs official protection and this is granted in the recognition of the union as a marriage.

The young must also learn to observe our social standards. The difficulty is that youth with its compulsion towards sexual activity has to learn within a short time what has taken centuries of cultural development to become the norm in society. Only if young people have already had help (see p. 42 ff.) in regulating their development can they adapt themselves fairly easily to this standard and identify themselves with it.

The problem in modern education is that the system is no longer one of command and obedience but of attempts to obtain conformity with the existing order by other and more democratic methods. It is therefore necessary to deepen the understanding of adolescents for the maintenance of order and at the same time to show them that in our society monogamy is an aid to self-realization. Because the period between the beginning of physical maturation and the manifestation of mental and emotional maturity has become longer and therefore more difficult to deal with, new ways and methods must be sought to achieve the goal of monogamy. These new ways must be accepted by parents and teachers.

Falling in love and its disappointments
The goal of sex education and of sexual maturation is the complete encounter of husband and wife in marriage; on the way, incomplete phases are passed through. The risk for the whole enterprise is that a transient phase may be taken for the end goal because a complete encounter of husband and wife cannot as yet be comprehended in terms of experience (see p. 155). If a transient stage is mistaken for the goal the whole thing will go wrong. The exercises involved however do not start in puberty and adolescence but reach back into early childhood. The better they are worked through then, the easier will the next stage be for the young.

At puberty there is a wide gulf between sexual wishes and the ideal goal. On the one hand there is an enthusiastic adoration of individual persons (usually older persons at first) of the other sex. On the other hand there is a need for sexual release, relieved by masturbation. It is still impossible to think of the adored object sexually, and indeed this would seem like an insult. Gradually sexual desire becomes of less importance than the erotic feelings of love and respect (cessation of masturbation at the end of puberty), only to reappear later as sexual desire for the love object striven for (now a person of like age). At this time sexual desire is almost exclusively directed at personal satisfaction. Love is still an expression of the wish to be loved and made happy by the surrender of another. With this is associated a scarcely attainable longing for a happiness which it is expected or hoped will solve all problems. This is what makes sexual demands so pressing at ages between 17 and 21.

In addition, at this age the partner is greatly idealized. Out of a wealth of impressions formed so far in life, a mental picture of an ideal partner has been constructed. The material used to construct this mosaic has been contributed to by the parent of the opposite sex, particularly loved teachers of the opposite sex, siblings of opposite sex and childhood friends, the object of pubertal adoration, and last but not least prevailing views on beauty and other qualities of maleness and femaleness. At the beginning of adolescence this picture gains in imagination and is looked for in reality. The search for one's 'type' among those of similar age begins and appears to succeed but this is only an illusion. The person found is not seen as he or she really is but as the other would have him or her. If the searching youngster finds among the great choice of his acquaintances of the opposite sex an individual who displays one characteristic reminding the searcher of something known the latter may fall victim to the illusion that the person found has all the qualities desired in his type. This discovery is intoxicating and enchanting. This is the moment of the first great love, of the intoxication of infatuation. This transfer of an idea to a person (projection) cannot be seen through by the individual in love although outsiders may occasionally ask what has led to this incomprehensible fascination and come to the conclusion that love is blind. If the lover's view of the other is questioned, the projection will only become more fixed while the reality is overlooked. He will consider himself as admirably suited to the other and possibly behave as if this were so. In this way an inextricable tangle of mutual projections and identifications with the ideal picture of the other may arise; this seldom corresponds to the real personal qualities and even more seldom leads to the maturation of the personality. It is therefore necessary to have had previous talks (at the beginning of adolescence) with the young about the consequences of falling in love, so that they already have some insight into the condition, for it is impossible or nearly so to get any sense out of someone in love.

Every partner relationship begins with a fascination, for this is the reason for seeking closer contact, but every fascination dies after a shorter or longer time, and disappointments always lead to its death. These essential disappointments arise because at last the partner has been at least partly seen as he is. Such a disillusion may and should be helpful for development of personality and for the partnership. It is helpful when it is recognized that the disillusion means the end of an illusion about the partner; this recognition can lead to a real relationship involving the whole person of the partner. Disillusion is only a disadvantage when it is made the ground for reproaching the other person. The danger of a long-lasting infatuation may lie in the possibility that the young couple will marry, without knowing each other even in part. When disillusion comes later the disappointed one no longer has the full freedom to decide to get rid of the partner. It is not uncommon to find that sexual intercourse although it comes to orgasm is unsatisfactory, because emotionally it has not been carried out with the actual partner but with a phantom, an emotional *fata morgana*. This however merges into a flesh and blood being with its own characteristics and reactions. There is mutual incomprehension and mutual disappointment but usually nobody has the courage to admit it. On the contrary, the illusion maintains its power for a while to cover up the misunderstanding, because it is closely related to personal vanity. There is no real love for the partner but only for a personal ghost of wishes and ideas thrown like a cloak over the real person; the disappointed one loves himself in the other.

If the disappointment is used to reproach the partner, this means that the ideal picture has been maintained. Either there is an attempt to re-educate the partner or the partner is abandoned in favour of a new object for one's personal projection. Heigl's remark applies to these cases, that 'falling in love is like catching measles without becoming immune'. Moreover the disease is not related to age, for it can recur just as long as the deception has not been worked through positively. Hence under the banner of 'the love of one's life' a person can fall in and out of love regularly without ever achieving a real partnership. In fact he can continue to do so when and after he marries, so that there are a series of marriages and divorces. These immature associations and their failure are a tragedy for the children, and this behaviour is not much of an example for them.

The positive working through of a disappointment begins with the recognition that the deception comes not from the partner but from oneself, in that it is the end of an illusion. If such illusions are given up and the projections taken back a real partnership may follow. Nor does this imply the search for a new partner, for the partner one was in love with may now be seen as a real person, approved of and loved as such. To understand one's partner 'completely' needs a long life together and the understanding is probably never really complete. Love begins when infatuation ends and the chosen partner is accepted as he or she is. For this there must be capacity for love instead of just the wish to be loved.

'Love is the ability to bestow upon one's partner responsible care, respect and understanding. Care means looking after the loved one and aiding the latter's growth and development' (Heigl). In contrast the infatuated person wants the other to be as he imagines her and does not want her to behave in accord with herself and her peculiarities.

'Responsibility means readiness to respond to stimuli, expressions and needs of the partner and to every manifestation of animation in the other. Responsibility therefore means making oneself available for the other' (Heigl). In contrast the infatuated person wants to perceive and respond only to the stimuli which are in accordance with his wishes. He wants the other person to be available to him. 'Respect means that one must have regard for the other and take into account his qualities, loving him not only for his good ones (this is usually easy) but also his shortcomings and weaknesses. Respect means recognizing the other as a person' (Heigl). The infatuated person wants the other as the object of his wishes, wants to bend the other to his intentions, wants to use the other.

'Understanding means knowledge of the essence of the other, with a sense of attraction for the other's personal characteristics which grows with increasing knowledge' (Heigl). The infatuated person thinks he understands the other but those personal characteristics which do not fit into his picture irritate him; on these characteristics his disappointment feeds, and they become a matter for reproach. The more the enamoured one knows about his partner the more he retreats, unless he abandons his infatuation as an illusion and begins to love in earnest.

Bases of partner choice

Choice of a partner is determined by a multiplicity of motives of which many are unconscious. There are however a whole series of points which should be taken consciously into account. The most significant basis for a happy choice of partner is equality of level. The following will make this phrase clear:

1. The difference in ages should not be too great. Otherwise there is in some circumstances a risk that a true partnership may be impaired through unreal expectations. (The girl may marry a man as a father figure or as a boy she has to bring up; the man may marry a woman who reminds him of his mother or of a little girl he wants to educate or to play with.)

2. Intelligences should be fairly equal. Anyone who feels he cannot tolerate an equally intelligent partner should ask himself whether he is simply making a marriage to exercise his absolute authority.

3. Educational levels should be similar. This is the only guarantee that both partners can really understand each other at the same level.

4. The circles from which the partners come should be similar. This is true both for cultural environments and for religious and social backgrounds.

Here we encounter the problem of mixed marriages. These may be either confessional or racial, cultural or social. Where encounters are continuous and direct as is the case in marriage, nobody can deny his origin however much secondarily acquired education, knowledge, or professional or social success he has to his credit. This is particularly so in marriages with racial or cultural mixing. Every young person who falls in love with someone from a foreign race and culture should ask himself seriously whether this love is not based on a projection. Marriages between people from different confessions are also problematic. Those who are closely integrated into their own religious circle are not likely to overcome the differences of opinion in their marriage which the confessions or religious groups have not yet overcome themselves. However those with no close religious ties who are willing to leave leadership to a more religious partner have an easier time, provided they are willing to recognize the authority of the other in these matters.

The significance of social and family origin is nowadays (unfortunately) often overlooked or devalued. Yet the imprint of the parental home is the decisive factor in later attitudes to life in all its areas. False attitudes can be corrected, of course, but there are no means of entirely obliterating the influence of the parental home or reversing it. Manners and customs in daily living have been imprinted from there and can be changed with great difficulty if at all. To demand change from a partner when he does not want to change is to impose too great a strain.

5. The partners should be free of hereditary disease. Illness and frailty, even if not hereditary, should never lead to a marriage based on pity. Nobody, least of all the handicapped person,

is helped by this. The person with a severe illness or handicap should ask himself very seriously whether in view of his responsibility for the marriage and children he ought to share his love with another. If all he wants is to be looked after, he should abstain from marriage.

Premarital encounters and associations
Choice of a partner implies that there is really a choice, and so every opportunity should be seized for young people to meet and get to know one another spontaneously. This is a serious problem in modern society where the tendency is for very early attachments and intimate relationships. A very early attachment even when it has arisen out of genuine and illusion-free motives of attraction means loss of growth in experience, such as is possible in general encounters between the sexes, in group activities or in social life.

If a boy and a girl go steady they become isolated from their environment, which they now encounter only when alone at work or at school. Leisure meetings no longer mean contact with others but isolation as a couple with other similarly isolated couples. It is not surprising that friendships of this type very soon lead to intimate relations. In the first place the couple have not learned to occupy themselves together without sexual tensions, and secondly their own social maturity is not sufficient with the passage of time and in spite of all previous resolutions to prevent their yielding to the need for release of sexual tension. Finally the common opinion that the full joy of love can be found only in the total and unrestricted encounter of two persons reinforces the yearning for sexual experience in a friendship isolated from the rest of society. All this is supported by arguments such as the one that sex must be tried out to see if the couple are suited to each other, and that premarital experience is essential if one is not to fail miserably on one's wedding night. Since the ultimate goal of marriage now demands more than it used to—absolute fidelity and the ultimate in mutual satisfaction with strong emphasis on sexual orgasm—this has the logical consequence that exclusive attachments are formed early and that an attempt is then made to ensure a happy sexual life by premarital experiment. It is therefore not astonishing to find that early sexual activity is widespread now in all social strata of our culture. There are also a variety of attempts to find new ways to deal with the time between the onset of physical maturity and marriage.

With the growing recognition that sexual experience and experience of the emotional reaction of the partner in intercourse cannot be applied unconditionally to the future marital partner, the former practice of young men of acquiring experience with prostitutes has receded and been replaced by formation of friendships with a basis of deep affection and positive disillusion, and with sexual intercourse; these friendships may endure and ultimately lead to marriage. In spite of all negative prognoses in the past, such marriages often turn out to be happy ones. It is true that in many cases the appearance of a pregnancy has hastened on the date of the wedding, but there is a growing responsibility for parenthood in respect of the child's upbringing. This is expressed by the care taken over contraception before marriage. Even if contraception is practised only so that the physical and emotional enjoyment of sexual intercourse may be assured over a long term, the motive of these measures is to be welcomed, for it must not be forgotten that this indicates a correct appreciation of parenthood.

The above group does not of course include all those sexual relationships in which the partners are not concerned with permanence and are not aiming at an exclusive and total sexual encounter. To the latter belong the associations based on mutual desire for sexual release which the partners desire for their physical well-being. There are also relationships based on the view that one must learn sexual techniques on as many objects as possible. Finally there are those in which an illusory projection is involved. All these relationships fail in respect of personal factors and lead to frequent change of partner. The connection with disturbances in the areas of contact, possession and status may be recalled. Pregnancies in these cases often lead to tragic shotgun weddings. In most cases it would be better for the family and society to stop pressing for marriage and to use the disillusion which often appears during the pregnancy to effect a final separation. Forced marriages have been found to be exceptionally crisis-prone and liable to end in divorce within a few years. The resultant bitterness often leads to an unconsciously motivated repetition of such an association or to isolation. If the disillusion and rupture of the relationship had been used to work through the situation, a fresh orientation might have been possible.

At this point the question of the meaning of the term 'premarital' should be raised again. In the strict sense all sexual relations before the official and legal conclusion of a marriage are premarital but this term embraces in different cases situations needing very different evaluation. Relations based on mere release of sexual tension or mastery of technique must be rejected, but this rejection refers not only to the premarital period but also to the marriage; such falsely based attitudes are not better or legitimate because they are first encountered in marriage. Their correction depends on the offer and acceptance of guidance and information.

Assessment of premarital relationships aiming at permanence and at a total encounter must be different, for this aim is maritally legitimate. Condemning the couple on the grounds that they have had relations before marriage must give rise to some perplexity in their minds, for they cannot logically understand why the same aim should be permitted after marriage and forbidden before it.

It would be of practical assistance if society could arrange sufficient opportunities outside working hours for young people of both sexes to cooperate on emotionally neutral tasks. This would create a desexualized environment. It would also make it possible for people to make contacts of all sorts in the pursuit of mutual or complementary interests and to get to know each other in a non-sexual atmosphere of sport, music, literature, social and political, religious and similar occupations. In the search for a desexualized environment it should be remembered that men are mostly stimulated sexually by visual signals and women by musical signals. Naturally, suitable situations must give opportunities for comradeship, friendship, flirtation and even the development of first love. They must never be isolated from the rest of the world but must remain open to its influences and also reach out into it. In these open mixed groups, in which care must be taken to maintain a balance, participants will have the chance to test out partnerships in many settings apart from the professional, scholastic or academic, without the need for closer ties than the situation demands. In addition, every participant will be tested out by the group and thus obtain valuable criticism of behaviour leading to greater maturity. Through changes in friendship within the group the opportunity to mature will arise before firm commitments are undertaken. On the other hand, a firm association which already exists or has been introduced into the group can be tested out and adjusted by a variety of standards, since other partners are available.

It is a significant task for modern society and its members and organisations to create such opportunities for youth as exercise grounds for social interchange and as training grounds for marriage. This work needs appropriate direction and should find a place for the widest possible variety of interests among the participants. A properly directed group also creates possibilities for objective information on sexual matters and for integration of the members into social institutions. Occasional casually introduced themes or even more formal presentations can be of lasting value, since they can be taken up and discussed repeatedly. This type of group discussion has undoubted advantages over more formal seminars in preparation for marriage, particularly if the latter are conducted with separation of the sexes. In seminars or courses with numerous participants limited only by age, the difference in levels between individuals may present an insuperable barrier because they cannot discuss things freely, either because they do not know one another or because they are not in the habit of talking together. Free discussion of sexual problems is possible only when trouble has been taken to bring out other problems and deal with them first. When the sexes are separated the corrective influence of the missing sex leaves a gap, and these groups are unsuitable for adolescents because they stick at a stage of development which belongs to prepuberty or early puberty and ought to have been overtaken long ago if a further delay in maturation is to be avoided. This does not mean that occasional transient withdrawal from the opposite sex is undesirable, but it ought not to be required on moral grounds; it should occur by free choice of the individual who must remain able to choose to withdraw if he finds the demands of his profession or training or hobby more pressing (see p. 39). Here again the youth group gives opportunity for development in the sense of learning early to respect one another's decisions.

In these groups in which boys and girls can channel their sexual energies in preparation for their place in society without needing to use them actively, the virtue of abstaining from intercourse until the final decision to marry has been made can be consciously practised without any need to belittle sex.

At this stage the family home has no great significance any more. The young separate themselves from it and seek their own way. The parents must now leave their offspring free to find their own way without trying to impose partnerships upon them and without prohibiting relationships they do not regard as serious. This is the time when the young must gather experience of contacts with the opposite sex through friendships and be free to change without creating a family tragedy. Parents must accept all these friendships without at first either approving or rejecting them. Any decisions must lie with the young and they must later abide by them. If parents are asked their opinion directly or indirectly, they should give an objective answer without concealing their views, but should avoid any direct or authoritarian intervention. If they find themselves unable to accept their children's friends or associates they should ask themselves whether this may be due to some illusory expectations. They should then try to find out whether their child's choice is based on some disturbance in the areas of contact, possession, status or love, and if they decide that it is they should take steps to overcome the disturbance. The most important thing however is to help the child to learn even from its errors, and in no circumstances to reproach it for making a wrong decision and for the consequences. The child must also be helped to work through its wrong decisions in a positive way, and must not be deprived of adult status and have its decisions made for it out of misplaced sympathy.

Necking and petting represent other attempts to bridge over the gap between physical maturity and the conclusion of marriage. This will be referred to elsewhere (p. 140 ff.). This is a form of responsible sexual behaviour provided responsibility and thoughtfulness are mutual and the attitudes and needs of both parties are taken into consideration. Games of this sort are a proper prelude to marital behaviour if they are not made an end in themselves, and demonstrate the effectiveness of social customs which do not regard premarital intercourse as the best solution to the problem and which prize premarital virginity highly.

Masturbation in the young is another attempt to solve the problems of maturity, but it is always an incomplete solution to the conflict, because sexuality directed towards a partner must remain unsatisfied by masturbation (see also p. 138 ff.). Nevertheless for many young people it is now the only possible way to resolve the dilemma between sexual desire coupled with the impossibility of marrying or having premarital intercourse on the one hand and of friendship in a desexualized atmosphere on the other. It should certainly not be thought of as more moral than premarital intercourse, but it should not be despised either. Especially in brain workers and students of both sexes it seems to represent a positively motivated means of controlling sexual energy even if it is a makeshift in cases where marriage and sexual relations have been renounced. Whatever the situation, young people must be made aware that the drive to masturbation may conceal a deviation in development. This is particularly to be suspected when the subject becomes as dependent on and dominated by masturbation as others are by drives towards sexual intercourse based on one's own pleasure.

Deviations into perversions and all forms of homosexuality must be regarded as abnormal and in urgent need of corrective treatment for the behaviour problem.

Early marriage

In view of the above there is a need to look into the attitude of society towards so-called early marriage. A distinction must be made between forced and voluntary early marriages. The former are marriages between minors which have been imposed on them because sexual relations have led to pregnancy. The partners are still at an age in which development is incomplete, and their action will have made maturation more difficult. This type of marriage is very liable to storms and often ends in divorce. Thus the child for whose protection the marriage was designed comes off worst of all. On the other hand there are early marriages in which the partners want to marry before they have completed their training and before they are economically independent. The desire for marriage may stem from a wish to regularize a situation in which they are living together or they may advance the date of the wedding because contraception has failed. There may however be other grounds. After mature reflection both partners may have come to the conclusion that their common preparation for marriage has reached a final point where a further postponement of intimate relations cannot be justified. In both cases an early wedding is to be recommended since the prerequisites except for the financial one are no different from those present if marriage is contracted later. These marriages scarcely come within the category of early marriages, but they are nonetheless marriages in which the partners are still financially dependent. Thus an essential element of marriage, the economic independence from parents or social institutions, has not been attained. This should cause the couple to take particularly seriously the problems of responsible parenthood and family planning.

If at some future time it becomes possible to arrange for sufficient suitable places for youth to meet in an atmosphere of preparation for marriage and family life and introduction to the social order, the number of premature marriages between immature partners will drop. Early marriage between partners who are still socially dependent but mentally and emotionally ready for this step will probably remain unavoidable, for periods of training for professions are likely to become longer, so that many 24-year-olds will still not have reached social and financial independence.

The engagement

In present climates of sexual behaviour the period of the engagement appears to be of secondary importance. However for many if not the majority of young people it is still the only way of getting the future partner acquainted with the family circle in a relaxed atmosphere. In most families also this official announcement of the intent to marry makes it easier for the two families to come together. The engagement is a time of intense testing of the partners, after they have publicly announced their intention to abstain from seeking other potential conjugal relationships. Whereas a pair can be friends without abandoning their choice of other friends, engagement means an abandon of other choice, for a choice has been made. The parties proclaim with the announcement of their decision their mutual love and respect and put themselves under the protection of those around them, who are now bound to respect their decision and abstain from disturbing the relationship. The engaged couple should however try to win the approval of their families and then to deepen this relationship. It is foolish to imagine that the only important matter is the mutual attraction of the couple, and to argue that they are not marrying each other's family. It is true that since the solidarity of the old powerful families has loosened they have lost a lot of direct influence over the marriage of their younger members, but there is still a place for a common attitude of the couple (each respecting the judgment of the other) towards the two families, even if after marriage they are going to live far removed from the influence of the latter. This is even more important if they are going to live in the immediate neighbourhood or in spatial and financial dependence on one or other of the two families.

The engagement is the last testing period before marriage. Apart from testing out the family the partners should undertake an honest assessment of themselves to examine whether they are truly ready to love their partner with tenderness, responsibility, respect and understanding. At this time it is necessary to meet often, for with geographical separation of the couple this self-examination is hard to undertake; there is always the risk that reality will be overshadowed by illusions and expectations.

If one or both partners come to the conclusion that the result of the examination has been negative, they should have the courage to part. What is more, the families and society should accept completely this last freedom to annul a partnership. A broken engagement is of course a breach of promise but it is not equivalent to the dissolution of a marriage even if intercourse has already taken place.

If the results of the test of engagement are positive, if false expectations have been dissipated and common ground has been consolidated, the partners should have the courage to marry and should not shrink from this step into a new life.

In spite of all preparation, every marriage represents the challenge of a common life needing daily renewal. However good the education it cannot guarantee the outcome, though it can and should make young people ripe for the trial. Hence the subsequent chapters of this book will contain detailed information about the physical and mental relations of sexuality in the individual, and about sexuality, pregnancy and delivery, in an effort to help men and women to understand their sexuality better and thus to make the best of their common way as married people and parents.

II

Sexuality and Sexual Relations

Man and Woman

Differences and Similarities

The differences in physical build between male and female first become apparent with increasing sexual maturity. In the newborn only the external genitals are different. Adults who know the infant's sex will however interpret many of its features as either male or female, such as its facial expression or its movements. These interpretations are not objective but based on the adult's experience of what we in our culture regard as male or female. If an infant is clothed, we believe that we are able to say with certainty that it is a boy or a girl. Only an unprejudiced observer unfamiliar with the way babies are clad might wonder.

Because a child born with female genitals finds itself faced with the expectations and demands of the world, its parents and the environment that it should behave like a girl, it learns to do just this and nothing else. Similarly a child born with male sex organs quickly learns to behave as a boy because this is expected and demanded of him. It may appear self-evident that parents and adults make these demands, but they represent an influence which should not be overlooked.

This influence and its effect on the subject depend greatly on the relevant culture, as many comparative studies of a great variety of the world's races have shown. Every child develops in its environment either as a male or as a female. In spite of all the innate differences within a culture and all the peculiarities permitted within a culture there is a definite standard picture of a man or a woman to which all members of the culture, male and female, conform.

However, since every mind has an influence on its body, the expected sex-specific behaviour pattern will also influence physical development. Obviously the mind cannot affect the inherited body build, but it will modify the way in which organs are used to a large extent; it will affect mimicry and gesture, the care of the body, the cosmetic or fashionable accentuation or under-emphasis of certain anatomical features, the strengthening of certain organs, or encourage the inability even to use what is there, will affect all degrees of capacity for expressing one's feelings, and even the capacity for forming relationships with

78 other persons or things. The biological development of the body of a child with female genitals during the time of maturation and growth differs from that of a child with male organs, because hormones produced in the body lead to the typical body conformation which we regard as female or male.

This physical development runs roughly parallel with mental development, but there are periods when crises appear because in our society there are transitory imbalances between the tempo of emotional and physical maturation. These periods are characterized by internal and external insecurity and require particularly delicate handling.

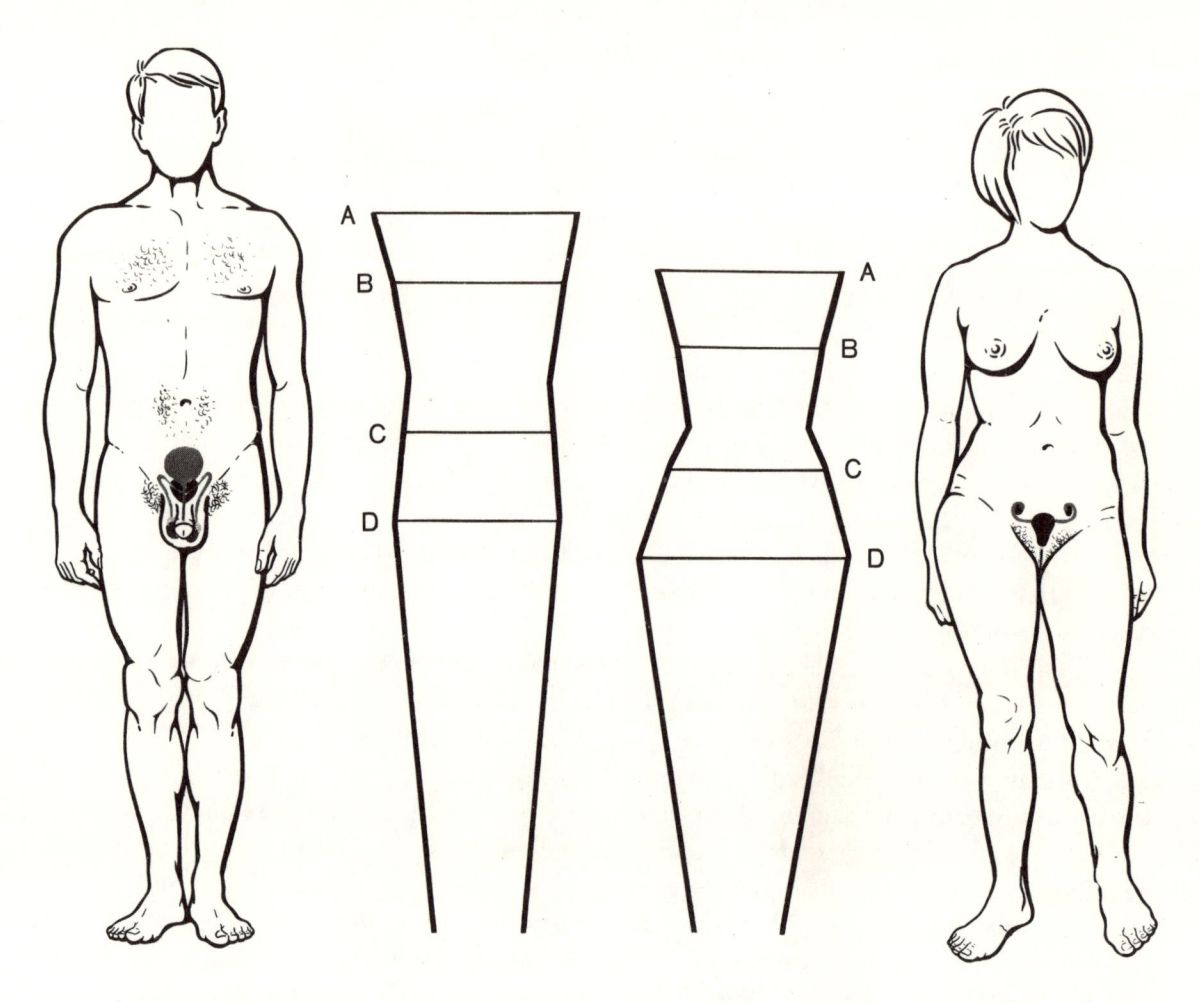

FIG. 2 *Body build of male and female. The sex organs and the typical sex characters are shown.*

A Breadth of shoulder girdle　　*B Breadth of chest*　　*C Breadth of pelvis*　　*D Breadth of thigh*

At the end of development the male or female body is completely mature, and its harmony reflects the unity of body, mind and soul. Such a unity can be attained at a wide variety of stages of development and in a wide range of ways.

The particular physical characteristics of male and female will now be discussed, bearing in mind however that this unity of body and mind is of great importance for the most intimate relations between the sexes. The basis of the differences between the sexes, apart from the impact of culture on them, is biological and consists in the differences in organs designed for different if complementary functions. We will therefore begin by describing these differences.

Male and female anatomy

On average the mature man is somewhat larger than the mature woman. The maximum width of the mature male body usually lies at the level of the shoulder girdle while that of the female lies at the level of the thighs. The female pelvis is generally broader and shallower than that of the male. The female bony pelvis (not shown in the diagrams) differs from the male one in that its upper surface is more everted to facilitate the descent of the baby during pregnancy and its passage downwards during delivery (see fig. 2).

In a general way the body of the mature female seems softer and more rounded than that of the male. This is due to the presence of a thicker layer of fat under the skin at the shoulders, chest and hips as well as the upper arms, and may make the subject appear flabby and fat at puberty. With increasing maturity and growth in height this unevenness, which causes some unhappiness to most girls, is smoothed out.

In the male the limbs appear longer than in the female, mainly because they are thinner and have less fatty tissue. Muscular development depends on the amount of physical activity. During puberty there may seem to be an isolated spurt in limb growth, so that the limbs may feel too long and unwieldy. Many boys at this age are clumsy in using their arms and legs, but this is only a temporary inconvenience.

Body hair

The hair distribution differs in the sexes. Whereas the length of hair on the head is dictated by fashion and in later years the male tends to lose hair sooner than the female (hence the predominance of baldness and receding hairlines in men), the distribution of body and facial hair is sex-determined. A mature woman usually has a delicate and almost invisible growth of hair on her face and body, while a man apart from his beard has a fairly strong secondary growth of hair on the trunk, principally on the lower abdomen in continuation of the pubic hair and on the upper part of the chest. Hair in the armpits is much the same in both sexes. The pubic hair (hair around the external genitals) in women stops at an upper horizontal line (mons veneris) while in men it continues upwards without a sharp boundary.

General sex characters
In the male the greater part of the sex organs is visible externally and only a small portion is concealed in the lower abdomen. In the female they are as good as invisible under the pubic hair, and for the most part lie within the abdomen. The sex organs of the female include the breasts, which make it possible to suckle the newborn child.

At this point the *erogenous zones* should also be mentioned; these are the skin areas where gentle touch leads to sexual stimulation (for details see p.153 ff.). In the male this zone is generally limited to the external genitals and their neighbourhood (upper and inner side of the thigh). In the female the whole of the skin is erogenous, especially the palm of the hand, the bend of the elbow, the outer side of the thigh, the inner side of the upper arm, the hairline at the neck, the dimple behind the ear, the breasts (especially the nipple and the coloured area round it), the inner side of the thigh and the pubic region itself.

Boys and Girls

External sex characters (see fig. 3)
These are already present in the unborn child by the third month of pregnancy and can be distinguished with certainty at the end of that month.

In boys at birth and up to prepuberty the penis is distinctly longer than the scrotum (in contrast to adults). The testicles or testes at birth can be felt as soft structures the size of lentils in the scrotum. At the end of the penis there is a protruding folded pocket of skin, the prepuce or foreskin, and if it is gently rolled back the rounded end of the glans penis with its opening of the urethra becomes visible.

By the second year of life boys learn to urinate while standing, holding the penis and pointing its aperture forwards and downwards. In girls the fissure between the adjacent major labia or lips is easy to identify but closed. When the child urinates with the legs apart in the squatting or sitting position (the adult position also) the opening of the urethra becomes visible between a pair of smaller lips (labia minor). Otherwise the very sensitive parts of the external genitals are hidden and protected within the fissure or vulva. These organs in both male and female have no sexual function until puberty.

Arousal of interest in sex organs
This interest is aroused in both sexes at an early age, though not earlier than the general interest in the child's own body and organs (such as the fingers, feet, nose, ears, mouth and anus) and their functions. The genitals are the object of particular attention because they are related to an interesting excretory function and are hidden from casual contact by the diaper. In addition, there is the regrettably widespread parental attitude and practice of

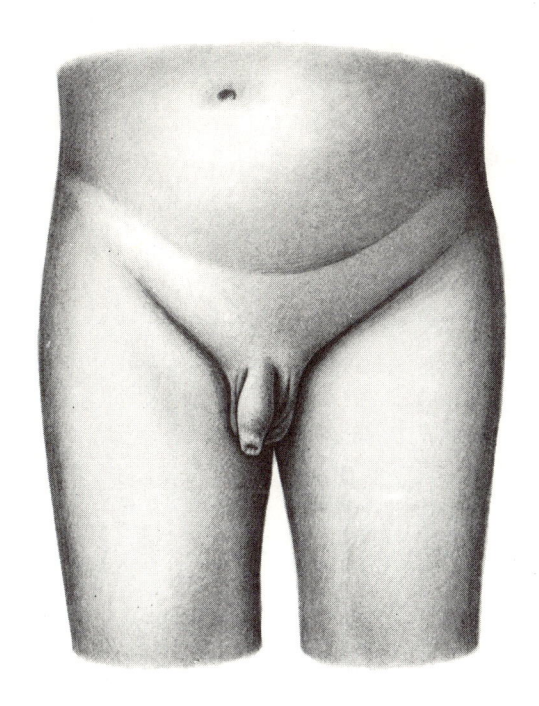

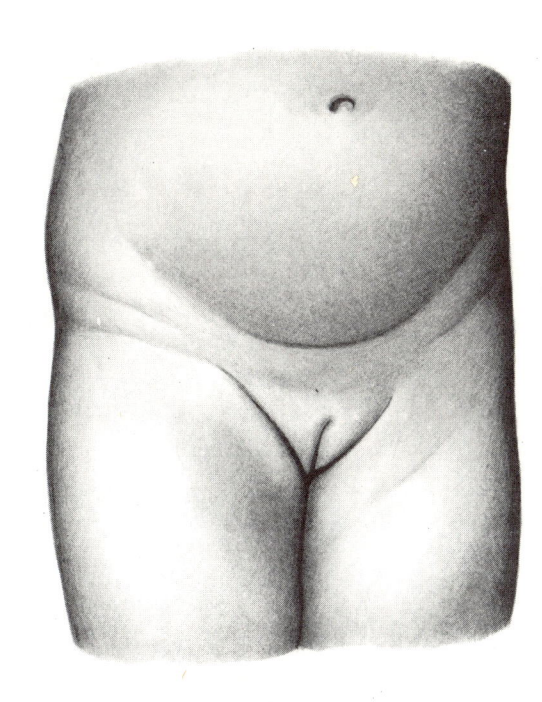

FIG. 3 *External sex characters of boy and girl before puberty.*

suggesting, at least in the child's presence, that the genitals are inferior organs with a value to be equated with the excretory products they expel from the body. Occasionally, a similar barrier between the child's person and his genitals may be erected on the basis that they are 'sacred' property.

Both attitudes and the consequent practice are wrong. As soon as the infant, whether male or female, begins to grasp things it should be given the opportunity to touch its genitals (for example when it is changed, in the bath, or when it is kicking around on a hot summer's day). These organs are commonly named in accordance with their primary function in childhood, urination, but it is advisable to give them their right names from the first—penis, vulva and so on (see p. 26 ff.).

When the infant discovers the difference between boys and girls (or men and women) his discovery should not be suppressed but explained in a matter of fact way. The sooner a child can grasp (both literally and otherwise) his sexuality without hindrance and can give names to the genital organs of both sexes, the less will he direct his conscious curiosity to them and the sooner will he be protected from the shock of later discovery and disclosure. He will learn to recognize sexuality as a natural property and how to come to terms with it, just as he must learn this with other organs. If however a child of either sex is forbidden to touch or to mention its genital organs by name, there is a danger of creating anxiety at puberty over his sexuality and that of others. Since nobody can live with anxiety over a long period, and in any case sexual anxiety is generally despised in modern society, anxiety must be repressed. In consequence the whole area of sexuality is rejected both consciously and unconsciously, often with prudery as the end result; otherwise, on the grounds that it is all 'natural', the subject becomes promiscuous, with sex simply enjoyed for itself and unrelated to the rest of life or to other interpersonal relations.

Adult Man and Adult Woman

External sex characters (see figs. 4 and 5)

At the onset of puberty under the influence of the specific male and female sex hormones, the typical secondary sex characters appear and the internal and external sex organs (primary sex characters) mature. This development and the final result vary greatly with the individual.

Hair distribution immediately around the genitals and in the armpits is the same in both sexes. The genitals of both sexes are also darker in skin colour than the rest of the body.

In general, the male is distinguished by the fact that his pubic hair continues on to the lower abdomen and occasionally up to the navel. Hair distribution on the trunk is very variable, but as a rule the individual body hairs are stronger and longer than in women. There may be a good growth of hair between the nipples continuing past the navel to join the pubic hair. Thighs and upper arms, but more frequently lower legs and arms, carry more hair than in the female.

The *genitals* increase in size during the time of maturation. The testes increase in size and weight so that the scrotum becomes longer than the penis, which in turn becomes stronger and thicker. Usually the foreskin recedes a little so that the tip of the glans penis with its urethral opening becomes visible. The male genitals are not covered in hair.

The female pubic hair is sharply delimited from the lower abdomen. The vulva and therefore the internal genitals, which have also increased in size during maturation, are completely hidden in the pubic hair. In women, body and limb hair is usually short and scarcely visible.

On maturation the *breasts* begin to grow and at first form the still firm and flattish budding breasts characteristic of adolescent girls, which gradually grow into the hemispherical breasts of the adult through increase in fatty tissue. Shape and size vary greatly. In the white and yellow races the hemispherical and slightly pendant breast predominates whereas in some Negro tribes the more prominent pointed or conical breast is commoner. In general the left breast lies somewhat lower than the right. The nipple and surrounding

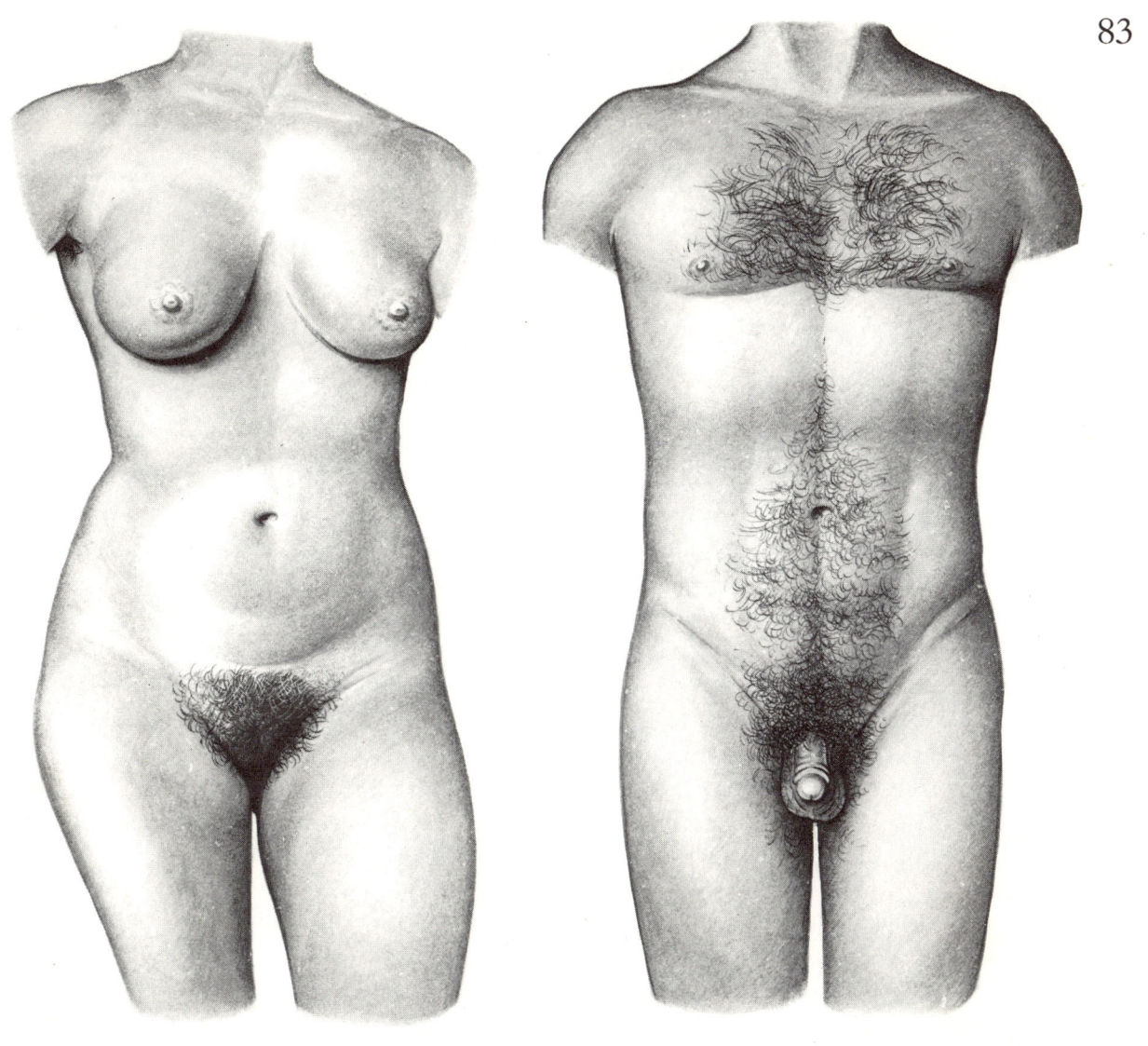

FIG. 4 *External sex characters of adult woman.*   FIG. 5 *External sex characters of adult man.*

areola are more prominent in women than men and darker than the surrounding skin. They look rather pink before the first pregnancy, and then usually turn dark brown. Malformations with flat or inverted nipples occur but need not necessarily interfere with breast-feeding later. The breasts commonly increase in size during pregnancy and at the beginning of lactation because glandular function augments. When breast-feeding ceases, the increase in size is maintained by substitution of extra fat for the shrinkage in glandular tissue.

As puberty begins and the sexual organs become functional, both male and female experience pleasurable sensations in the genitals with a desire to touch or rub them. These agreeable and occasionally almost overwhelming sensations prepare the body for sexual intercourse.

What is Modesty?

Some readers may find descriptions of the male and female body repugnant. Why? It will be said that it offends modesty and causes embarrassment. Is this true?

Modesty or the sense of shame is the concealment of one's intimate parts from other people, but what constitutes an intimate part of the body is always determined by the prevailing culture and society. Nowadays it is the genital area, but there have been times when it extended as far as the ankles. Modesty is concerned not only with physical landmarks but also with mental and emotional factors. Embarrassment is evoked when a stranger carelessly confides something of his secret thoughts if according to the prevailing culture he should not even have admitted to having them. The fact that modesty serves to protect one's privacy is true of all its areas, but we will discuss only specific sexual modesty. In the West, sexuality and all its expressions including the physical have long been taboo and regarded as shameful. By a distortion of the biblical message sexuality has been seen as sin and its exercise tolerated only for reproductive purposes. Discussion of the cause of this misunderstanding is beyond the scope of this book. The body has often been regarded as an inferior vehicle for the soul or the intellect, but since the Church has discovered that Christ died also for our bodies, it has recognized that the body with all its activities and functions, including those it shares with animals, is a very good work of divine creation, and that the Fall was primarily an affair of the spirit and not of sex.

Even as Christians we can rejoice in our bodies, though this should not be interpreted as either giving unrestricted licence to the so-called cult of the body or on the other hand as absolute rejection of it. This has been discussed elsewhere (see p. 32 ff.).

So modesty protects one's intimate life from strangers, but in the living relationship of husband and wife, which the Bible so simply and comprehensively describes as being one flesh, the partner is not a stranger and there should therefore be no shame. Yet people often fail to recognize that a couple do not achieve permanent unity; the process of rapprochement is a repeated one even though emotional and erotic relations are maintained. During the periods of relative separation modesty is again appropriate, not only as a means of tender flirtation but also for maintenance of individuality so that the whole person may be brought once more into the next act of love. Shamelessness would in such an instance remove the sense of distance and imperil the integrity of the personality. It is an illusion to suppose that in the WE of marriage the I and THOU must be submerged. A fresh WE is possible only out of the continuously regained I of one or the other partner.

A single experience of the nakedness of the other partner does not mean complete and final recognition (apart from nakedness in the emotional or mental sense). In the continuing and oft-repeated encounter of love both partners will continue to make fresh discoveries of each other with further pleasant or unpleasant revelations. Loving one's partner in spite of the unpleasant traits can arise only out of mutual respect.

It has been pointed out that the maintenance of a certain privacy until a man and a woman are one is of considerable significance. The abandonment of shame is an essential step on the way to unity of man and woman (this is the problem of nudism). Many men and women still come to the discovery of one another's body without knowing what there is to discover. To deal with what has been discovered without clumsily destroying the relationship through the 'joy of discovery' however requires knowledge that is no longer subconsciously present or handed down but has to be learned. The illustrations in this book are designed for this purpose; since the other person's privacy must be respected, this knowledge should not be obtained on their body.

Should these pictures be shown to children? Modesty requires the preservation of intimate areas from strangers. Are children and parents strangers? In a certain respect, yes; one's own child is a different and individual being who needs acceptance with all its unknown qualities after birth and later. On the other hand the child grows up in a unique confidential relation to its parents (more than ever in modern times) so that it loses all sense of strangeness.

For the child, the family is the area of privacy, and an intrusion into this family area is embarrassing. This would happen for example if mother opened the front door in her underwear, father met visitors in his pyjamas, or the child went on sitting on its chamber-pot in the presence of its playmates. The child's privacy must also be respected.

There is a point at which the child learns to say 'me'. Up to the time when it begins to be conscious of its own personality, and by an effort of will to separate itself off from the environment, it should be permitted unrestricted access to its parents' nakedness. It needs this access to discover that just as father also has a nose and mother ears, father also has a penis and mother a vulva while she has breasts and father has none. Just as the child learns everything else from repetition, it should learn these things by this method (see p. 29 ff.).

At this point the parents face a dilemma. They learned when young to conceal their intimacies from others, and although they abandon their modesty in their most intimate relations with each other, they never do so in the presence of a third party. Parents will always feel that the child is a stranger in the area of sex, even though they may not have noticed this in other areas. Whether they admit the child to their nakedness depends on their true attitude to their bodies, their sexuality, their states of maleness or femaleness and on how far this is insecure, disturbed, or inhibited. If they catch the child peeping through the keyhole to satisfy its understandable thirst for knowledge they are furious about its 'wicked' childish curiosity, although they themselves have frequently suffered as children from similar prohibitions. But all that happened long ago at a time they hardly recollect. It is perfectly natural for a small child to see its parents naked, and at this age such a parent–child relationship is not shameful. When the parents respect their child's privacy (leaving it to dress itself if it wants to, even if it appears with shirt or pants back to front; leaving it to wash alone even if neck and feet are not always quite clean) it will also spontaneously learn to leave its parents alone when they bath or dress.

To maintain this attitude is very hard for a lot of parents on account of their own upbringing. In the teaching materials used in school the human body is still mostly represented as sexless, and it is not surprising that many adolescent boys and girls in spite of all the public emphasis on sex and the erotic have never seen an adult man or woman naked, or for that matter been informed about the details. Since all children are on the road to maturity and it is easier to follow a road if the goal is known, these pictures should be shown to children.

The Man

Male Genital Organs

The male genitals are partly contained within the body and partly plainly visible. The penis and scrotum containing the testes lie at the base of the abdomen in front of the thighs; the internal sex organs (a major portion of the spermatic cord which conveys the sperm and some special glands, as well as the base of the organs which swell on erection) and the urinary bladder lie in relation to and behind the external organs.

Penis and scrotum in the mature male are framed in pubic hair but are themselves hairless apart from a relatively few hairs on the scrotum and the root of the penis; in contrast to the female external genitals they are therefore very obvious. Because of their situation the male external genitals, to which in a certain sense the testis and epididymis belong also, are more vulnerable to injury than the corresponding female organs.

Since, in the male, urine and semen are emitted through the same organ—the penis with its tube the urethra—and since urination from an early age is accomplished in the standing position, the male child must actively manipulate his penis quite early in life to urinate. Thus in contrast to the female, his attention is drawn very early to this organ, later of significance in sexual intercourse. Perhaps this is one reason why later sexual excitement in the male is almost exclusively limited to his genitals, whereas the female only gradually, and through accidental sexual contact, discovers the particular excitability of her more concealed genitals and is in fact almost equally excitable all over her body.

External Genitals

The external sex organs of the male consist of the penis and the scrotum (see fig. 6). The scrotum contains both testes or testicles and their appendages, the epididymides as well as the beginning of the seminal ducts. Usually the left half of the scrotum lies somewhat lower than the right. The temperature in the scrotum is about three degrees Centigrade (over five degrees Fahrenheit) lower than the general body temperature. This is a prerequisite for the healthy development of the sperm cells in the testes. Under the influence of cold, for example while swimming, the scrotum may contract, as it also does for another reason during sexual excitement.

Since the testes arise in the interior of the body and at first lie there, there may be a disturbance of development while the child lies in the womb, such that one or both testes do not descend into the scrotum but stick in the inguinal canal leading from the abdomen, and come to rest just above the fold of the thigh or at an even higher level. With this type of undescended testicle the scrotum or one half of it is empty. Such a condition requires medical supervision and treatment at an appropriate time in childhood (operation or hormone treatment, the latter being reserved for the years of puberty).

Male organ, the penis
The penis usually hangs down slackly and in the mature man measures 6 to 12 cm. (2½ to 5 inches) long. In the phase of sexual excitement it becomes stiff and erect, pointing upwards. In this state the penis increases in length to 10 to 20 cm. (4 to 8 inches), becomes thicker and is then able to penetrate into the female vagina or passage. When this happens, a small penis usually undergoes considerably greater increase in size than one which is already large at

FIG. 6 *External male genitals; left, with foreskin peeled back, right, with foreskin forward.*

1 Scrotum
2 Penis
   a Root of penis
   b Shaft of penis
   c Glans
   d Coronary sulcus
   e Foreskin (prepuce)
   f Urethra

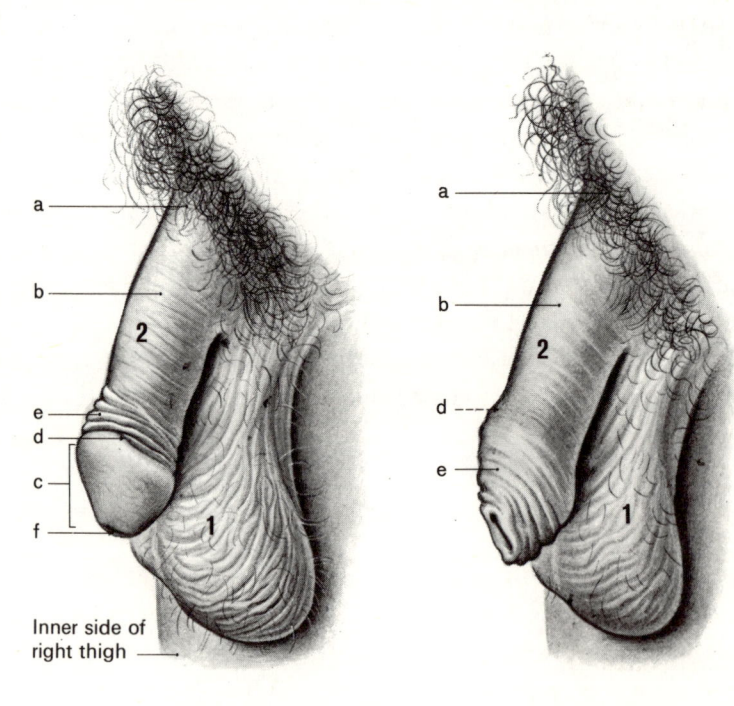

Inner side of right thigh

rest. When the penis enlarges the foreskin must peel back off the glans, which is exposed with its highly sensitive receivers mainly on the underside and in the furrow round the glans. These receivers (sensory receptors) are the nerve endings by which in the skin and mucous membranes touch, heat, and cold are perceived. Their stimulation on the male sex organ leads to an increase in pleasurable sexual excitement and finally to ejaculation of semen.

The foreskin is prevented from completely peeling back by a band, the frenulum, which begins at the under side of the urethral tube opening and runs back in a cleft on the under side of the glans. This band also contains many receptors and is particularly sensitive in the state of sexual excitement when the foreskin is peeled back and the band thus put under tension.

Foreskin (prepuce)
A relatively short foreskin may stay constantly peeled back in a mature male (see fig. 6) but in other cases it falls forward again over the glans when excitement has passed, thus protecting the latter from stimuli due to touch.

Glans penis
Through the scaling off of the outermost layers of skin the foreskin and glans penis make a greasy substance, smegma, which must be carefully removed by washing, otherwise it may give rise to undesirable irritation through its decomposition, and later even to ulceration or cancer of the penis.

The hygiene of the penis (smegma removal) seems to be significant in the origin of cancer in the female sexual organs, quite apart from its unpleasant odour which may upset the woman during sexual intercourse. At any rate statistics show that in races in which circumcision (removal of the foreskin and therefore of the principal source of smegma) is common and ritual washings of the genitals precede sexual intercourse, women rarely if at all suffer from cancer of the vagina or neck of the womb. On the other hand, it seems certain that where general personal hygiene and thus hygiene of the male genitals is neglected, these types of cancer are commoner.

Circumcision is customary among the semitic races, being carried out at an early age, sometimes as a ritual as in Jewry. In the U.S.A. it is also commonly done on hygienic grounds.

Phimosis
During the development of the penis at about the third or fourth month in the embryo the foreskin adheres to the glans, only to free itself again just before birth. However the adhesion may persist, either in the form of fine strings between the inner surface of the foreskin and the glans or in the form of a narrowing of the opening of the prepuce. This state is called

FIG. 7 *Penis and scrotum of older boy; left, normal, right, with phimosis. The figure on the left shows the normal situation of the foreskin in a boy before puberty. Both figures show that the left testis hangs a little lower than the right in boys as in the adult.*

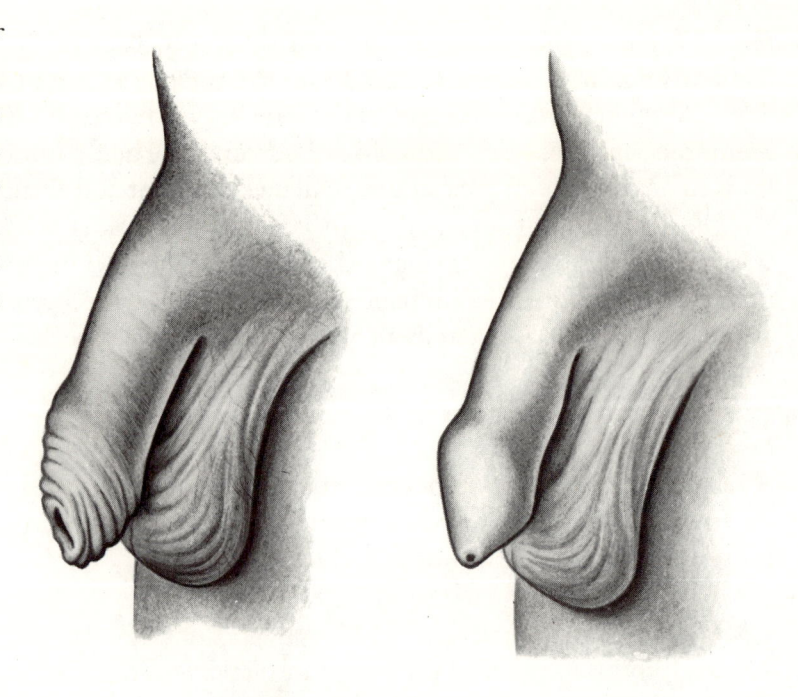

phimosis, and in it the foreskin can be peeled back either not at all or at the most only partially. A relatively marked phimosis is not so rare as the laity often believe (see fig. 7).

Normally the foreskin after birth should be capable of being peeled right back to the furrow behind the glans. Since many if not most parents and unfortunately midwives too neglect this elementary examination and are satisfied to establish that the boy is 'complete', i.e. has a penis and scrotum (often failing to notice an undescended testicle (see p.88), a phimosis is often overlooked.

The reason for this illogical behaviour of adults is likely to be found in their own disturbed or inhibited attitude to sexuality, so that their personal knowledge of the significance of intact sex organs is unconsciously repressed; moreover they want to regard the infant as sexually neutral so that they have no wish to examine it closely. Phimosis is therefore in many cases discovered only much later when the boy is out of diapers and compares his penis with those of playmates, or else suffers from itchy inflammation under the foreskin because of decomposing remains of urine. If the boy, taking his cue from his parents, is sexually inhibited he may notice his phimosis only during adolescence or even when he first attempts intercourse. If a sexually mature young man discovers during masturbation or an attempt at intercourse that his foreskin will not go back, the result is relatively harmless apart from mental trauma or feeling that he is abnormal. More dramatic are the occasions on which a tight foreskin can be peeled back but then constricts the glans penis at the corona so that increased swelling of the glans due to trapping of blood further prevents the foreskin from going forward again. In these cases of paraphimosis rapid medical intervention is usually needed; all attempts to reduce the mechanically trapped excess of blood in the glans by application of cold commonly fail. Many parents are annoyed because their younger sons 'play with themselves' and forbid this, without ever examining the boy to determine whether his behaviour is due to a phimosis with urinary decomposition underneath and intolerable itching in consequence.

In every case phimosis requires surgical treatment. Shortly after birth, most adhesions can easily be separated without operation but later this becomes harder as the thin strings between foreskin and glans gradually grow together and form bridges of tissue. When the foreskin is narrowed to a high degree (see right-hand picture in fig. 7.) an operation similar to ritual circumcision is needed. The doctor will of course decide on this, but it is better for the emotional future of the child if any necessary operation is carried out within the first years of life. If possible, operation should be avoided between the years of three and seven, an age at which the boy begins to test out the efficiency of his penis on a childish scale by showing how high he can urinate. He also during these years becomes increasingly interested sexually in his penis, comparing it with the adult penis and not wanting it to be mutilated. If an operation in this period becomes unavoidable on medical grounds and a portion of the foreskin must be removed, the boy must be carefully prepared for this by repeated assurances that he will be more of a man afterwards and will be better able to use his penis later. This needs emphasis even if the child is over seven, but the older child will already have a better idea of the limitation of function and be interested in gaining better function.

Apart from operation in infancy or in toddlers, the next best age for operation for phimosis is the first year after the onset of puberty, after the first seminal emission has taken place; the only snag here is that the child must not be allowed to regard his operation as punishment for masturbatory activity.

Internal Genital Organs

The seminal cells are formed in the right and left testes, the male sex glands (for structure and function of the testes, see p. 96). The epididymis serves for maturation and storage of seminal cells (see figs. 8 and 9). During storage the spontaneous mobility of the spermatozoa is increased chemically to save energy. Seen from the front the epididymis appears to sit like a cap on each testis but a lateral view reveals it as an elongated body attached above and behind the gland (see fig. 8).

The mature spermatozoa at the culmination of sexual excitement are sucked out of the seminal duct and through its tapering end and squeezed out into the urethra, which here becomes a common duct for urine and semen. The seminal ducts lead from the scrotum into the abdominal interior. For their passage there is an oblique gap in the abdominal wall muscles, the inguinal canal (in fig. 8 the inguinal canal is shown schematically on one side only).

Through this gap in the muscles the testicle during its development passes from the abdominal cavity into the scrotum. In some persons, great exertion involving the trunk muscles including those of the abdominal wall, and therefore increasing intra-abdominal pressure, can also force loops of intestine through the muscle hiatus into the inguinal canal and even into the scrotum; this is the so-called inguinal hernia or 'rupture', and it requires surgical treatment. The inguinal canal is also present in women but the gap need not be so wide open and hernia is therefore less common in women.

The *seminal ducts* or vasa deferentia (see fig. 15) pass backwards alongside the urinary bladder, shown in moderate filling in both diagrams, and open through a fine orifice into the upper part of the urethra. Between the urinary bladder and the urethra there is a constricting muscle or sphincter (not shown in the diagram) which prevents the outflow of urine, also during sexual intercourse.

The *seminal vesicles* open into the back part of the seminal duct. They lie behind and to the side of the bladder. Their name arises from the false belief that they store semen, though it is now known that they are of little importance in man, like the appendix in the bowel. However they play a part in rodents in which they supply a substance which sticks the vagina together after coitus to prevent semen from flowing out. In man their secretion is emitted during ejaculation of semen and helps to maintain the spontaneous movement of spermatozoa.

Prostate gland
The seminal duct passes through the prostate gland shortly before it opens into the urethra. This gland consists of a middle and two lateral lobes and is apposed to the urinary bladder. It produces the greater part of the seminal fluid, and its secretion is emitted through a good many small ducts opening into the urethra near the seminal ducts, to join with the spermatozoa and the secretion of the seminal vesicles.

With ageing the lobes of the prostate may grow larger (hypertrophy). If the middle lobe grows too much it can bulge into the bladder and prevent the outflow of urine, causing difficulty in urination in older men. The semen consists of sperm cells or spermatozoa together with seminal fluid (mostly from the prostate but also from the seminal vesicles). The prostatic secretion confers the characteristic odour on semen; the secretions of prostate, seminal vesicles and Cowper's glands increase the mobility of the spermatozoa.

FIG. 8 *External and internal male genitals seen from the front.*

1 *Scrotum*
2 *Testis*
3 *Epididymis (head)*
4 *Seminal duct*
5 *Inguinal canal (shown on one side only)*
6 *Seminal vesicle*
7 *Prostate*
8 *Urinary bladder*
9 *Urethra*
10 *Cowper's gland*
11 *Penis*
12 *Coronary sulcus*
13 *Glans*

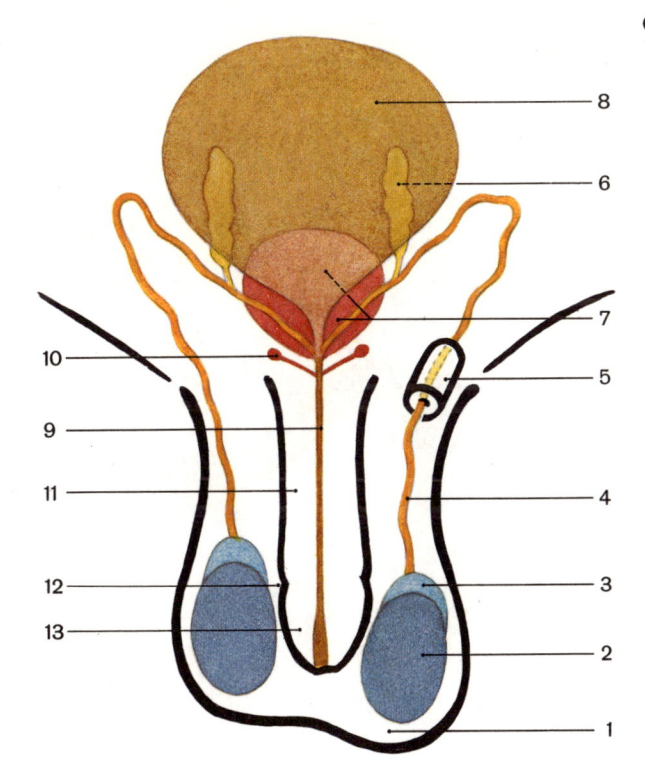

Erectile or cavernous tissue
In the male penis there are three sets of erectile tissue (see figs. 9 and 10) with the property of swelling up when full of blood. These are the two corpora cavernosa and the unpaired corpus spongiosum, which surrounds the urethra completely. Stiffening and erection of the penis is caused by these three bodies, which contain a rich network of blood vessels. During sexual excitement there is a greater blood flow than in relaxation, and at the same time the outflow is throttled down, so that the three bodies are filled to capacity and take up the position which affords greatest possible stretching. This causes the penis to rise and increase in circumference and length.

In the corpus spongiosum on the under side the restriction on blood outflow is not so great as in the corpora cavernosa. Since this corpus surrounds the urethra and also forms the glans into which the two other corpora penetrate from behind, even in the stage of maximum excitement or orgasm when the semen is ejaculated the urethra remains patent for the semen and the glans stays comparatively soft. The fact that the glans is softer preserves the function of the sensory bodies situated there, and protects the vagina from injury.

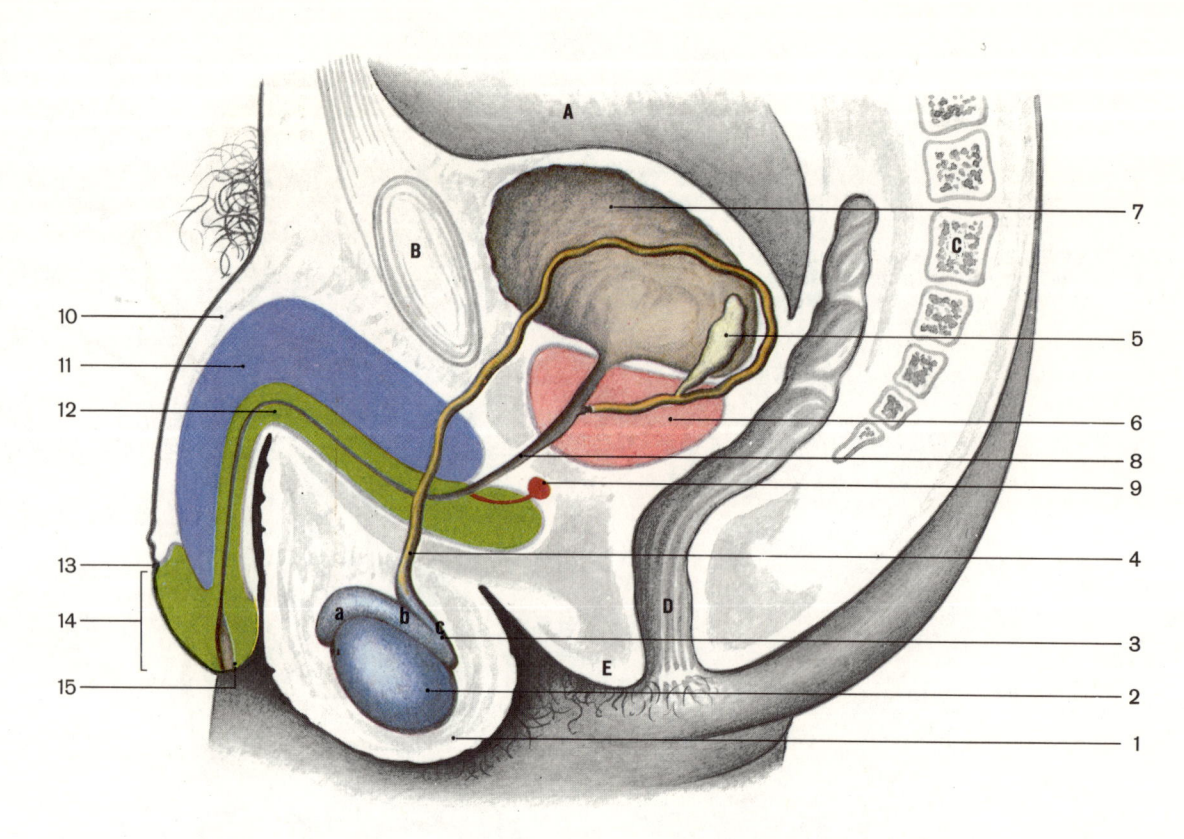

FIG. 9 *External and internal male genitals: section through pelvis, seen from the side.*

A Peritoneal cavity   B Pubis   C Vertebral column (coccyx)   D Rectum and anus   E Perineum

1 *Scrotum*   2 *Testis*   3 *Epididymis (a head, b body, c tail)*   4 *Seminal duct*
5 *Seminal vesicle* 6 *Prostate*   7 *Urinary bladder*   8 *Urethra*   9 *Cowper's gland*
10 *Penis*   11 *Corpora cavernosa (paired)* 12 *Corpus spongiosum (unpaired)*   13 *Coronary sulcus*
14 *Glans*   15 *Urethral orifice*

Cowper's glands

These are small glands at the hind end of the corpus spongiosum, which is penetrated by their ducts before the latter open into the urethra. Their secretion is excreted at the beginning of sexual excitement, often long before the semen. It serves to lubricate the urethra and glans and also the vagina. It also counteracts chemically any harmful effect of traces of urine on following spermatozoa.

In intercourse which follows relatively rapidly upon a previous act, the emission of secretion from Cowper's glands may include viable spermatozoa left behind in the urethra. This is not infrequently the reason why a woman becomes pregnant if her partner has ejaculated more than once, even if he has been careful to withdraw before ejaculation each time.

Injection of the semen into the urethra causes the seminal vesicles to secrete as well. At this stage, which the man can sense, he can still by an effort of will arrest the process, for example if his partner is still far from reaching her climax or orgasm. However he will partly forfeit his erection for the time being. He must then wait until the next wave of excitement when the seminal duct has recovered sufficiently to suck up sperm cells once more and eject them into the urethra. This mechanical process will then set ejaculation off again.

Ejaculation of semen
Very soon after the seminal ducts and the seminal vesicles have ejected their products into the urethra the further march of ejaculation can no longer be arrested. The prostate then powerfully contracts the muscle around its gland and ejects its secretion in turn through fine ducts into the urethra. These powerful movements of prostate muscle stimulate other muscles between the prostate and the corpora cavernosa, which now force semen through the urethra by four to eight intense contractions, which can no longer be restrained voluntarily. The man consciously experiences this rhythmical ejaculation during intercourse and it imparts a last surge to his feeling of ecstasy. Since all the lower abdominal muscles are involved in this excitation, there is also a last increase in filling of the corpora cavernosa and usually a jerking movement of the penis in the vagina. The woman experiences all this movement and excitement, occasionally even feeling the impact of the semen against the posterior wall of the vagina, and this accentuates her own sensation.

FIG. 10 *Transverse section through penis: left, slack; right, erect.*

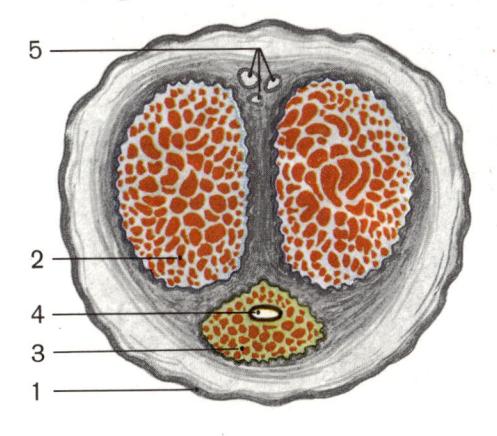

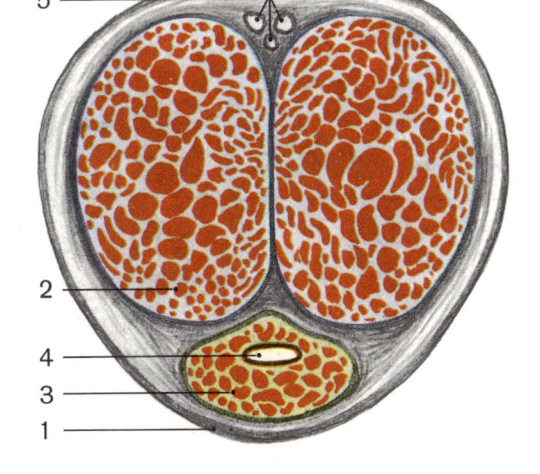

| 1 Skin | 2 Corpus cavernosum with blood vessel network | 3 Corpus spongiosum with its blood vessels |
| 4 Urethra | 5 Blood vessels supplying the penis | |

96 After ejaculation male excitement subsides more or less rapidly and his erection also subsides, and can be repeated only after a prolonged interval (recovery phase of all the nerves, muscles and glands involved in sexual excitement).

Testis and epididymis
Both testes (see figs. 6–9 and 11) already lie in their halves of the scrotum at birth. In the newborn they are the size of a lentil to a bean and undergo their last increase in size during puberty. In mature males they are about 3 to 5 cm. (1¼ to 2 in.) long, i.e. the size of a plum, oval and rather flattened laterally. Each testis is enclosed in a tough shell. The testes

FIG. 11 *Testis and epididymis.*

1 Capsule of testis
2 Septum
3 Lobe of testis with seminiferous tubules
4 Seminiferous tubule teased out
5 Rete testis
6 Head of epididymis
7 Body of epididymis
8 Tail of epididymis
9 Efferent ducts
10 Epididymal duct
11 Beginning of seminal duct

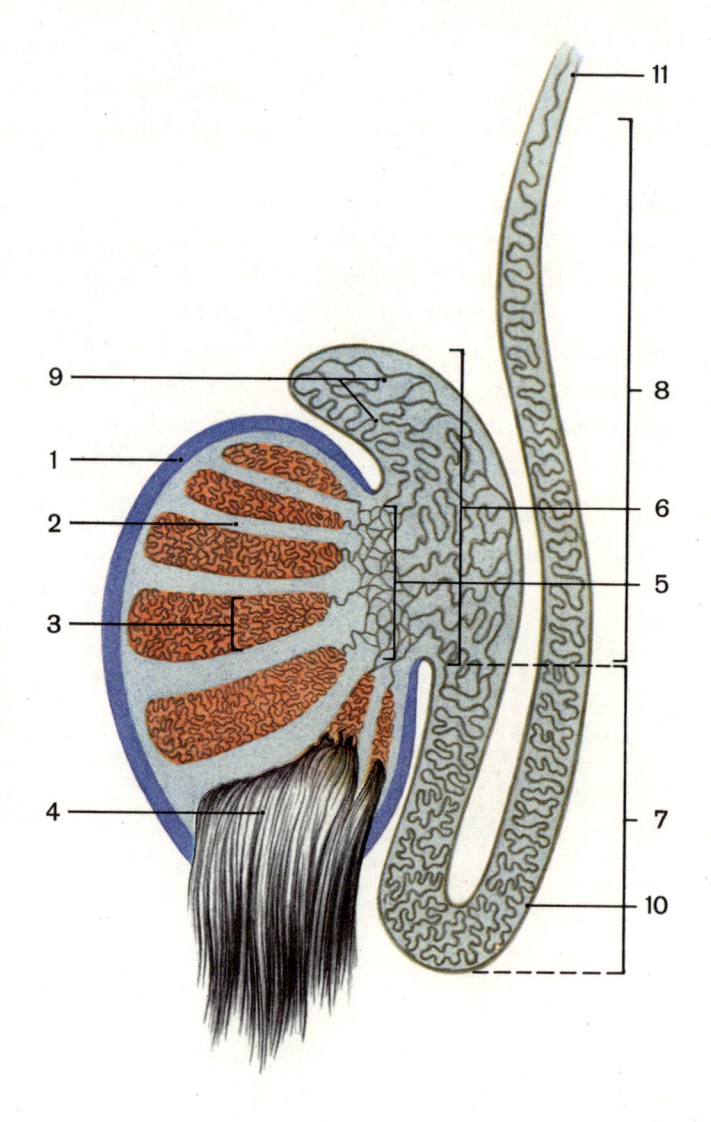

are divided up by fibrous walls into 200 to 250 lobules, in each of which there are 2 to 4 thread-like coiled-up seminiferous (semen-bearing) tubules. The total length of the 400 to 600 tubules in one testis is said to amount to between 200 and 800 yards. Thus the total length of all the tubules in both testes is well over half a mile.

Between the tubules lies the so-called interstitial tissue containing interstitial cells which produce the male sex hormone (see especially fig. 13).

The tubules open into a network of canals, the rete testis (testicular net), from which 12 to 15 efferent ducts pass into the head of the epididymis where they end in the epididymal duct, about 3 to 4 yards long. This duct by its convolutions fills up the body and tail of the epididymis and continues as the seminal duct.

The sperm cells are formed in the testis. Their final maturation takes place in the epididymal duct, where their movements are inhibited chemically with the object of saving energy. When the cells are ejaculated, other chemical processes brought about by secretions of other glands will liberate this energy, so that the cells can move freely within the female body.

Regulation by the pituitary

The production of sperm cells and of male hormone in the testes is regulated by hormones from the pituitary. Hormones are substances formed in the body by glands but not passed out through the ducts; instead they pass directly into the blood stream, through which they reach all organs; however they exercise their function only at places where, like a key, they find a corresponding lock. Thus every hormone has a definite action only on certain organs or on certain functional areas within particular organs.

The pituitary, about the size of the kernel of a hazel nut, lies almost in the middle of the base of the brain from which it is suspended in a small bony cup open above. It is closely related to the part of the brain lying above it, the hypothalamus. Between the hypothalamus and the pituitary there is a close functional relationship, assured by nerve paths and also, as has recently been shown, by a ductal system containing hypothalamic hormones. Through the hypothalamus the functional unit of hypothalamus and pituitary is in turn connected with the cerebrum, so that the latter influences the regulatory functions of the pituitary. Since in the human body all regulating systems are also influenced by feedback, the lower parts may in turn affect the cerebrum.

The pituitary forms hormones with an effect on the testes and ovaries. We now distinguish three such hormones, which are formed both in men and women. Because they and their effects were first recognized in women, they are named accordingly. Their different effects are due to the different functions of the end organs on which they act.

We will first discuss the actions of these hormones on the male reproductive glands, though it has been shown that one of the three hormones (although formed by the male pituitary) has no effect on these glands or on the male breast. We will return to this in later discussion of the female body (see p. 242 and fig. 73). Another pituitary hormone, the so-called follicle-stimulating hormone or FSH, acts on the seminiferous ducts and brings about maturation of sperm cells. The third pituitary hormone, the so-called luteinizing hormone or LSH, or more recently interstitial cell stimulating hormone, ICSH, acts on the interstitial tissue in the testis and thus stimulates formation of male sex hormones. In its turn, male sex hormone leads to maturation of male genitals and appearance of secondary sex characters (hair growth, breaking of the voice, etc.), and also regulates production of sperm cells by the seminiferous ducts.

In both boys and girls the pituitary begins to secrete its sexually active hormones only at the beginning of puberty. Until then not only is this branch of pituitary function inhibited but also the reproductive glands themselves are little if at all receptive to their hormones. It should be mentioned that the adrenal cortex in both male and female also makes a male sex hormone, which is apparently of little significance in amount in either sex but can in pathological conditions lead to external (not mental) masculinization of women.

The following working diagram (drawn without feedback effects) is a condensed and simplified account of the situation in the male:

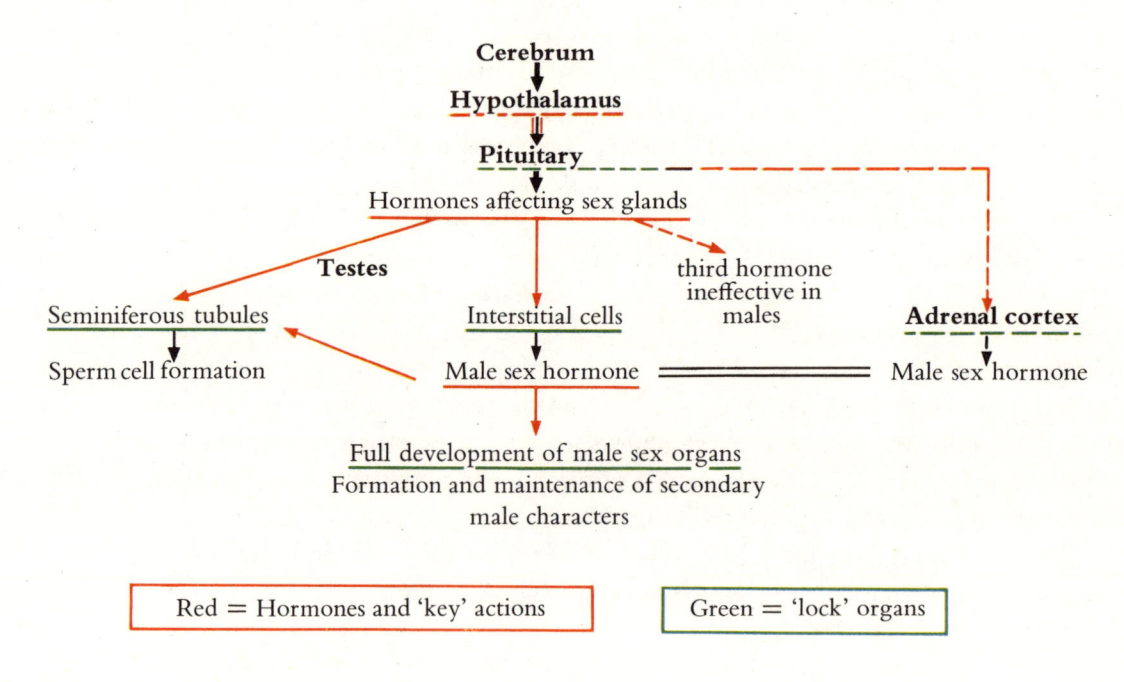

Cerebrum
↓
Hypothalamus
↓
Pituitary
↓
Hormones affecting sex glands

Testes

Seminiferous tubules　　Interstitial cells　　third hormone ineffective in males　　**Adrenal cortex**
↓　　　　　　　　　　↓　　　　　　　　　　　　　　　　　　　　　　　　↓
Sperm cell formation　　Male sex hormone ══════════ Male sex hormone
↓
Full development of male sex organs
Formation and maintenance of secondary male characters

| Red = Hormones and 'key' actions | Green = 'lock' organs |

Semen and sperm cell maturation (see figs. 12–14)
The sperm cells are formed in the seminiferous tubules which are about half a mile long

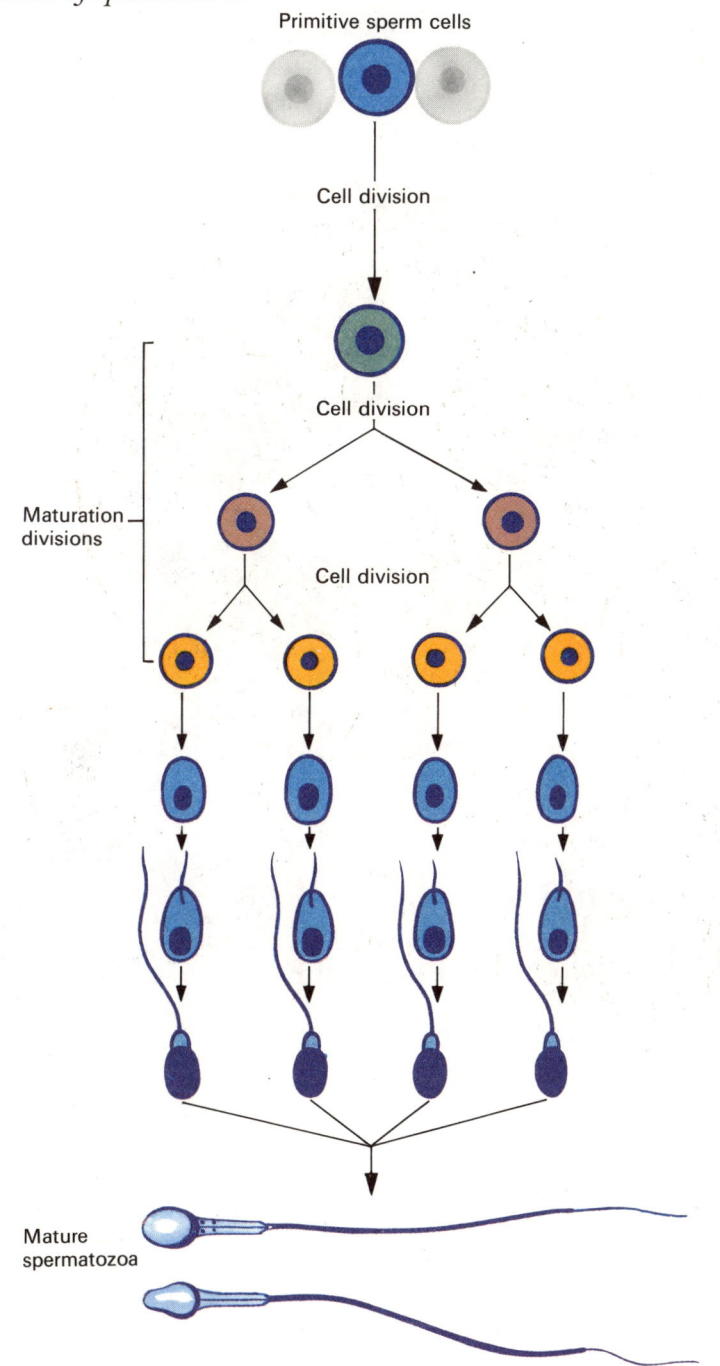

FIG. 12 *Maturation of spermatozoa.*

99

Primitive sperm cells

Cell division

Cell division

Maturation divisions

Cell division

Mature spermatozoa

100 (see especially fig. 13). On the walls of the tubules lie the primitive sperm cells or spermatogonia, which multiply only until puberty. So long as no sperm cells are being produced the tubules are relatively narrow and in the resting state. This resting state may also occur during mature sexual life (from puberty up to extreme old age) either if there is no great need for spermatozoa (sexual abstinence with simultaneous absence of mental sexual stimuli such

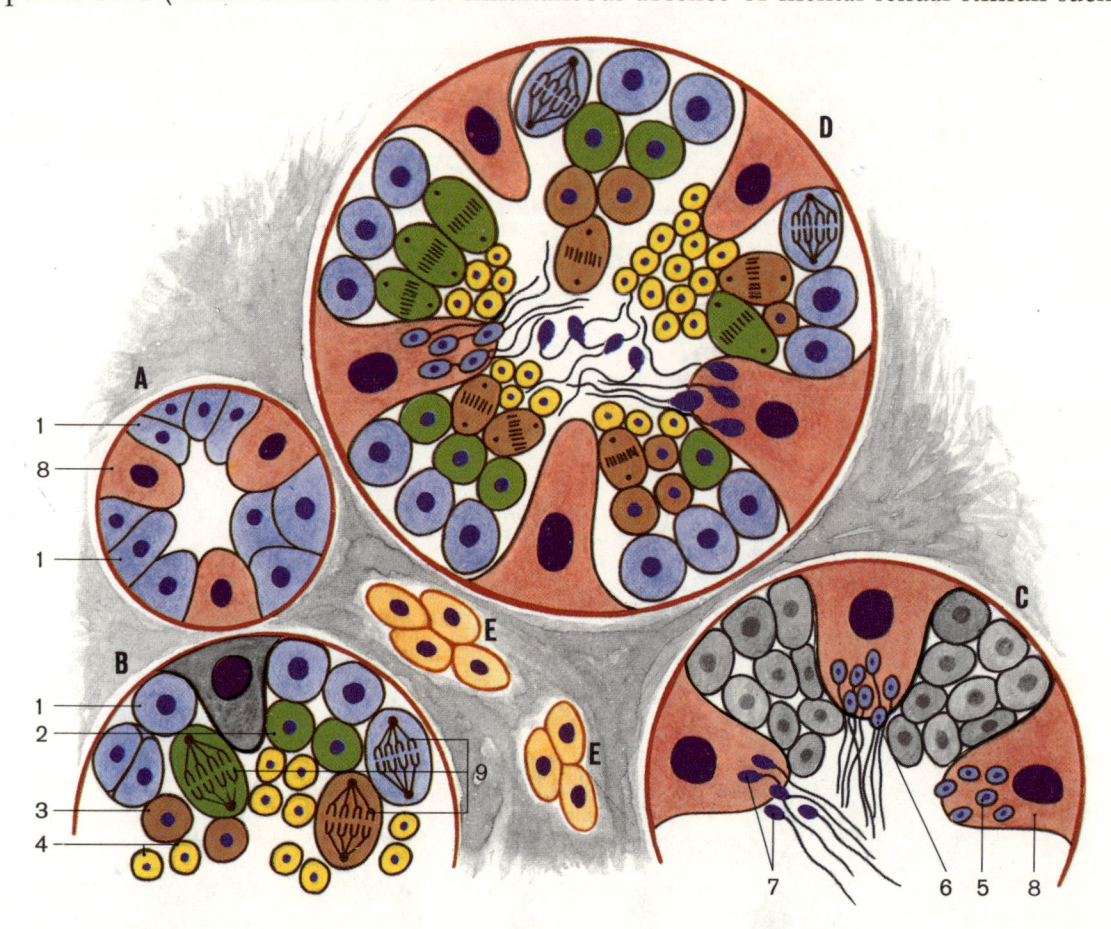

FIG. 13 *Seminiferous tubule.*

A *Resting tubule*
B *Part of a tubule showing sperm cell division*
C *Part of a tubule showing maturation of sperm cells within supporting cells*
D *Section through a fully active tubule. The number of sperm cells has been reduced for the sake of clarity*
E *'Interstitial cells' producing hormone*

1 *Spermatogonium*
2 *Primary spermatocyte*
3 *Secondary spermatocyte*
4 *Spermatids*
5–7 *Maturation stages of sperm cells*
8 *Supporting cells*
9 *Cell division (mitotic) figures*

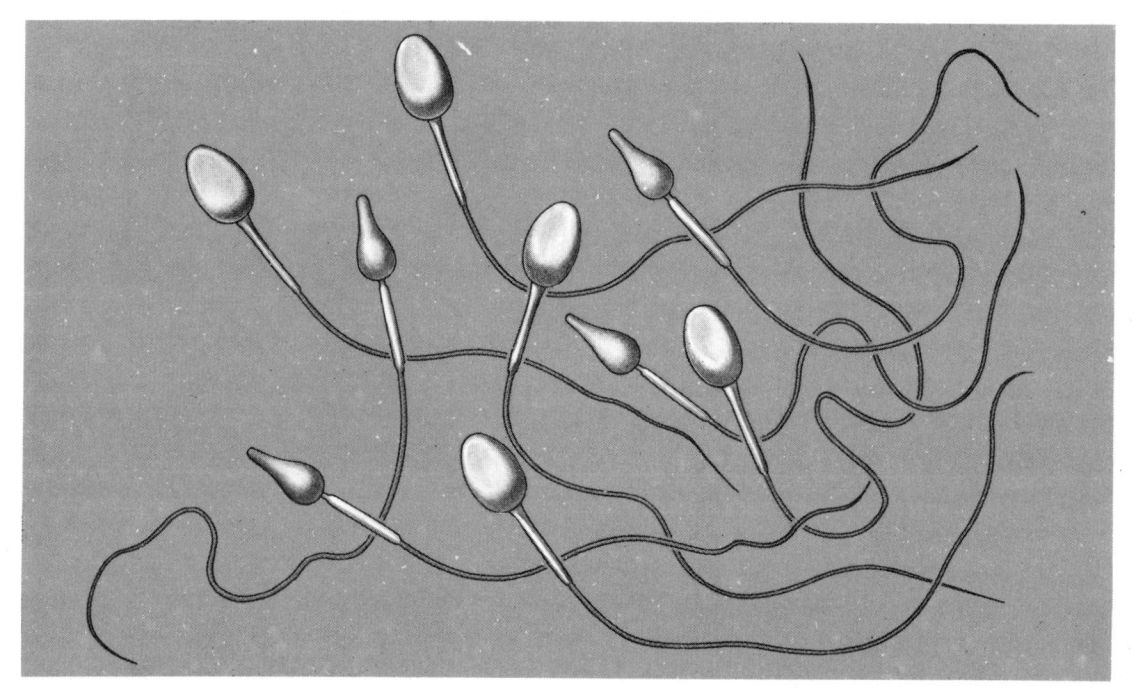

FIG. 14 *Mature spermatozoa. Length 0·04–0·06 mm., about two-thirds the diameter of a hair. Tennis-racquet-shaped seen full face, pear-shaped seen from the side.*

as imagination, pictures and so on) or if as a result of major anxiety (for example, in criminals before judgement) central regulation goes wrong.

The activity of the seminiferous tubules is unaffected by either overnutrition or undernutrition, in spite of folk myths to the contrary. In fact, the capacity to produce semen is lost only when there is extreme lack of protein sufficient to endanger life. However in the usual and fairly regular sex life within marriage there are always some sections of the tubules at rest or in a recovery phase. Theoretically the primitive sperm cells or spermatogonia maintain their capacity for division until extreme old age. Out of this division the next stage of cells form; these are the two primary spermatocytes, which again divide in two giving four secondary spermatocytes. These divide once more, giving rise to immature spermatozoa or spermatids.

The latter gradually intrude into the lumen of the tubule and are nourished by the so-called supporting cells, which extend from the wall into the lumen. For a while the immature sperm cells embed themselves into these nutrient cells (similar cells are present during maturation of the ovum) as they undergo a complicated change, from which they emerge as almost mature spermatozoa. Thence they travel into the epididymis, where they finally achieve their mature shape.

The duration of development from the first division of the spermatogonia to the maturation of spermatozoa has been calculated as 19 to 20 days. Since however millions of these processes are taking place simultaneously there are usually enough mature cells in the tail of the epididymis.

The mature spermatozoon is 0·04 to 0·06 mm. long (see fig. 14) and has a head, body and tail. Seen from the front the head is oval and in profile pear-shaped and about 0·003 to 0·005 mm. long. It carries the genes which are responsible for hereditary characters. At the tip there are chemical substances which aid the further movement of the sperm within the mucus of the internal female genitals and its penetration into the ovum. The body or connecting piece contains the necessary elements for forward movement as well as the necessary stimulus for the first division of the fertilized ovum. The tail serves to move the cell actively along by its whiplike undulations. As a result the spermatozoon can swim against the stream and the ciliary current.

The life span of the spermatozoa depends on the chemical composition of their environment. It is of significance to know that in the epididymis they are chemically inhibited in their movements to save energy, and then reactivated by the secretions of the prostate and other glands. They can live for only about two hours in the vagina, but in the fallopian tubes or egg ducts, the site of fertilization of the short-lived ovum extruded from the ovary, they can live for about 2 days.

Seminal duct

This is the continuation of the tail of the epididymis and opens into the upper part of the urethra which thus becomes a conduit for both semen and urine (see figs. 8, 9 and 11). The seminal duct is about 3 mm. thick and has a lumen of only $\frac{1}{2}$ mm. Especially at its beginning it is markedly coiled, and if stretched out would measure 50 to 60 cm. (20 to 24 in.) long. It passes through the inguinal canal into the pelvis accompanied by the vessels and nerves which supply the testis and epididymis.

This duct (see fig. 15) consists of a mucosa, a muscle layer and an outer coat. The muscle layer is thick and powerful and consists of spiral muscle bundles coiling both right and left; these bundles climb steeply inside and outside but climb very little in the middle, so that a transverse section gives the impression that there are outer and inner layers of longitudinal muscle with a middle layer of circular muscle in between.

If the muscle contracts, the lumen widens because of the arrangement of muscle fibres, and the seminal duct shortens. As a result the contents of the epididymis (sperm cells) are sucked in. With further contractions of the muscles the lumen contracts and there is a rise in pressure which expels the semen. Acceleration is further imparted to the sperm cells because the far end of the seminal duct tapers off into an ejaculatory canal.

Sterilization of the male is a surgical operation in which the seminal duct is exposed at

FIG. 15 *Seminal duct.*

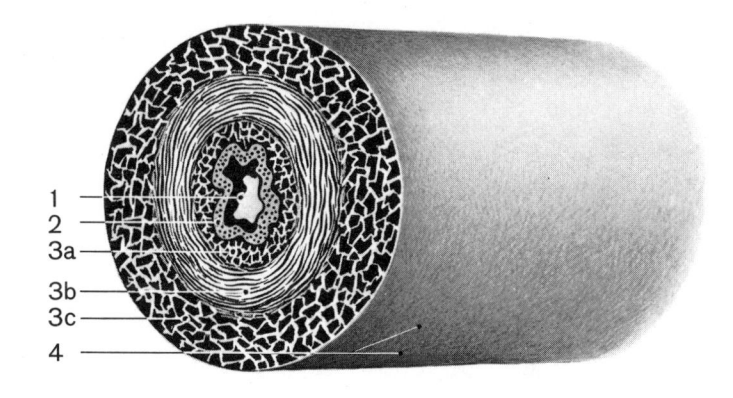

1 *Lumen containing spermatozoa*
2 *Mucosa*
3 *Muscle layer*
   a *Inner longitudinal layer*
   b *Middle ring layer*
   c *External longitudinal layer*
4 *Outer coat*

the point in the inguinal canal where it runs close to the surface of the body, cut and the two ends tied off. This operation can be performed on out-patients and it results in incapacity to produce children. In rare cases such an operation is needed for a medical reason but in most cases the object is simply to make the man infertile. An attempt can later be made to render him fertile again but the prospect is very poor. The use of this measure to prevent the conception of more children in a marriage is discussed on p. 176.

Ejaculation
The average volume of semen ejaculated is 2 to 6 cubic centimetres, and in each c.c. there are between 60 and 90 million sperm cells. Thus one ejaculation includes 120 to 540 million cells. A certain percentage of these are infertile and therefore though they are often deformed they cannot cause malformation in children. However about 80% of the sperm cells are usually normal in form and function. If the number of sperm cells with disturbances of form or function rises above a certain percentage, the fertilizing capacity of the entire semen is questionable. Further limitations on fertility of semen may arise through disturbances in composition of the seminal fluid.

Infertility in marriage
In such cases a marriage may be infertile (see p. 173). We now know that the cause of an infertile marriage lies in about 40% of cases with the husband, in another 40% with the wife and in the remaining 20% either in both or in an unknown cause. Hence investigation of the cause must include examination of the husband, whose infertility can sometimes be cured by appropriate treatment. For the sake of completeness, it might be added that there are other causes for male infertility such as mechanical blocks to the exit of semen.

Impotence
The above forms of infertility must not be confused with impotence. The latter is the

incapacity of the man to carry out the sexual act because he cannot get an erection when he encounters a woman and therefore cannot introduce his penis into the vagina. This sort of disorder may occur even though the man is able to have erections apart from intimacy with women, as for instance in dreams or on masturbation. There are some cases in which the man is impotent only with a certain sexual partner but not with other women. A conscious wish for an erection is as a rule a barrier to success.

A further disorder medically related to impotence is that of *premature ejaculation*. Here the man ejaculates either before or immediately on introducing his penis into the vagina, so that his erection subsides and his wife remains unsatisfied in her sexual excitement and expectations. Impotence and premature ejaculation are both due to neurotic disorders which in severe cases are based on erroneous sex education and failure to prepare the man for maturity; in milder cases there may be unconscious rejection of the present sexual partner with whom impotence or premature ejaculation exists. Rejection may be present in spite of conscious feelings of love. Since these disorders are emotionally caused they can be overcome only by psychotherapy. Unfortunately the area of sex is still taboo in a fair-sized proportion of the population, so that men with these disorders prefer to endanger their marriage rather than go to a doctor and obtain treatment, though the earlier treatment is begun the better the prospects of success. It should be pointed out that there are also combined disorders of potency and fertility, in which a combined drug and psychotherapeutic approach is needed.

The Woman

The Female Genital Organs

In contrast to the male, the internal genital organs of the female lie essentially within the lower abdomen (see fig. 16). Entry to them is reached through the external genitals which in the mature woman lie hidden under the pubic hair and behind the vulva. The entry itself lies in the front third of the area between the thighs. The whole area of the external genitals in the woman is known as the pudenda (Latin: 'of which one should be ashamed').

The vagina represents the link between external and internal sex organs. In relation to the body axis it is directed obliquely from below upwards and backwards. It serves to admit the male organ and semen, and as an exit for the menstrual flow and the child.

The uterus or womb, which because it exists to protect the new life within it, must lie inside the body, bends forwards at an angle to the vagina so that when pregnant it may grow without hindrance in the abdominal cavity. The two fallopian tubes connect the womb with the ovaries and serve to transport the ovum or egg from the ovary where it is formed to the uterus, and to transport the sperm cells from the vagina to the ovum.

FIG. 16 *Position of female genitals (three-quarter view).*

1 Vagina   2 Uterus   3 Tube   4 Ovary

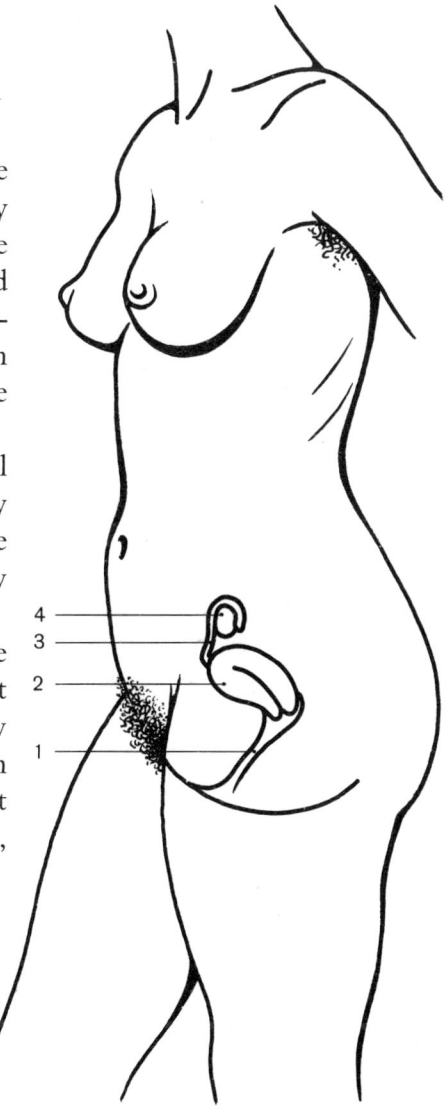

106   The body profile of the woman generally contrasts with that of the male in the softness of its contours. The breasts accentuate the upper part of the trunk in relation to the relatively small shoulder girdle. The profile is further conditioned by the fairly prominent rounding and softness of the hips, thighs and buttocks. The woman's lap, the soft area between lower abdomen and thighs, conceals access to the external genitals in the sitting position with the legs together; in this position the upper limit of the pubic hair with the mons veneris is just visible.

External Genitals

The female external genitals are visible only when the thighs and the greater lips (labia majora) are separated.

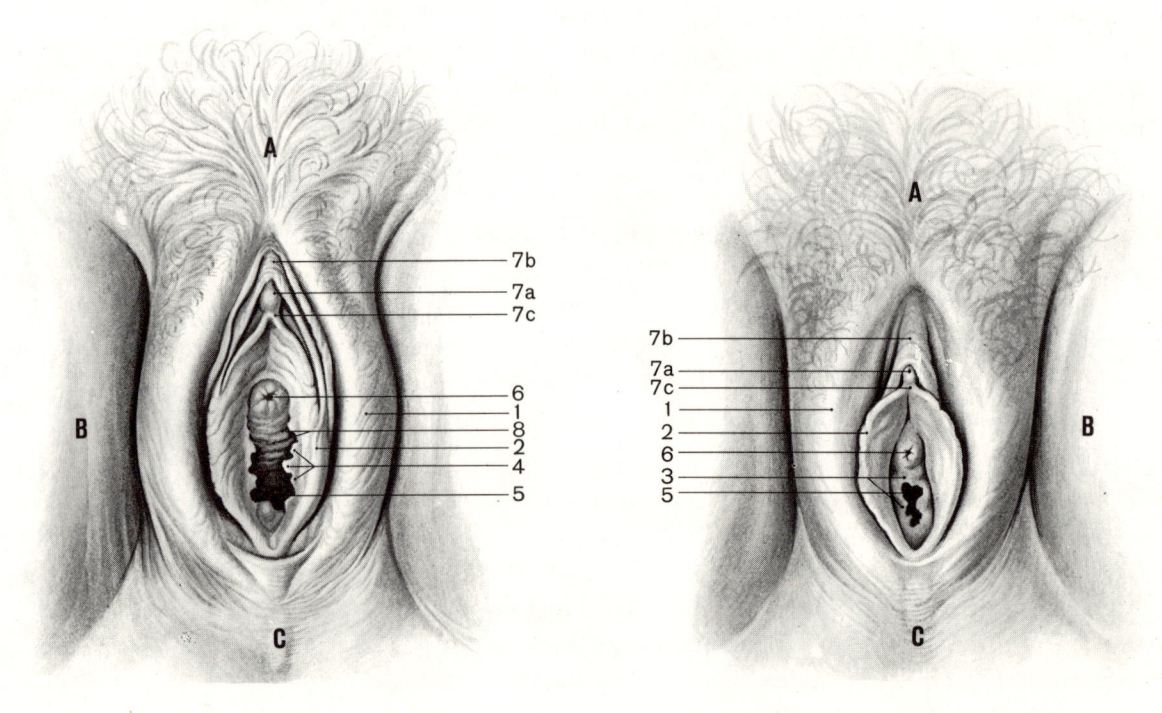

FIG. 17 *Vaginal entrance, with walls separated. Left, after delivery; right, with intact hymen.*

A Mons veneris	1 External labia majora	5 Vaginal entrance
B Thigh	2 Internal labia minora	6 Urethral opening
C Perineum	3 Hymen	7 Clitoris (a glans, b prepuce, c frenulum)
	4 Tags of hymen	8 Transverse ridges on front wall of vagina

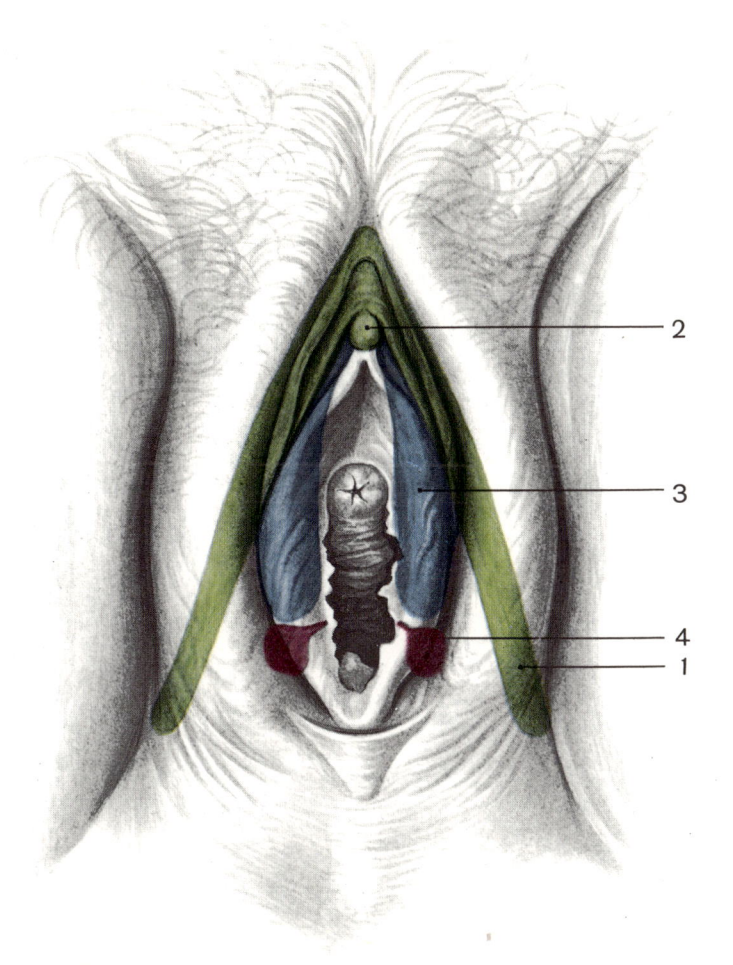

FIG. 18 *Erectile tissue of the female genitals.*

1 *Corpora cavernosa of the clitoris (lying deeply in the labia majora)*
2 *Glans of the clitoris*
3 *Corpora cavernosa of the vagina (lying under the labia minora)*
4 *Bartholin's gland with excretory duct on the inner side of the labia minora*

Labia majora and minora

The greater lips or labia majora (see figs. 17 and 18) are two folds of skin enclosing a pad of fat; they are hairy on the outside and provided with glands, and lie in apposition in normal postures, having a pudendal cleft about 3 inches long between them. Developmentally they correspond to the two halves of the scrotum in the male. They are connected behind through a transverse skin fold separating the vulva from the perineum, an area between vulva and anus.

In the front, the two labia majora end in the mons veneris. If they are separated an area is seen into which both the urethra and the vagina open. This entrance lies between two smaller lips, the labia minora, which are delicate and hairless and of varying thickness and size (a few mm. up to over an inch) in different women; they are often asymmetrical and contain numerous very sensitive sensory receptors and a network of blood vessels. They are responsive to touch, and on contact grow firmer because their blood vessels fill; this causes the pudendal cleft to widen a little so that they can be seen as moist skinfolds in the latter. In playing with the genitals or in the love play preceding intercourse the labia minora are commonly touched; if this stimulation is prolonged and habitual they may eventually enlarge into long thin lips.

On the inner side of the posterior third of the labia minora the excretory ducts of Bartholin's glands open (see fig. 18). These are paired structures varying in size from a pea to a bean, and correspond to Cowper's glands in the male. At the beginning of sexual excitement they secrete a mucous greyish-white fluid which serves to moisten and lubricate the vaginal entrance so that entry of the penis into the vagina is facilitated. At the beginning of puberty when the genitals are being reoriented towards their later function, there may be so much secretion from these glands that it amounts to a discharge, as in some women immediately before sexual intercourse.

In love play before intercourse this moistness of the external genitals is a signal to the man that his partner has reached an advanced stage of excitement. Since at the same time the labial glands are working harder and secreting a fluid with an agreeable and stimulating smell, his own excitement is also increased.

Immediately behind the labia minora lie the two corpora cavernosa of the vagina (fig. 18). These fill up as the woman becomes more excited so that two soft pads appear, narrowing the vaginal opening; these will hold the penis gently but firmly and thus increase pleasure by their contact with it during penetration and intercourse and the consequent mutual nerve stimulation.

At the back the labia minora are connected by a small band, the fourchette, which is also provided with sensitive receptors but usually tears with the first delivery. At the front, each labium minus splits into two folds, of which the two inner ones join as the tiny but exquisitely sensitive band or frenulum behind the clitoris. The two external folds unite over the clitoris to form its prepuce or foreskin.

The clitoris

This corresponds to the glans penis and is formed by the ends of two large erectile bodies or corpora cavernosa clitoridis, which arise from the lower arches of the pubic bones and are bent outwards and united in front. The clitoris (see fig. 18) is the most sensitive organ of the female genitals and is the organ which, acting in conjunction with the posterior part of the vagina and an assorted collection of sensory receptors within the genitals, is mainly responsible for the pleasurable feelings associated with copulation and orgasm (clitoris orgasm). The name clitoris comes from the Latin for a key, indicating that doctors in Roman times regarded this organ as the key to sexual pleasure in the woman.

Like the male penis, the clitoris varies in size, but in white women it is usually between 4 and 15 mm. (one-sixth to one-half inch) long. In states of excitement its length may double as a result of filling of its corpora cavernosa with blood, so that it comes in intimate contact with the shaft of the penis during intercourse. Because the prepuce of the clitoris allows only the glans to protrude even on extreme excitement, the organ is always pointed downwards, so that it is directed to the vaginal entrance between the labia minora.

As in the male, there are numerous sebaceous glands under the prepuce, and together with the glands on the labia majora these cause the characteristic smell of the mature woman; this smell varies in intensity and usually excites the male.

The opening of the urethra is about one inch beneath the clitoris on a small raised papilla. This papilla is also very sensitive sexually in many but not all women. In its neighbourhood there are several very small glands, which on sexual excitement secrete fluid moistening the vaginal entrance; they probably also neutralize any traces of urine near the urethral orifice.

Hymen

Immediately below the urethral opening lies the vaginal entrance which is narrowed in virgins by the presence of a membrane, the hymen, usually to a size admitting only a little finger. The hymen (or maidenhead) may be ring- or sickel-shaped or sieve-like or fringed or dentate (see fig. 17b). Its thickness and extent are also very variable. In rare cases it entirely encloses the entrance and must therefore be opened up by operation at the onset of puberty to let the menses out; failure to do this may lead to dangerous damming up of the menstrual blood into the fallopian tubes.

The thickness of the hymen lies between 0·1 and 2 mm., but it is exceptional to find this an obstacle to the first introduction of a penis. This usually tears the hymen and often results in the loss of a few drops of blood. This process of defloration plays a significant part in all civilized races. Defloration is rarely painful and then usually only if intercourse is carried out against the will of the girl. Otherwise the sexual excitement and tension as well as the stimulation of the external genitals are so intense that the momentary tearing is scarcely felt.

The first delivery further injures the hymen so that only a few warty remains persist; the front wall of the vagina with its transverse folds then becomes plainly visible if the labia minora are parted.

Vaginal entrance

The entire vaginal entrance (see fig. 17) is surrounded at a deeper level by muscles which can be tightened voluntarily so as to narrow the entrance on intercourse and thus bring the labia minora and clitoris into closer association with the penis and heighten the penile erection. Every woman can learn to contract these muscles rhythmically during intercourse and thus increase her own satisfaction. Contraction also brings the male more smoothly and rapidly to his orgasm. Recent studies seem to confirm that stimulation of these muscles causes a *vaginal orgasm* in distinction to a clitoral orgasm, for the high point of vaginal sensitivity lies at their inner edge about 1 to 2 inches from the opening. This knowledge means that the male is in a position to pay special attention to this zone during intercourse and to increase stimulation by penile movements against the vaginal walls. Comparatively slow and gentle movements are most helpful, for too violent and rapid movements and too deep and violent penetration by the penis may upset the woman and cause her excitement to subside.

Frigidity

Muscle spasm at the entrance of the vagina as an expression of emotionally conditioned defence may prevent entry of the penis or else grip the latter powerfully and cause pain. If such cramp persists during intercourse medical aid may be needed. This disorder, often associated with dryness of the female genitals, is an expression of a deep and unconscious emotional rejection of sex or of the partner concerned. This type of attitude, which may exist in spite of conscious love for the man, is called frigidity. Dilating the vaginal passage represents only an incomplete type of treatment, because the crucial point is the defensive reaction and this is not an organic spasm due to a narrow vagina but a predominantly unconscious event. The commonest forms of frigidity are the above mentioned vaginal cramp or vaginismus, and failure to achieve orgasm in intercourse. In yet another type the dryness of the vaginal passage due to emotional inhibition of glandular action makes intercourse painful. Since all these types are emotionally caused, they require appropriately timed psychotherapy, just as impotence in the male does.

Internal Genital Organs

The internal genital organs of the woman (see figs. 19 and 20) consist of two ovaries, two fallopian tubes, a uterus and a vagina. The ovaries are the reproductive glands of the woman. They are flattened oval organs and during the reproductive life of the woman are about the size of a plum (average $1\frac{1}{4}$ to $2\frac{1}{2}$ in. long). There is considerable variation in size but the glands shrink with loss of function on ageing.

The ovaries lie on the side wall inside the lesser pelvis below the fallopian tubes and at some distance from the uterus. They contain ova from birth on, and the latter throughout that period of life when reproduction is possible, usually from the fourteenth to the fiftieth year nowadays, mature and leave the ovary when they are ripe.

The fallopian tubes, about 4 to 8 inches long, unite the ovaries with the uterus. At the outer end, open to the ovary and the abdominal cavity, they widen out like a trumpet and

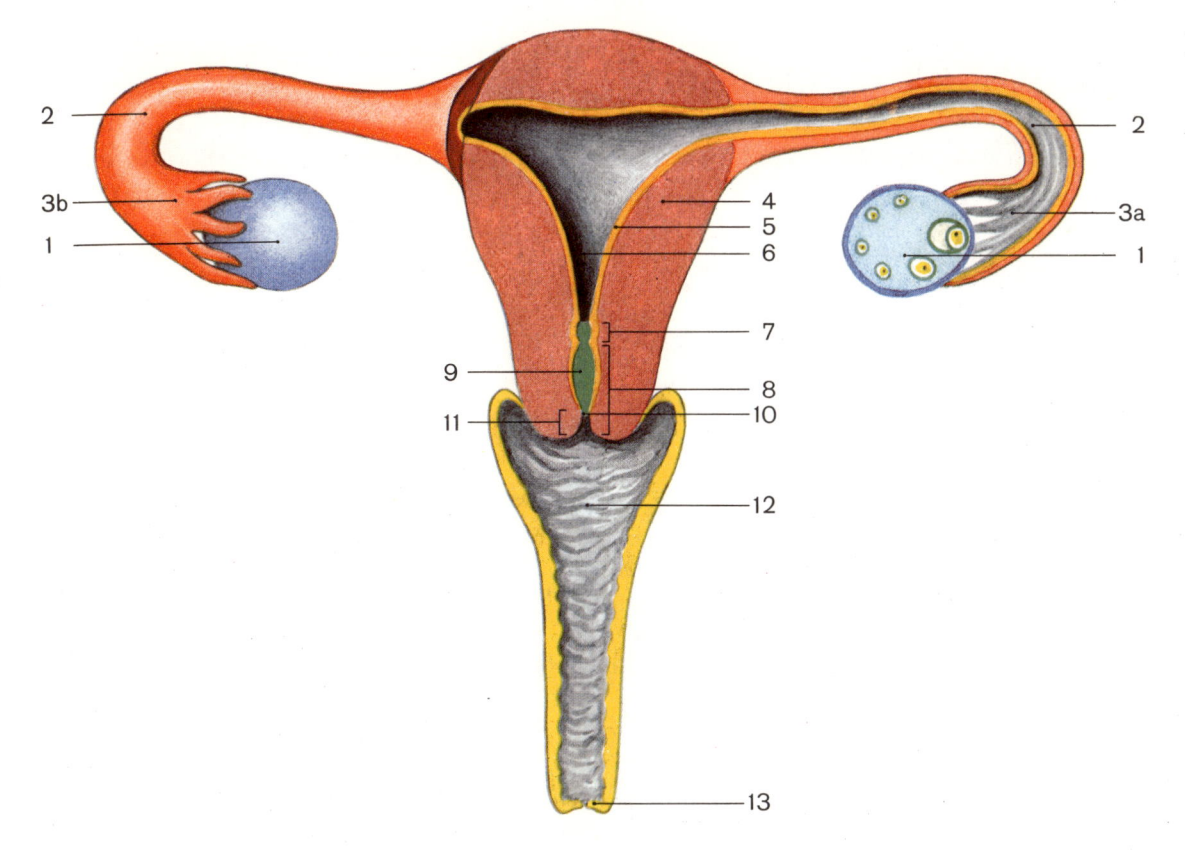

FIG. 19 *Female internal genitalia seen from the front. For simplification tilting and kinking of the uterus are disregarded.*

1 Ovary—sectioned on right to show follicle
2 Ovary, sectioned on right
3 a Funnel-shaped end of fallopian tube, open to peritoneal cavity and to ovary
  b Fimbriae of tube embracing site on ovary where follicle will rupture
4 Body of uterus (muscles)
5 Mucosa of uterus (endometrium)
6 Cavity of uterus
7 Constriction between body and cervix
8 Cervix of uterus
9 Mucus plug in cervical canal
10 External os
11 Vaginal portion of cervix
12 Vagina
13 Hymen

have an edge with finger-like fringes or fimbriae of varying sizes, the whole resembling a carnation. At its open end the fallopian tube is about 1 cm. wide while at the uterine end it is only 2 mm. wide. During the period when ova are extruded from the ovary, the tube arranges itself in relation to the latter in such a manner that any emerging ova will be taken up by it.

112 The uterus is a powerfully muscular hollow pear-shaped organ, about 3 inches long in the non-pregnant woman. It lies between the urinary bladder and the rectum and is kept in place by highly elastic tendinous ligaments. The vagina, flattened and tubular, unites the uterus with the external genitals. With loss of elasticity, the position of the uterus may change. It may protrude into the vagina, turning the latter partially inside out. This is called a prolapse of the uterus and requires operation.

Uterus
The uterus is not only responsible for delivery of the pregnant woman but also for the maintenance of the fertilized ovum, to which it affords all the necessary conditions for living;

FIG. 20 *Female pelvis and genital organs; longitudinal section.*

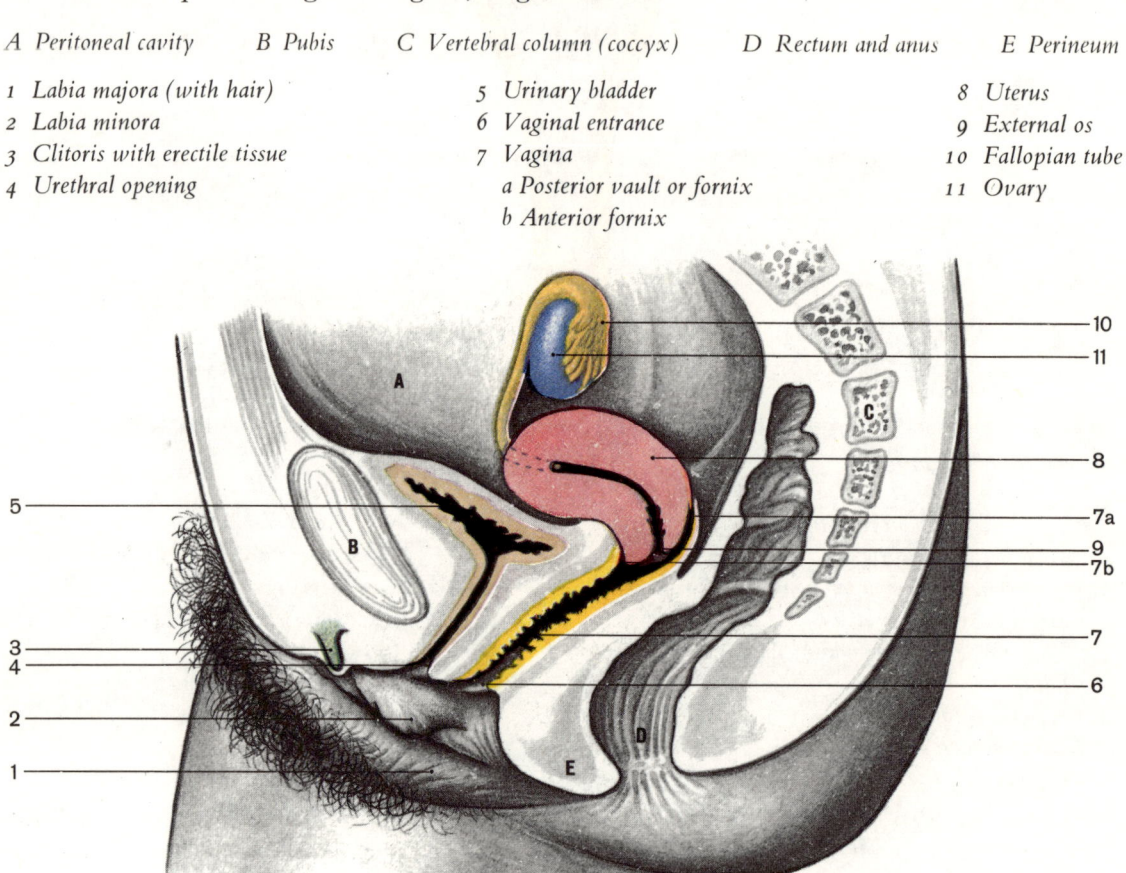

A *Peritoneal cavity*	B *Pubis*	C *Vertebral column (coccyx)*	D *Rectum and anus*	E *Perineum*
1 *Labia majora (with hair)*		5 *Urinary bladder*		8 *Uterus*
2 *Labia minora*		6 *Vaginal entrance*		9 *External os*
3 *Clitoris with erectile tissue*		7 *Vagina*		10 *Fallopian tube*
4 *Urethral opening*		a *Posterior vault or fornix*		11 *Ovary*
		b *Anterior fornix*		

previously it has played an active part in receiving the semen and allowing spermatozoa to proceed into the fallopian tubes. It is also the organ which carries out intense movements at the height of orgasm, contributing considerably to the woman's pleasure. Lastly it is the organ responsible for menstruation, though this function is closely allied to its function as a receptor for the fertilized ovum.

In the uterus the upper part, the particularly muscular *body*, is separated from the lower neck or *cervix* by a constriction about one-fifth of an inch long. Part of the cervix protrudes into the vagina and on this prominence lies the external os or mouth, which is dimpled in women who have not yet borne children but later tends to become somewhat fissured or star-shaped.

The cavity of the uterus is triangular and lined by a mucosa called the endometrium which undergoes rhythmical changes as long as pregnancy does not take place. In the cervical canal there is a tough glassy plug of mucus which shuts off the uterine cavity and thus the abdominal cavity from the exterior. If it were not for this, the abdominal cavity in women would be directly connected with the outer world via the tubes, uterus and vagina. This plug of mucus has however other functions than the protection from infection of the inside of the body, and in pregnancy the developing foetus. At the height of sexual intercourse through uterine muscular action the plug is partially expelled into the vagina and then returned. If male and female orgasms coincide, semen will be taken up into the cervical canal, thus affording the most favourable situation for insemination.

This process is however not absolutely necessary for insemination, fertilization and pregnancy. Without an orgasmal reflex on the part of the woman, and in fact sometimes when semen is merely deposited on the external genitals of a virgin, sperm cells may migrate actively towards the ovum.

The process of sucking the sperm cells into the cervix does not mean that these cells mixed with cervical mucus are directly shot into the uterine cavity. They migrate by their own efforts through the plug of mucus, undergoing en route a chemical cleansing from all adherent substances including the other elements of the semen.

In *artificial insemination* the initial attempts were made by injecting semen with a syringe and hollow needle directly into the uterine cavity past the mucus plug. In most cases this led to serious local reactions which were sometimes so painful that the woman went into shock and was in danger of dying. These reactions were not due to a hypersensitivity to sperm from a given donor but to the general intolerance of the uterine mucosa to semen. So the semen is now usually introduced, either diluted or with the sperm cells suspended in a non-irritating fluid, only into the outer layer of the mucus plug, whence the spermatozoa must find their way up under their own power.

In a view from the side (fig. 21), the uterus is seen to be 'normally' tipped forward and also bent forwards at an angle with a kink at the boundary between body and cervix.

FIG. 21 *Tilting and kinking of uterus.*

1 *Vaginal axis*
2 *Axis of cervix*
3 *Axis of body of uterus*
4 *Angle of tilt*
5 *Angle of flexion*

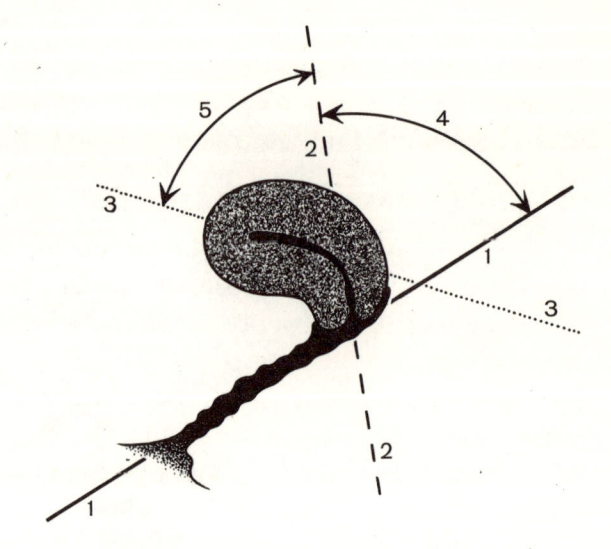

  This tipping and kinking of the uterus are necessary to bring the opening of the cervical canal into relation with the posterior vault of the vaginal canal into which the semen is deposited at intercourse. This facilitates penetration of the spermatozoa into the uterus. The position of the uterus also permits the organ during pregnancy to enlarge into the abdominal cavity unimpeded by the bony pelvic girdle.
  The vaginal portion of the cervix is tough and about as firm as the glans penis during sexual excitement. With deep penetration during intercourse the male glans and the female cervix come into contact. This contact not only increases male stimulation but also acts indirectly on the woman by raising the whole uterus up. The process leads reflexly to a reversed muscular contraction in the uterus, which is similar and supplementary to the general reflex contraction on copulation. However, sexual enjoyment does not depend on the ripening of ova and the associated hormonal changes in the ovary, or on the rhythmical contractions of the uterus or its other functions. The capacity for sexual satisfaction depends only on the presence of the pituitary hormones which act on the sex organs, and on the general attitude to sexuality and to sexual intercourse. It is also dependent on the response of the external genital organs and the vagina to stimuli. A woman who has lost both ovaries and the uterus can have an orgasm if she is mentally prepared for it and her husband lovingly cooperates. However both partners often need some time to practise together after such an operation, just as they do immediately after marriage.

Vagina
This is a tube from $2\frac{1}{2}$ to 6 inches long, the length depending on the situation of the uterus in

the pelvis. It is equipped with a tough mucosal wall outside which runs a relatively thin spiral muscular layer; the vagina is folded and extremely distensible. It serves for the reception of the penis in intercourse and the passage of the baby at delivery. The breadth and diameter of the vagina are hard to determine because it stretches so much. At rest the lumen appears as a narrow transverse fissure in the shape of a capital H.

The cervix protrudes into the upper reaches of the vagina, and because of the normal tilting of the uterus this leaves a short front vault and a longer hind vault. The latter is also in a straight line with the vaginal axis.

Below, the vagina opens into the vestibule, and the hymen or its remains marks the line of transition.

The inner wall of the vagina is tougher than other mucosae and is arranged in many transverse or ring-like folds which stand out on both front and back walls and increase contact and friction with the penis as well as making adaptation to any size of penis possible. (Thus there is no need to try out intercourse before marriage to see whether the sex organs fit one another.) These folds enable the vagina to stretch enormously at delivery, so that the baby's head, the most solid part of the child, can pass through. A few weeks after delivery the vagina has not quite returned to its original elasticity, so that for a while it feels bigger and more roomy on intercourse. After a large number of deliveries—in some women with poor elastic tissue, after only one—there may be a permanent loss of elasticity of the vagina. In these cases it is advisable during intercourse to adopt those positions which promote more effective and sensitive contact between penis and vagina. This includes all those positions in which the woman closes her legs after introduction of the penis, as well as those variations in which the two pelvic girdles lie a little out of the parallel line so that the axes of the penis and vagina do not correspond and either the front or the back wall of the vagina (and also the upper or lower surface of the penis) is increasingly stimulated. If elasticity of the vagina is lost to a greater degree the surrounding organs (bladder, uterus, rectum) may protrude so far into the vagina that they push the vaginal wall out and beyond the normal; this is a vaginal prolapse which needs operation.

The superficial layers of the vaginal mucosa contain large quantities of a certain type of carbohydrate and readily scale off. From this carbohydrate certain bacteria which are normal inhabitants of the vagina can form lactic acid. This acid is a normal protective agent, and builds a barrier between the genitals and any bacteria entering from the exterior. However lactic acid is harmful to spermatozoa, and so the acid effect is always temporarily neutralized by the seminal fluid.

The vaginal mucosa is practically devoid of glands, its moistness being ensured by a small quantity of uterine mucus and by fluid permeation of the wall.

The relatively weak muscle layer in the vagina reinforces by its contraction the sexual stimulation due to mutual contact of penis and vagina. Other powerful muscles which surround the vagina but belong to the pelvic floor further accentuate stimulation, since during intercourse they contract rhythmically and usually spontaneously and help the penis into the vagina; their alternate contraction and relaxation can often be felt by both partners and increases their excitement. After orgasm this excitement only gradually subsides in the woman, so that most women are grateful if the man remains for a while with his penis still inside them.

Sensory nerve endings are less common in the vagina than in the female external genitals, but it would be a mistake to think that because of this the vagina plays little part in sexual enjoyment and the arousal of orgasm (for orgasm, see p. 148 ff.). Under the influence of the sexual stimulus the mucosa of the vagina swells up to varying degrees. The rhythmical alternation of extension, contraction and vaginal swelling cause a special form of excitement, and in some women this alone suffices to cause extreme pleasure. An orgasm achieved by this means is called a vaginal orgasm. Whether vaginal orgasm represents a higher degree of sexual maturity in women remains controversial. Recent studies have shown that vaginal and clitoral orgasm are independent of the sexual experience of the woman. They are much more dependent on the individual excitability of these zones and on the woman's special relationship to her partner; in other words they depend on the particular partner and his technique. Nevertheless there is no doubt that at the beginning of her sex life the woman derives her stimulation mostly from the clitoris and only acquires vaginal orgasm through experience. In addition, a woman experiences physical and mental fulfilment through the consciousness of having a penis within her. This increases her pleasure in conjunction with the total experience of male wooing.

The ovaries

The germinal cells of the woman, like the primitive sperm cells of the man, arise from division of certain cells during development of the embryo. They can be demonstrated in an embryo only 1·5 mm. long, about three weeks after conception. Towards the end of the fourth month of pregnancy they are already firmly embedded in the tissues of the ovary. Whereas the primitive sperm cells in the walls of the seminiferous tubules retain their capacity for division into old age, the primitive ova divide into mature ova only up to the birth of the girl. At this point the girl has about 400,000 to 500,000 ova (about 200,000 to 250,000 per ovary).

While the female embryo is still developing in the womb, one-layered coats are being laid down from surrounding tissue to cover the individual ova as they lie in clumps near the surface of the ovary; these are the primary follicles. Most of these ova will perish during the woman's life—even before she reaches the reproductive years. Final maturation is reached only by about 400 to 550 ova (this means about 12 to 14 ova a year during the reproductive years between about the fourteenth and the fiftieth year, not counting pregnancy). At the beginning of the reproductive age there forms around the previously resting ova a cell layer, first one cell, then two cells and then several cells thick. Among these, fluid forms between the cells so that finally a follicle or vesicle about 5 to 8 mm. in

FIG. 22 *Ovary. Diagram showing follicle rupture.*

1 Resting ova, lying in clumps under the surface of an ovary in the newborn
2 Resting ova at the beginning of sexual maturity (in clumps)
3 Ova surrounded with several layers of follicular cells, and early follicle formation
4 Larger follicle
   a Follicle cells
   b Hillock (cumulus oopherus) with ovum
   c Follicle with fluid (follicular hormone or oestrogen)
5 Maturing follicle elevated above ovarian surface
6 Rupture of follicle
   a Expelled ovum with coronal cells
   b Escaping follicular fluid
   c Individual follicular cells escaping
7 Corpus luteum with traces of blood
8 Corpus luteum in regression
9 Functionless remains of corpus luteum (corpus album)
10 Scar stage at ovarian surface

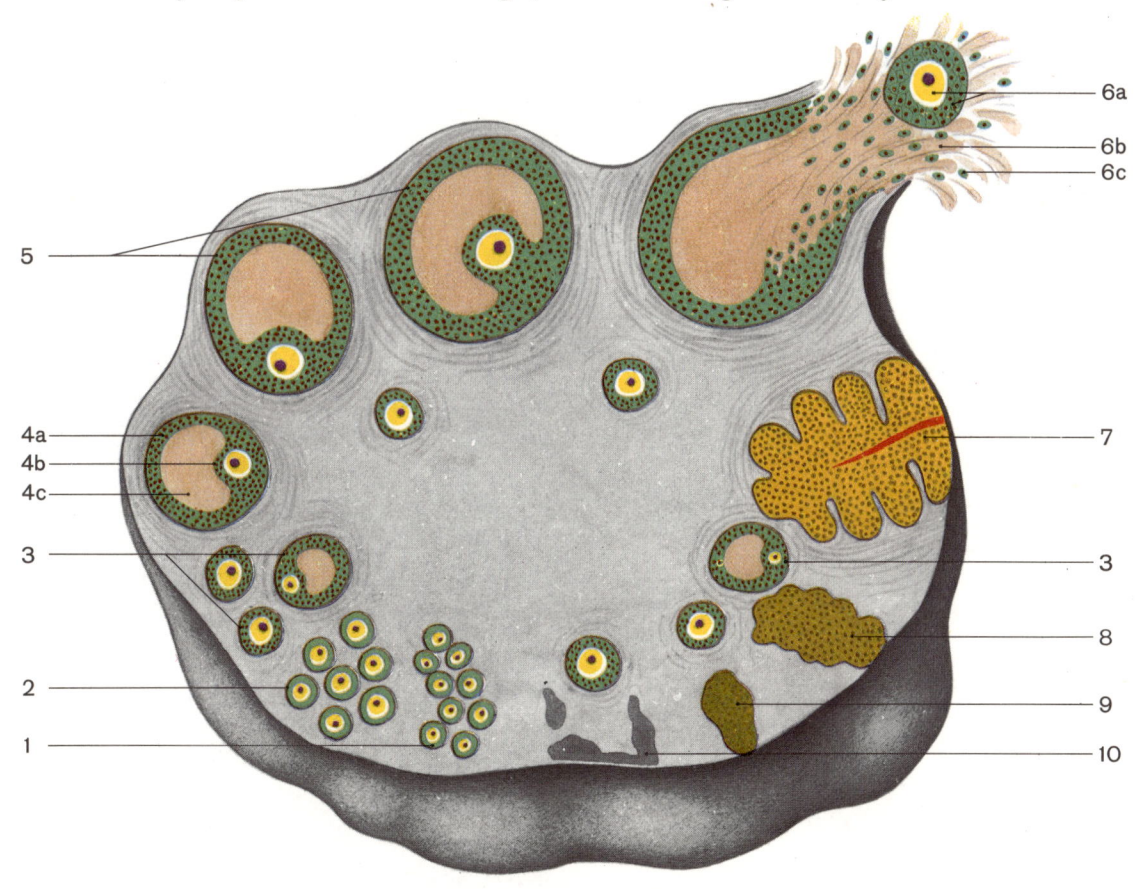

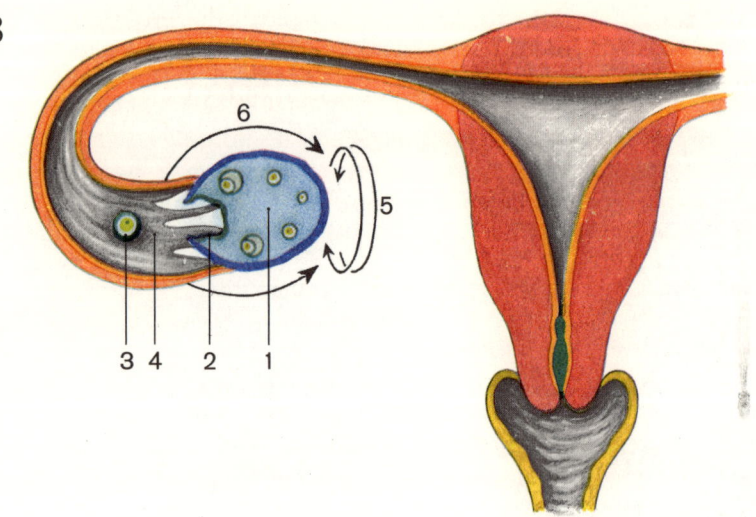

FIG. 23 *Diagram showing mechanism of uptake of ovum.*

1 Ovary
2 Ruptured follicle (remains of follicle)
3 Ovum surrounded by coronal cells in
4 Funnel of tube
5 Direction of rotation of ovary on its long axis
6 Direction in which tube seeks contact with ovary

diameter appears. These vesicles, which were formerly thought to be the human ova themselves, contain the resting ovum in a mass of other cells; they may remain at rest, die or mature, but only one at a time. Meanwhile a cell wall has been built round the ovum which is particularly well adapted to let spermatozoa through. Each vesicle is surrounded by a dense network of small blood vessels which ensure the nutrition of the vesicle and also take up the hormones arising there.

The maturation of a follicle containing an ovum is shown in Figure 22, where development proceeds clockwise. The early follicle consists of a round object in which several layers of cells and a little fluid surround the ovum. Under pressure from the growing follicle the other ovarian tissues around it build a capsule, and as the cavity containing fluid increases in size the ovum comes to lie on a hillock on the inner wall of the fluid vesicle. The ova remain the same size but their follicles grow within a few days to the size of a cherry (about $\frac{1}{2}$ to $\frac{3}{4}$ in. in diameter). The mature follicle now causes a bulge on the surface of the ovary, and through its internal pressure as well as chemical degeneration in its capsule it finally bursts. Through the resulting hole, about the size of a pinhead, the ovum escapes with its surrounding follicular cells, the corona radiata, floating in the follicular fluid. This process is known as rupture of the follicle or of the ovum. The word 'rupture' is a misnomer, for the ovum escapes very slowly on account of the high viscosity of the fluid. (Sensitive women are occasionally aware of the rupture of the follicle because they feel pain in the right or left side of the lower abdomen halfway through their menstrual period, the so-called Mittelschmerz.)

Mechanism of uptake of ova
One might imagine that when the follicle ruptured the ova would escape freely into the

abdominal cavity, but this is not so. Just before the follicle ruptures the ovary and the fallopian tube concerned move towards each other to facilitate uptake of the ovum (see fig. 23). The open end of the tube sweeps rhythmically over the ovarian surface, and at the same time the ovary turns periodically on its long axis. Thus every two minutes the whole surface of the ovary is swept over and the ovum leaving the ovary is directly taken into the fallopian tube without any contact with the free abdominal cavity. (We must remember that the ovum only lives two days after leaving the ovary, and can only be fertilized during this time.)

Corpus luteum

Those follicular cells left behind in the ovary after rupture undergo a characteristic change. First the wall of the follicle collapses in folds because it has lost its fluid and contains only a little blood from the vessels torn at rupture. The follicular cells no longer divide but undergo a change with storage of an orange-yellow substance, to whose appearance the follicle now owes its new name of yellow body or corpus luteum. This yellow body has its own hormonal function (see below). About 2 to 10 days (opinions about this are very varied) after follicular rupture the corpus luteum has reached maturity and measures $\frac{1}{2}$ inch or so in diameter. If the ovum is fertilized and pregnancy ensues, the corpus luteum persists until the end of pregnancy and at the same time prevents the maturation of another follicle. If the ovum is not fertilized, about 12 days after follicular rupture the corpus luteum begins to regress. Finally, all that remains is a small scarred body under a dimple in the ovarian surface, indistinguishable from the other follicles which have perished. The disappearance of the corpus luteum makes it possible for the next follicle to develop, though there is no regular alternation of the two ovaries as regards maturation of ova.

The ova

The ova which arise from primitive ovular cells (see fig. 24) first lie in clumps near the ovarian surface and may assume different forms. Usually an ovum with its nucleus lies in a primary follicle (fig. 24, 1 and 2), but some of the ova have two nuclei (3); cells with three nuclei are exceptional (4). However two complete ova can lie in one primary follicle (5) and this suggests one possibility for the origin of binovular twin pregnancies. There are also follicles with three ova (6), which might form the basis for a multiple pregnancy with three ova. A mixed form is possible but rare; one follicle may contain two ova of which one has two nuclei (7).

Since it has been observed that multiple pregnancies can occur in families through the female succession (grandmother, mother, daughter, etc.), the recent finding of the presence of two and three ova in one follicle (perhaps through division of primitive ovular cells) may be of hereditary significance. If this type of follicle with several ova predominates, the

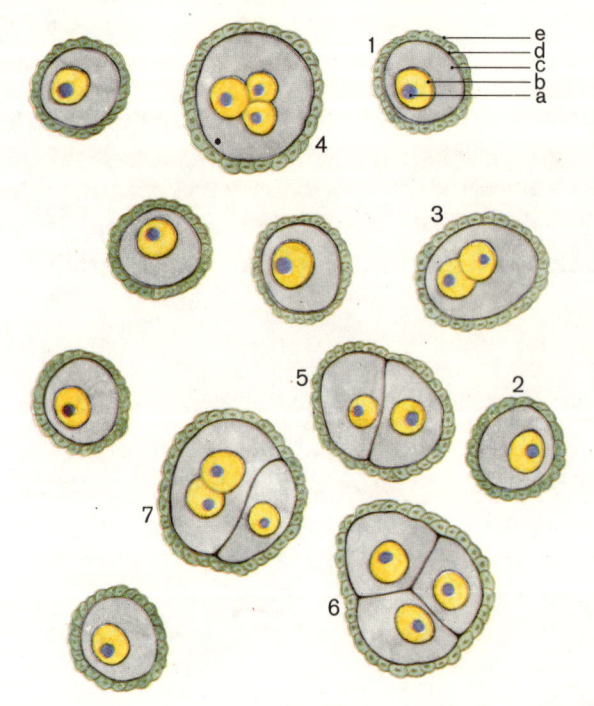

FIG. 24 *Various forms of ovum in ovary.*

1 *Ovum: a cell nucleus; b yolk area; c cell substance; d capsule; e surrounding cells from ovary, later becoming coronal cells*
2 *Single cells in a future follicle (almost all follicles start thus)*
3 *Ovum with two cell nuclei*
4 *Ovum with three nuclei*
5 *Two ova in a future follicle (may lead to binovular twins)*
6 *Three ova in future follicle (rare, but may cause triple-ovum triplets)*
7 *Two ova in future follicle, one with two nuclei (very rare)*

Because every nucleus must be separately fertilized by a spermatozoon, to set in motion cell division and thus the development to a foetus, no uniovular multiple births can result from cells with several nuclei.

probability of its maturation and multiple fertilization of its contained ova must be greater than if uniovular follicles predominate. We have no certain knowledge of the fertilization of human ova containing two or three nuclei.

The resting ovum found at the beginning of reproductive age and measuring 0·04 to 0·05 mm. in size consists of general cell substance, yolk material, and the vesicular cell nucleus, 18 to 20 microns in diameter. The nucleus and the yolk substance may lie excentrically near the border of the cell, which is surrounded by several layers of capsule, and these in turn by follicular cells. The latter are later separated again by a capsule from the rest of the ovarian tissue.

The yolk area is so-called by analogy with the corresponding component of birds' eggs and has a similar function, namely to nourish the ovum during its first cell division after fertilization, before the latter can obtain nourishment from the maternal tissues.

As the ovum grows before leaving the ovary the yolk material also grows considerably, the remaining cell substance to a lesser degree, and the cell nucleus least of all.

Maturation of the ovum
As the follicle itself matures, the ovum also ripens (see fig. 25). In the male the primitive sperm cell divides twice to give rise to four cells, and a similar event occurs with the primary oocyte

FIG. 25 *Maturation of the ovum.*

Early stages of ova before sexual maturity

First maturation division of ovum

Second maturation division of polar body

Second maturation division of ovum

Mature ovum

In the ovary

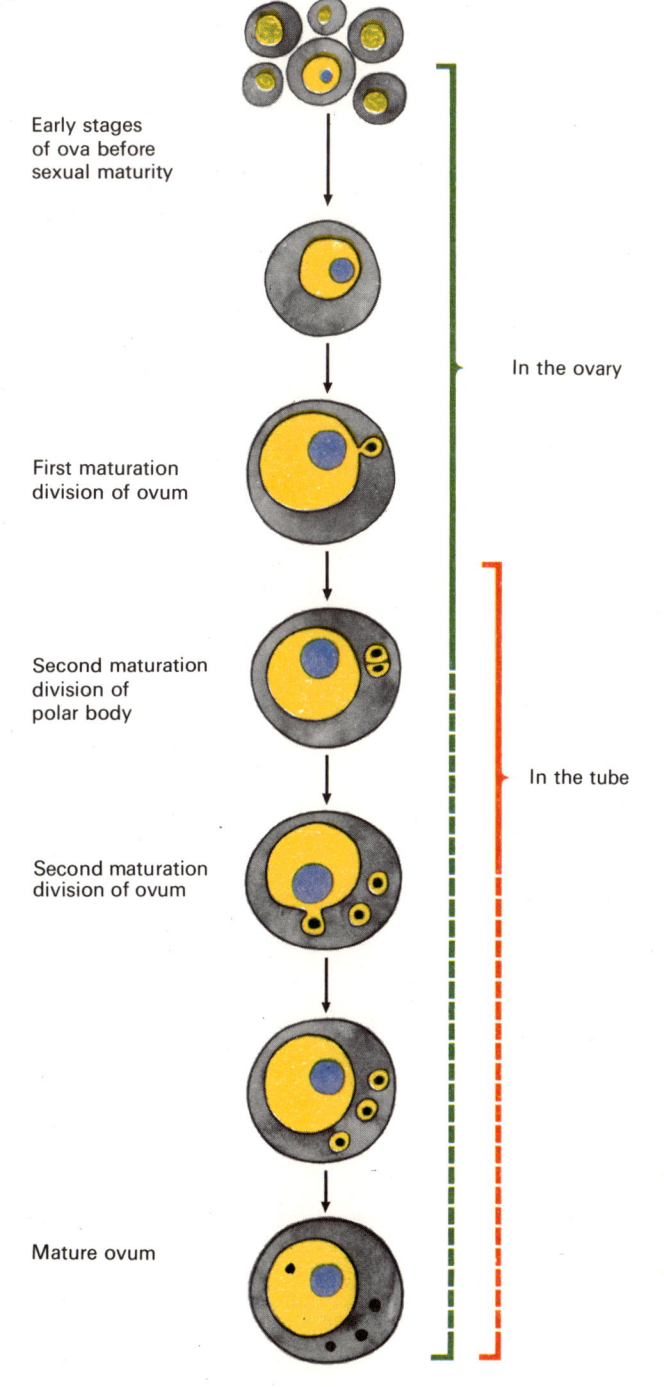

In the tube

or egg cell, but in contrast to the male the oocyte produces one large cell and three tiny and almost invisible ones. Not all the cell divides, but only the nucleus together with a little yolk substance. The three tiny cells are extruded into the cell substance as polar bodies but cannot leave the follicle on account of the capsule. This first maturation division produces a secondary oocyte plus one polar body. These then divide again and produce a mature egg plus three polar bodies which usually perish. The primary maturation into secondary oocyte and polar body occurs while the ovum is still in the maturing follicle within the ovary.

The second maturation division occurs as a rule after the secondary oocyte has got into the fallopian tube and been penetrated by a spermatozoon, but before the two nuclei have fused. One curious feature is that the polar body tends to divide before the secondary oocyte. These maturation divisions are of special significance for the distribution of hereditary characters, and this point will be returned to in discussion of heredity (see chapter on germ cell maturation and inheritance, pp. 159–160 and figs. 37 and 38).

The diagram below (fig. 26) compares the maturation processes in the spermatozoon and ovum:

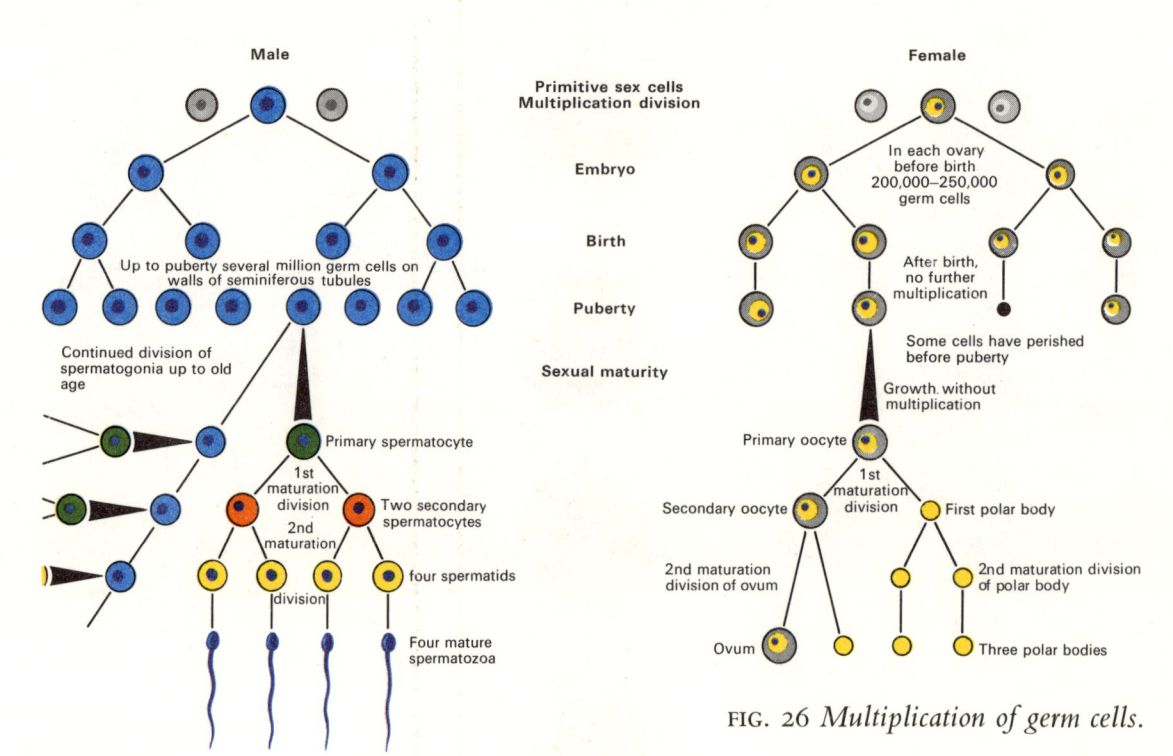

FIG. 26 *Multiplication of germ cells.*

Mature ovum

The mature egg (fig. 27), without its surrounding follicle or corona radiata, is only 0·10 to

FIG. 27 *Mature ovum. Diameter of ovum (without corona radiata) 0·1 to 0·15 mm., about that of a needle point.*

1 External elastic layer
2 Yolk area
3 Cell nucleus, corresponding to head of spermatozoon
4 Remaining cell substance
5 Three polar bodies
6 Surrounding cells of corona radiata
7 Process of coronal cell penetrating ovum
8 Remnants of coronal cells

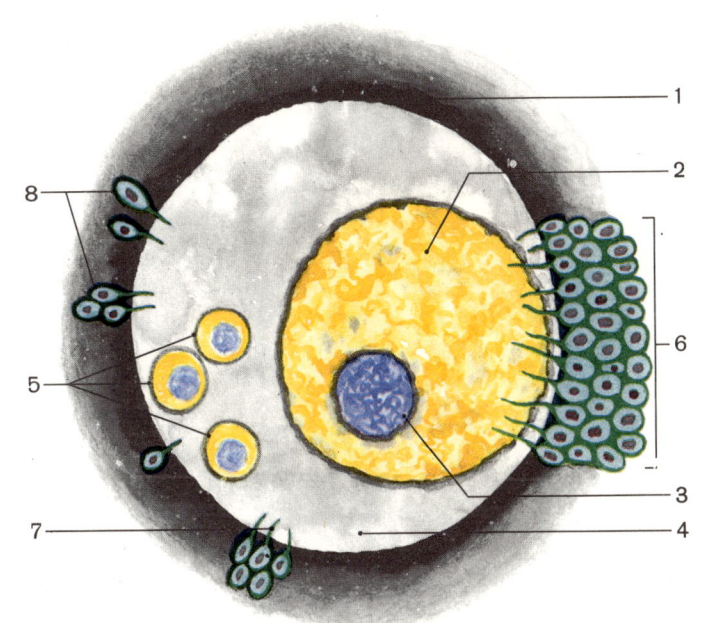

0·15 mm. in size. The outer elastic coat is closely related to the enveloping follicular or coronal cells after the egg has left the ovary. These 3000 to 4000 follicular cells have a special function. They send out cell processes into the ovum and these penetrate the yolk material at points where it lies near the surface of the egg, emptying their contents into the ovum. They are also interconnected by branches like the tributaries of a stream. This clearly has to do with the nutrition of the egg during its growth in the ovary.

When the ovum has entered the fallopian tube, the coronal cells are very rapidly (within a few hours) separated off by the fluids of the tube. This separation of the corona radiata is a prerequisite for penetration of the ovum by the spermatozoon. Human spermatozoa have been shown by special microscopical studies on living ova not to be able to pass through the corona to the egg, in contrast to other animal species.

Fallopian tube and egg transport
The fallopian tube, which is about 4 to 8 inches long and unites ovary and uterus, consists of a mucosa, a thin layer of muscle and an outer coat; the mucosa is much folded at its open end and less folded near the uterus (fig. 28). The mucosa is composed of cells with hair-like processes or cilia, which set up a rhythmical wave motion in the direction of the uterus so that a total view of the mucosal surface would suggest a field of corn waving powerfully in one direction. Between these cells there are mucus-producing cells, both the ciliary stream and the mucus stream helping to transport the egg to the uterus. This mucus also has special components for dissolving off the corona radiata.

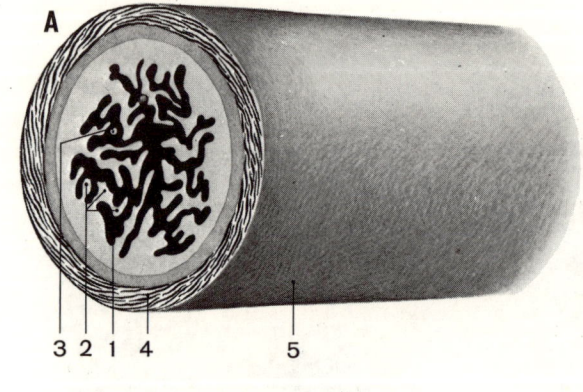

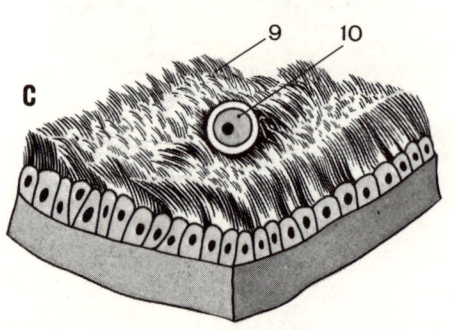

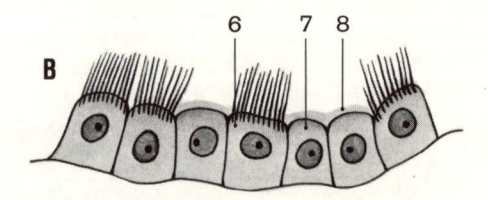

FIG. 28 *Fallopian tube and ovum transport.*

A Transverse section, greatly enlarged
B Mucosal surface
C Mucosal function

1 Lumen
2 Mucosal folds
3 Ovum
4 Muscle layer
5 Outer coat
6 Ciliated cell
7 Mucus-secreting cell
8 Mucus
9 Wave motion of ciliae in direction of uterus
10 Passively transported ovum

The arrangement for egg transport is supported by appropriate movements of the intrinsic tubal musculature, which consists of two spiral systems running in opposite senses. An outer tubal muscle layer is responsible for the grosser movements of the tube during the functioning of the mechanism for egg uptake.

The ovum must traverse a distance several times the outer length of the tube on its way to the uterus, since it has to wander over hills and valleys among the mucosal folds. Transport of the egg lasts for about five to six days, from rupture of the follicle (not fertilization) until the embedding of a possibly fertile egg in the uterine mucosa. If it is not fertilized, the ovum dies within 48 hours, is dissolved by the digestive juices in the mucus of the tube and soon disappears from view.

Sterilization in women involves a surgical operation with opening of the abdominal cavity, cutting through of the tubes and tying them off. This makes union of egg and sperm impossible, and the woman can bear no more children. In contrast to male sterilization, the patient must be in hospital for this operation. Sterilization may be needed for certain illnesses but may be done simply to render the woman infertile. An attempt may later be made to render her fertile again but it is associated with a certain amount of risk and the prospects of success are small. One recent operative technique consists in displacing the open end of the tube which takes up the ovum and concealing it in a fold of the abdomen so that the tube itself is not injured. Theoretically the previous state of fertility can be restored by a second operation at any time, replacing the tube where it was originally. So far we have not sufficient experience with this technique to say whether such replacement succeeds in practice. For a discussion of sterilization of women as a method of contraception see p. 176.

Menstruation

During maturation of the ovum and growth of the follicle in the ovary and during transport of the ovum through the fallopian tube, the uterine mucosa makes characteristic preparations for the reception of a fertilized egg.

Uterine mucosa (endometrium)
The endometrium grows and stores up nutrients so that it can if required embed a fertilized egg and provide favourable conditions for its development. But most mature ova die unfertilized, and the preparations made for embedding the egg in the mucosa are therefore superfluous. The prepared bed is shed so that fresh preparations can be made later. This is because the nutrients stored in the mucosa will not remain indefinitely unchanged, so that the mucosa must be cleared of these perishable goods to start afresh with a new store.

The superficial layers of the endometrium are cast off, the uterine muscles contract fairly rhythmically and powerfully, and the cast off and mostly dead masses of mucosa are propelled out of the cervix into the vagina, where by the force of gravity they reach the exterior. The mucus plug in the cervical canal is also cast off at this time. The whole process is called *menstruation* because the menstrual periods of bleeding take place at about one month intervals (Latin: mensis = month).

The menstrual discharge from the vagina is brownish-red, occasionally mixed with tags of mucosa, and does not clot. It has no smell unless the air gets at it, when it decomposes and gives rise to a characteristic odour. The amount of menstrual loss and its duration vary greatly from woman to woman, and also vary during the individual lifetime of the individual woman.

As a rule, menstrual flow is greatest in the first two days and lasts altogether three to five days, though only a little secretion appears in the last couple of days. It has been customary for women to absorb the menstrual flow with an absorbent binder or sanitary towel attached to a belt. In the interests of hygiene the towels have to be changed several times during the days when secretion is greatest, and the woman should wash or douche the external genitals at least once daily. Women who have had intercourse or given birth can use tampons instead of towels. These are specially prepared cylinders of absorbent substances which are inserted

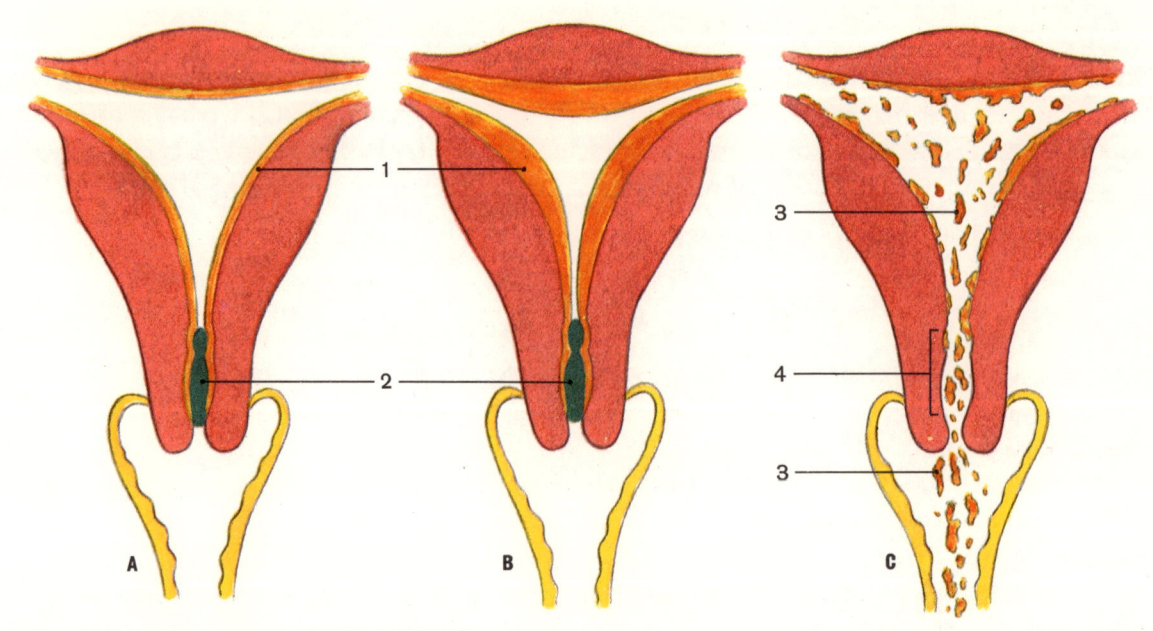

FIG. 29 *Uterine mucosa (endometrium).*

A Growing endometrium after menstruation
B Endometrium ready for ovum implantation (grown and fortified with nutrients)
C Breakaway and expulsion of endometrium in menstruation

1 Endometrium
2 Mucus plug sealing off uterus
3 Detached endometrium being shed
4 Unplugged area

into the vagina. They swell upon contact with fluids so that they seal off the vagina and retain the menstrual flow until the tampon is changed. Although there are various sizes of tampon (because of the varying elasticity of the vagina, not the varying size; a vagina can take anything up to a baby's head), many women prefer to use towels or pads during the first days of the period, because the latter take up the flow more reliably. Girls with intact hymens should not use the tampons or they may find difficulty in removing the swollen tampons.

The first menstrual period (menarche)
The menarche ushers in the reproductive period of a woman's life and occurs relatively early nowadays. Girls who begin to menstruate in their ninth year are no longer a rarity in Europe. In general, however, the menarche occurs between the twelfth and fourteenth years (average age $13\frac{1}{2}$ years).

Girls who have not menstruated before the sixteenth or seventeenth year must be medically examined, whether or not secondary sex characters have appeared, such as growth of pubic hair or breast development. There are a great variety of causes for absence or delay of the menarche. Most commonly there is inadequacy of hormonal regulation, associated with persistence of the internal genital organs at the infantile stage; medical treatment at the appropriate time can restore the situation to normal. If the period of growth has ended (around the twentieth year) medical measures will no longer succeed and the disturbance may not be curable. The result is permanent infertility. Other disorders may be responsible for absence of menarche, such as the already mentioned imperforate hymen. In this case the menstrual blood is dammed up in the vagina and periodically causes pain. Should the condition not be relieved by operation, severe changes in uterus and fallopian tubes may follow.

The reproductive period of life ends with cessation of menstruation at the *menopause* between the fortieth and fifty-fifth year. This epoch is often preceded by a two to three year period during which menstruation becomes irregular, and this time of change is known as the climacteric. The years of change are often accompanied by major changes in emotional mood.

Cycle and menstrual calendar
Since menstruation depends directly on maturation of ova it occurs, like maturation, at regular intervals about 12 to 14 times a year. The interval of time between the beginning of a period and the last day before the subsequent one begins is called the *period* or *cycle*. This cycle is usually very irregular in the first two years after the menarche, so that it is not really a cycle at all. The female body has not yet learned how to carry out the necessary processes smoothly. Later and until the years of change, every girl and every woman achieves her own individual rhythm, though the latter may not be invariable throughout life. It changes for example after pregnancies, severe illnesses, change in climate, severe physical stress, severe mental stress or even without warning, but it still remains characteristic for any woman apart from a few deviations. The average length of cycle may change quite considerably during the life of a woman. Careful recording on a so-called menstruation calendar (figs. 30 and 31) reveals considerable stability of the cycle between the twenty-fifth and fortieth years, with almost equal intervals. Yet deviations of three to five days are considered normal, and it is erroneous to talk as if the average cycle amounts to four weeks. This may be true of statistics for thousands of women, but the statistically average woman as an individual is a very rare person. Women who do not keep a calendar are apt to get very false ideas of their cycles. It has been shown that women with an average cycle of 21 days are just as normal as those with an average of 35 days. The two calendars illustrated in Figures 30 and 31 clearly show the various changes and deviations. In the Figure 31 the 28-day cycles, as well as the shortest and longest cycles in each year, are specially marked. Note the increasing stabilization of the cycle from the twenty-fifth year on.

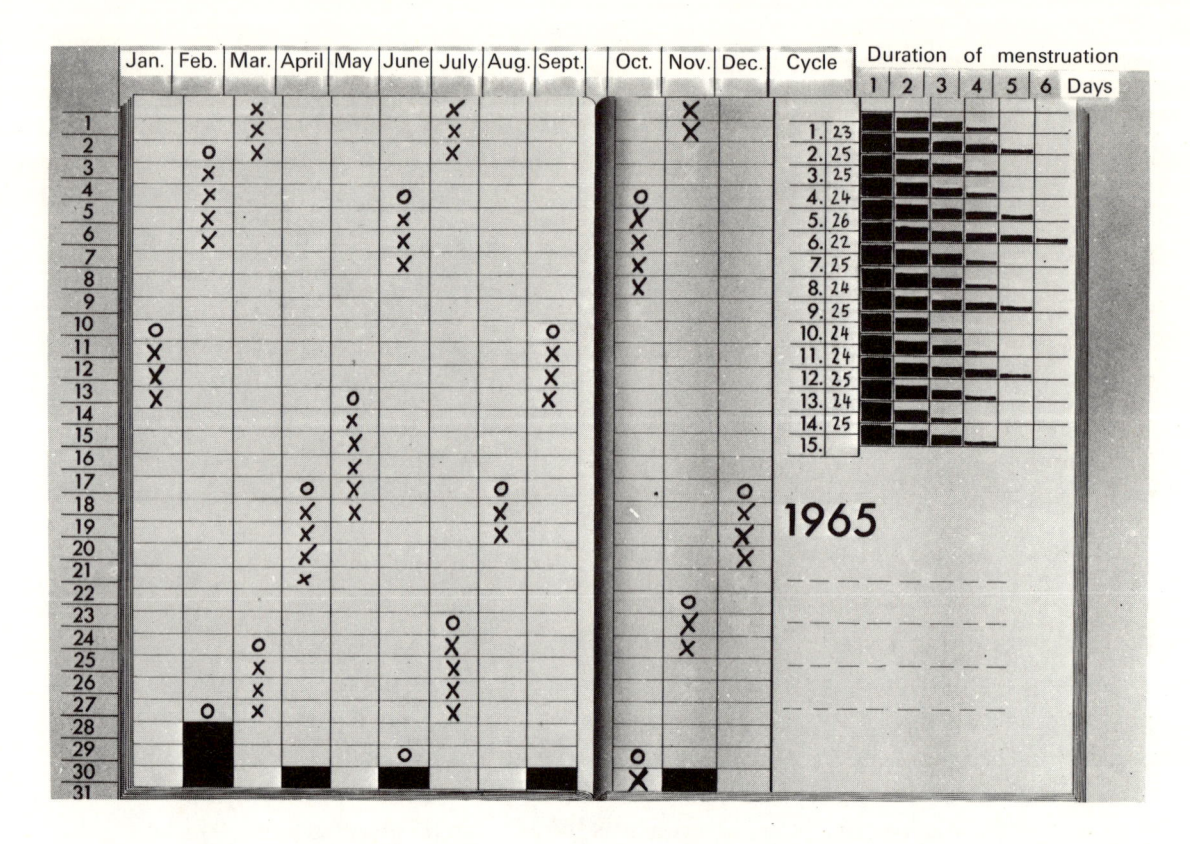

FIG. 30 *Example of menstrual calendar; any woman can keep one and every one should.*

Hormonal regulation of menstruation

Ovarian function is regulated by the pituitary hormones (see figs. 32 and 33). This gland in turn is under the dominance of the sexual nerve centre in the hypothalamus, and the latter is also subject to the cerebral hemispheres.

It should be pointed out that severe anxiety (as may occur with rape) can completely inhibit maturation of the ovum and lead to a so-called secondary cessation of menstruation which may even be permanent. There are also other causes for failure to menstruate (for example, pregnancy). In every case a medical examination is called for. Happier events and stimuli may also affect the regulating function of the pituitary and change the cycle so that 'as desired' a follicle may rupture and fertilization be made possible.

It should be repeated that, as with hormonal effects in the male, the secretions of the pituitary (the hormones acting on sex organs) are responsible for the response of genital

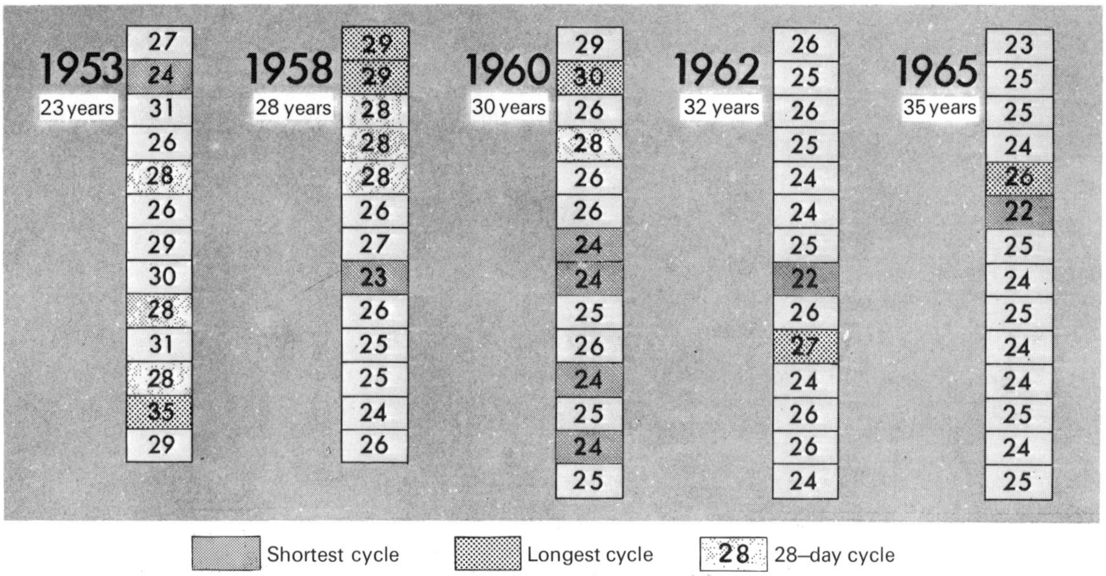

FIG. 31 *Summary of five years of cycles in a woman born in 1930.*

organs to exciting stimuli. Secretion of these hormones is increased at the beginning of puberty and the climacteric.

The female pituitary forms the same types of hormones directed at the sex organs as does the male gland. The differences in effects are due to the fact that the receptor organ in women is the ovary and not the testis.

One pituitary hormone acts on the follicle of the ovary, promoting its growth and fluid secretion, and is therefore called the follicle-stimulating hormone (FSH). A second hormone acts on the corpus luteum and is therefore called luteinizing hormone (LH), lutein being the yellow substance formed by the corpus luteum. The third hormone of the pituitary causes growth and activity of the breasts; although it is also present in males it is without action in them. Clearly its effect depends on the presence of hormones arising in the ovary. In turn, the ovarian follicle secretes a follicular hormone (oestrogen) and the corpus luteum a luteal hormone (progesterone).

Follicular hormone (secreted even by follicles which do not mature) causes the onset of secondary sex characters (pubic hair growth, deposition of fat on breasts and hips) even before menstruation appears, and collaborates with the third hormone of the pituitary in promoting breast growth. It also affects uterine muscular contraction during menstruation. This last effect is overcome by any corpus luteum hormone present either in the second half of the cycle or in pregnancy. Follicular hormone also acts on the fallopian tubes and ovaries

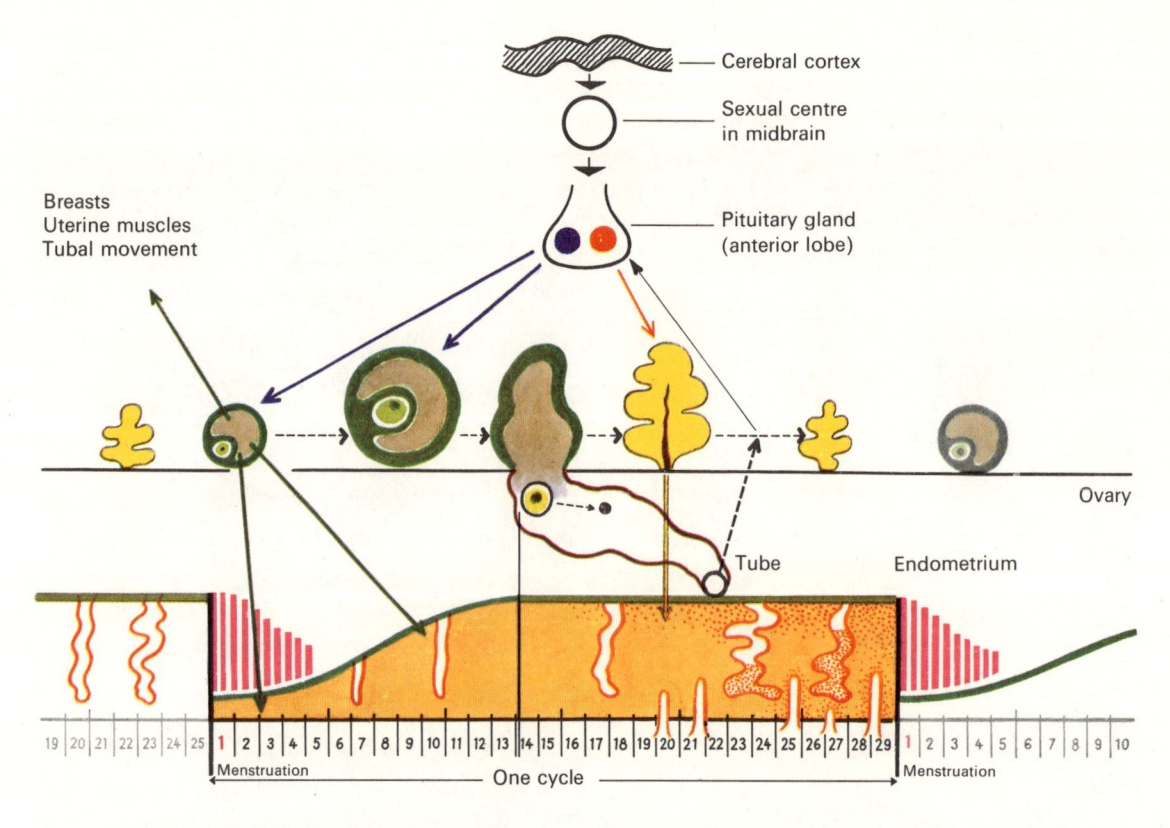

FIG. 32 *Diagram of ovarian function and menstruation. Follicular rupture is not regular but may occur any time between the twentieth and fourteenth days before menstruation.*

and facilitates uptake of the ovum. Its most obvious effect is however on the uterine mucosa, which it stimulates into growth (proliferation phase). Under its influence the tubular glands of the mucosa increase in length.

Shortly before rupture of a follicle, when the latter is fully distended, this hormone is found in decreasing amounts in the blood, and the same ovarian cells are encouraged to begin secretion of luteal hormone, though the level of follicular hormone never falls to nil as does that of luteal hormone. Even the corpus luteum still secretes some oestrogen, while during the reproductive phase of a woman's life there is always some oestrogen present from a follicle in process of development (see fig. 33).

Luteal hormone essentially promotes storage of nutrients in the uterine mucosa (secretory phase) and prevents the break-up of the latter. Under its influence, the uterine mucosal glands assume a serrated appearance and fill with protein. On the surface of the endometrium there is deposition of readily soluble sugars, while the loops of vessels which grow in from the base bring in fat. Thus all the nutrients needed for a fertilized ovum are present in easily accessible form. If the egg dies a further hormonal stimulus essential for the process fails to appear, and the corpus luteum abandons its function.

If an egg is fertilized and pregnancy follows, a hormone produced by the maternal and foetal tissues in the uterus stimulates the pituitary to secrete more luteinizing hormone and thus maintain the function of the corpus luteum. In the absence of fertilization this does not happen, and as a result levels of luteal hormone (progesterone) and its constant companion, follicular hormone (oestrogen), sink in the body.

The simultaneous fall in levels of the two hormones with an effect on endometrium has two results: First of all, the pituitary is stimulated to form more follicle-stimulating hormone and thus cause another follicle to ripen, so that oestrogen again accumulates in the blood. The rise in FSH in blood is also responsible for the increase in sensibility shortly before menstruation. Secondly, the fall in progesterone and oestrogen levels when fertilization fails leads to degeneration in the endometrium, and to a sloughing off of the mucosa about two days after the two hormone levels have fallen. All but a small basal layer of the mucosa is cast off, and out of the remains new growth takes place.

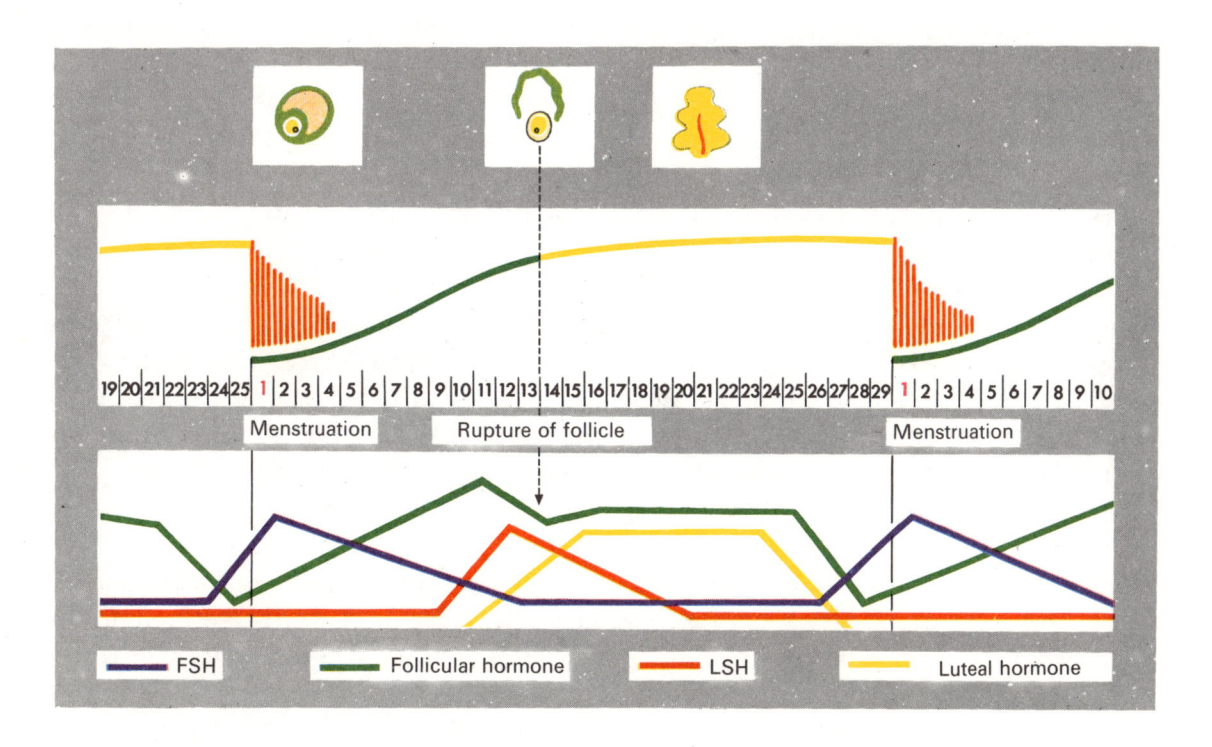

FIG. 33 *Hormones and menstruation.*

When menstruation begins there is an immediate reconstruction of new mucosa under the influence of fresh oestrogen, and the whole cycle begins once more.

The cycle is counted from the first day of endometrial reconstruction, which is also the first day of bleeding, to the last day of endometrial existence, the day before the next bleeding. The variable length of the cycle has already been mentioned, and it remains to add that follicular rupture happens 20 to 14 days before the next menstrual period. It is important to establish this, because the old and inaccurate rule of Knaus and Ogino, who first studied menstrual cycles to any extent, stated that the corpus luteum hormone phase lasted for a constant 14 to 15 days in every woman. As a result of serial estimation of hormones associated with recordings of electrical activity from the lower abdomen (electro-vaginograms), this is now known to be incorrect. The calculation of 'fertile' and 'infertile' days as the basis of a method of contraception will be discussed later (p. 178).

There are some cycles in which a follicle does not rupture and therefore no fertilizable egg appears in the fallopian tube between menstruations. The causes for this may lie in disturbed function of the ovary or of the pituitary. The commonest cause seems to be that the mature follicle cannot rupture and persists until it finally shrinks with age. As a rule these cycles without follicular rupture are somewhat shorter than the others in the same woman. In the early years after menarche these so-called anovulatory cycles are much commoner than normal ones, but even at 18 to 20 years they still form about 20 to 30% of all cycles. Between the twentieth and fortieth years however they are at their lowest (about 3 to 10%) apart from the periods after delivery or after nervous stress. This failure of ovulation must not be relied upon however after a delivery. In the years of climacteric, the anovulatory cycles become commoner once more and become as frequent as in the years after the menarche.

Demonstration of such a disturbance in the cycle is usually easy with the aid of *basal temperature measurement*. The technique depends on the fact that one or two days after the follicle ruptures a woman's temperature rises by some tenths of a degree. In an ideal case the picture would be as follows. During and immediately after menstruation the basal temperature lies below 98·4°F. and may still show a tendency to fall, to say 97·5°. After rupture of the follicle there is a rise lasting about two days to values over 98·4°, maybe to 99·2°. This level is maintained for a while and then drops again to 98·4°F. shortly before the next menstrual period. It is important to note that the jump in temperature takes place one or two days after follicle rupture. If the cycle is anovular and no follicle ruptures the temperature does not rise, so that from the temperature chart one can tell whether a follicle has ruptured or not. This method has been applied to contraception but is not suitable in every case because temperature charts are influenced by both physical and mental stresses as well as infections and inflammations. It should be added that about one woman in ten does not show this classical temperature chart (see p. 180).

That a menstrual period follows even if no egg has left the ovary is due to the fact that the endometrium, which has proliferated under the influence of oestrogen but has not been stored with nutrients, breaks away as it grows older and is cast off.

Emotional experience of menstruation at the menarche and during the reproductive age
Science has clearly shown that menstruation has nothing to do with the phases of the moon. This idea, still superstitiously believed in, is merely an expression of the ancient wisdom that the whole life of a woman proceeds rhythmically.

The most extraordinary experimental arrangements have been set up to prove that menstrual blood is 'bad' blood or even contains poisons, but all these experiments have failed. This is a somewhat dangerous and perverted inference deriving from the ancient rule that shortly before and during menstruation a woman is sexually taboo, 'sacred and untouchable', because she needs to have this time to herself. This rule has been almost completely abandoned by modern woman to her detriment, because her services are in constant demand either in a household or in a job; she can no longer withdraw into solitude away from her husband, her children and the world. She can still however acknowledge the rhythm of her femininity (see p. 135).

Girls should not be allowed to reach their menarche unprepared, and every mother should give her daughter some preparatory advice well ahead of the onset of menstruation. The transition from girl into woman can be very seriously affected if she is left to face the shock of discovery of her bleeding and her sexuality, a shock that may cause her to hate her own femininity. If however she has been correctly informed about the structure and function of her own genital organs, she can rejoice in the onset of menstruation as an essential step on the way to womanhood. Acceptance of female sexuality includes a positive attitude to menstruation; women should not regard this as a curse which men are spared, or reject it. On the other hand it is an equally false attitude to pretend that the days of the menstrual period do not exist. Spurious advertising for towels and tampons may foster such an attitude.

Menstruation is not directly related to capacity for sexual enjoyment or orgasm. This is particularly emphasized by the fact that after the menopause a woman remains perfectly capable of orgasm until old age, although as in the male the need for sexual enjoyment in old age gradually falls off and is finally replaced by a wish for tenderness in general. However, the events of the menstrual period, so long as they continue, do exercise some influence on all this.

In general for a few hours or days before menstruation, women undergo a change of emotional mood and yearn for rest, safety, protection and tenderness, not necessarily sexual. Environmental influences hostile to this need are felt as disturbing and bothersome. At this time those personal characteristics and attitudes which are otherwise concealed for social or intellectual reasons come to the surface. There is also heightened sensibility coupled with heightened response to external stimuli, disturbing or challenging. This rise in sensibility and the associated swings in mood result in greater liability to fatigue. Finally, it must be recalled that the menstrual period may be awaited with mixed feelings. Both a vain desire for a child and fear of possible pregnancy can make a woman look forward to a menstrual period with anxious expectations, tension and restlessness. Unconscious wishes may battle with conscious ones and create an apparently inexplicable conflict situation.

A feeling of tension in the breasts and a heightened sensitivity in the nipples, due to their involvement in the hormonal changes at menstruation, may be experienced as pleasant. Readiness for sexual intercourse varies greatly and may be either increased or diminished during these days. Presumably the causes for this lie also in the area of the emotions.

Thus every woman before menstruation tends to live more than usually from within outwards. If she battles against this because she erroneously believes that a modern woman ought not to give way or let this event interfere in her competition with men, with whom for some ill-understood reason she would like to be equal, she will not infrequently experience organic disorders during her period. These may range from cramp-like pains in the lower abdomen, sometimes severe enough to lay her out, through migrainous headaches to insomnia. This does not mean that menstruation normally passes unnoticed, but by her attitude of resistance she has exaggerated the usual sensations.

Experienced gynaecologists know that at least 80% of so-called menstrual complaints are of emotional and not organic origin, like the common complaints of girls after the menarche. Apart from poor instruction or failure to prepare the girl for the menarche, current circumstances often play a vital role. Every girl (and every young man) must come to terms with the fact that from one day to the next a girl becomes a woman capable of being fertilized. Acceptance of this takes a long time and menstruation is first accompanied by uncertainty, especially if, as often happens, the congestion of the genitals leads not only to malaise but also to sensations of pleasure which may be regarded as forbidden (this will be discussed later). Out of her insecurity with its need for love, understanding and sympathy from her environment, the girl may also want to reject any adult help because, alongside her growing consciousness of sexuality, she feels the rivalry between her and other women (mother, sister, etc.). An understanding mother and family will not become indignant over this but make a proper place within family and society for the newcomer. With sexual intercourse it is quite otherwise; a girl has no innate requirements for this and must first undergo further mental and emotional development before intercourse can be more than a piece of false evidence of womanliness, or satisfaction of curiosity, or a desperate but halfhearted union which may undermine further maturation of her personality. After menstruation most women experience a burst of mental activity, an increase in joie de vivre and a better design for living; all this may reach a peak at the time of rupture of the follicle.

The more the modern woman learns to recognize her cyclical changes and rejoice in her womanhood, the better she will be able to accept them in her heart and to live positively. She must shed her resistance and its pathological consequences, or her worrying ignorance as well as her usually unconsciously ambiguous resignation to her feminine fate. Women can learn to channel their natural rhythm and thus regain access to the lost wisdom of ancient cultures.

If we put together what we have learned about hormone effects, with special reference to their harmonious relationships to the mental changes during the menstrual cycle, the following picture emerges:

Menarche. The increased secretion of follicle-stimulating hormone by the pituitary during puberty leads, as with all other hormones directed at the genital glands, to sensitization of response to sexual stimuli. The girl is in consequence made aware suddenly of sexual stimuli she had overlooked. With the increasing maturation of secondary sex characters (due to follicle formation in the ovary) she will also find herself desired by young men. Finally FSH and LH together with oestrogen and luteal hormone, and the subsequent follicle rupture, lead to the menarche. Thus the girl experiences her onset of fertile womanhood as well as a genital congestion that calls out for contact. Her mental and emotional insecurity leads to her typical ambivalence of attitude, by turns wishful and defensive.

Menstruation. Rise in FSH level is associated with heightened sensory perception but also with general edginess. The simultaneous fall in LH and corpus luteum hormone and oestrogen levels (see fig. 33) leads to diminished excitability of the erogenous zones, such as the breasts which are under the special influence of oestrogen itself, and thus to a general resistance to sexual excitement. Hence before menstruation a woman has an ambivalent attitude to sexual intercourse.

After menstruation, the rise in FSH and thus of oestrogen level (see fig. 33) leads to stabilization of the emotional situation and makes possible a positive attitude to life with increased sexual response and activity. The rise in LH before rupture of the follicle, which in similar manner raises the sensitivity of the genital organs and erogenous zones, causes just before follicular rupture a marked readiness for sexual intercourse with the biological goal of fertilization. However at the same time the corpus luteum hormone level is also rising and stabilizing not only the endometrium but also the emotional state. The result is that after follicular rupture the desire for sexual activity becomes less acute and finally disappears shortly before the next period, whereupon the whole cycle begins again.

Hormones for prevention of ovum maturation (see also p. 187 ff.). Contraceptive pills provide an even and undeviating supply of oestrogen and/or corpus luteum hormone and therefore after prolonged administration they level out the hormone secretions from the pituitary and hence may diminish sexual excitability and the desire for intercourse. On the other hand, there are no sudden drops in hormone levels such as occur before ordinary menstruation and thus sexual intercourse is not completely rejected. As a whole the heights and depths of sensation in a woman's life are abolished and the result is a more equable approach to sexual intercourse. The woman's attitude over the long term will come to depend more and more on her individual basic attitude, and thus there may be all variations from positive acceptance of coitus to general indifference or even rejection of intercourse. The contraceptive pill will merely bring the fundamental emotional attitude of a woman into prominence. Relative indifference over a long term will imply lessened desire for coitus and this may be considered a nuisance, especially by the husband.

Climacteric. It is well known that for some cause not yet explained there is an increase in secretion of gonadotropic hormones (i.e. hormones directed at the sex organs) at the beginning of the years of change. This increase in secretion leads, as it does at the beginning of puberty, to a rise in sensibility and an increase in sexual receptivity. The rise in sensory perception also naturally causes the woman to be touchy and hence to undergo mood swings. However, when more FSH and LH are secreted there is now no feedback effect from the ovary (because the latter is functionally disordered with persistence of follicles and failure of corpus luteum formation), and the stabilizing action of the luteinizing hormone is absent. Thus the artificial supply of certain hormones may heighten the emotional situation at the climacteric.

Menopause. With the extinction of all ovarian function the feedback effect from the ovaries on the gonadotropic hormones of the pituitary remains absent. Therefore at first the pituitary forms more FSH and LH and causes once more an increase in sexual response. In other words, sexual drive is at first heightened at the menopause. The swings in mood however cease because of lack of feedback and because of a constant secretion of pituitary hormones. It is only in later life that the excess production from the pituitary slows up, so that there is a general and gradual reduction in sexual desire.

Sex Life

The Development of Sex Life

In the introduction to this book it was pointed out that, in the developmental process to male or female maturity, not only are adult structure and capacity for function of the genital organs involved but also a knowledge of the functional processes in sexual intercourse; this knowledge is also important for the better mutual understanding of the partners. Also important are personal, mental and emotional attitudes to one's own sex and the opposite sex, maturity and capacity for responsibility in partnership, and care of and respect for the other, if the relations between husband and wife are to be properly formed. In the life partnership of monogamy, which in our culture represents the best possible chance of finding and experiencing a total encounter with a partner of the opposite sex, both husband and wife increasingly expect from it a continued and satisfying fulfilment of the sexual side of human life. For this reason it is important not only to consider mental and emotional preparation for marriage but also training for sexual expression.

Every training period passes through incomplete stages which, seen in isolation, may obscure the whole. The danger is that any one of these stages may be mistaken for final fulfilment. Another danger in training for sexual expression is that the trainee may regard this as the only thing worth striving for and thus fail to achieve the highest level.

This problem may be encountered with masturbation, necking and petting. Prohibiting or deprecating these practices may actually cause fixation at that point, for they all too readily become a goal without further advance to higher forms of maturity.

The training stages of sexual expression are necessary stages of development, and their duration varies greatly with the individual. Yet every boy and every girl should be made aware at this time (and not later) that they are only stages on the way and only meaningful as a step on the way towards sexual training. Apart from this they are without purpose. This is important because the powers unleashed in training must be correctly harnessed. Since all sexual drive should be centred on the partner, harnessing it means taking note all the time of the wishes and needs of the partner; drive centred on the self is certainly misdirected. This direction should therefore be practised at an early enough stage, instead of giving way to every personal inclination. Partnership depends on constant mutual respect and this is achieved better if the two partners have previously learned to subordinate their own wishes and needs.

Masturbation
Boys and girls early discover that touching the penis or the pudenda with pressure on the clitoris (girls are relatively slow to find this out by themselves) leads to a peculiarly pleasant form of titillation, which because of this pleasure is readily repeated. This discovery, which is made at the latest at puberty and mostly before that, is harmless for both sexes. What is harmful to both is parental disapproval or condemnation as sinful of either the discovery or repeated production of the pleasant sensation. These experiences are simply training of the body and senses for the sensual event of sexual intercourse, and of the appropriate organs for the function assigned to them in the most intense expression of love between man and woman. This preparatory training is just as normal as the fact that infants first kick, then crawl and finally practise standing up before they can walk upright. If an infant were prevented from kicking or crawling, it would never be able to walk or run or learn to dance. It is often overlooked, sometimes deliberately, that the sexual feelings which boys and girls experience first as children and later at puberty can only be integrated into love if they are permitted. If they are despised or forbidden, further development in use of the organs and the feelings their activity generates becomes impossible. All later sexual events will remain linked to the early childish or early pubertal stage, so that physical and sensual sexuality becomes the only goal, isolated from all responsibility, care, respect and sacrifice.

Thus a faulty attitude of parents and teachers reinforces the progress of the situation which began with forbidding a small child to touch or to refer to its genitals. The untouchable cannot later be correctly used and the unmentionable remains anxiety-ridden and unrelated to the rest of the body even if it is anatomically a part of it. A situation that started as a false one remains so, but ironically enough the fruits of a situation created by parents and other adults will be regarded by them with sorrow or opposed with moral righteousness. This does not help and it is therefore necessary to return to a discussion of relief of desire and tension by masturbation, since so many parents and teachers regard it as shameful and inappropriate behaviour, especially in adolescence (see pp. 25, 46, 58, 72).

This form of sexual activity may appear incomplete since no partner is involved, but this is usually wrong because during the activity there are wishes and fantasies directed towards another person of the opposite sex. In small children this person is originally the parent of the opposite sex. Because such a wish cannot be fulfilled in our society and is indeed disapproved of—the daughter cannot marry her father or the son his mother, while parents are prevented by the incest taboo from giving way to such wishes—the original idea is prohibited, is accompanied by feelings of guilt, and finally given up. But this does not mean that the basis of the wish, the desire for sexual activity, is bad. On the contrary, the wish, which will appear unconsciously in all kinds of play activity and can be recognized by attentive parents, should be taken seriously by parents and teachers and reoriented towards a future possible partner outside the family. This will retain the power behind the wish and make it available for progress towards adult life (learning, growth, maturation) without associating it with an earlier prohibition which would bar it from use in other contexts.

At puberty, sexual drive towards activity and practice will seek new goals, though the proposed sexual partner will at first be unattainable. This characterizes the plight of girls and boys at this phase. In addition to the above need for experience, our culture which frowns upon early sexual activity for both sexes tends to prolong the period during which boys and girls obtain their sexual satisfaction through themselves. Because of the earlier onset of puberty (ninth to tenth year) and the prolongation of the period of learning before the individual is socially independent, both boys and girls are often put in a position where they cannot marry and fulfil their sexual wishes for ten or fifteen years, that is, assuming they do not have premarital relations.

In contrast to former generations, the modern girl is permitted to have and strive for sexual pleasure. Even if her information is faulty and she has had no proper sex education, she has a mother who also claims the right to sexual pleasure. This maternal attitude is enough to create an environment in which the daughter can formulate her own demands and regard them as justifiable. As a result, girls today pay more attention to their sexuality than formerly, and, as boys have always done, discover the satisfaction to be obtained from masturbation and practise it. The tradition that boys masturbated but not girls is no longer valid.

In education therefore it should be pointed out that the sexual pleasure and release from tension obtained by auto-erotism is consciously or unconsciously aimed at a partner from this time on. Because the partner is unattainable the desire is of course only partially satisfied. If the process is simply directed by the person at himself, it will persist later on the same narcissistic lines as during the short transitional phase at the beginning of puberty when masturbation mainly serves to train the organs. This represents a deviation in development due basically to a faulty attitude—prohibition of sexuality. Nor can masturbation be replaced in development by advising the adolescent to indulge in sexual intercourse, for intercourse early in puberty means in our society the involvement of immature and unprepared individuals who cannot experience the act as an expression of a comprehensive partnership but only as a means of relieving sexual tension. This lack of responsibility for the partner is likely to render habitual a type of sexual behaviour that later hampers maturation, yet if the couple stay together a real partnership may develop out of a relationship at first purely physical. There is always the danger however that purely physical enjoyment may lead to dissatisfaction in the long run so that a change of partner is sought; the experience will remain unsatisfactory until an attempt is made to find emotional and physical harmony in mutual responsibility, respect and care. Thus in our culture we cannot avoid the phenomenon of masturbation continued over long periods. We will have to learn to regard this, both in the small child and the boy or girl around puberty and adolescence, as a method of dealing with the conflict between a justifiable desire for a sexual partnership and the personal and social difficulty of obtaining a partner.

Petting

Even if masturbation is related in imagination to a partner, the person remains alone and isolated. Since human beings seek relationships with others and are in fact concerned to construct a society, they tend to value a relationship higher than a physical satisfaction. In individual development the sex organs mature first. Thus a prerequisite is created for directing personal wishes towards a partner and hence towards society. Development of sexual maturity means that after the physical capacity to carry out sexual intercourse has been reached there comes later the capacity to make a comprehensive relationship, for the individual is a unit of body, mind and soul and therefore seeks reciprocity in these three areas in his encounters. Until a man or a woman is mature enough to create a full relationship in this sense, he or she is not ready for a complete and lasting relationship.

A person takes some years to reach this stage. In the introductory chapter of this book we noted that it is important during this period to carry on with the obvious tasks of preparing for a profession, concentrating on specific goals and practising general formation of relationships within a group of both sexes in daily work and leisure time. There will be sports, music, literary, political and other activities, everyday contacts with men and women, experience of sympathy, comradeship and friendship, assumption of duties and responsibilities at home, in industry, in religious and in political circles and so on. The adolescent boy and girl can bring their energies to these areas and use them in preparation for their role in society. In spite of all our modern permissiveness there is no doubt that anyone who has been able, through insight, to deal with the period between puberty and marriage without giving way to the natural desire for sexual intercourse has chosen the better and easier way to reach complete sexual maturity. The deciding factor in such a line of conduct should be a growing insight with advancing years into the complexities of the problem and not a taboo on sexual activity.

While relationships are developing it is not uncommon for a man and a woman to seek a common way to maturity as a result of mutual liking and exercise of responsibility. This has nothing to do with illusions or infatuation. Since even a mental and spiritual relationship between a man and a woman cannot wholly exclude the physical but can only set it aside or postpone it, the partners as they get to know each other better will naturally feel the need and desire for physical contact. However there is often no immediate possibility of marriage for social or financial reasons. The pair are therefore faced with the alternatives of indulging in premarital intercourse or intensifying their exchanges of caresses. This more intense exchange of caresses is referred to as necking and petting. It was mentioned in European literature at the turn of the last century, long before the two American terms passed into common usage. It includes repeated passionate embrace with arousal by kissing, touch and stimulation of the female breast and other erogenous areas, followed usually by mutual touch, fondling and stimulation of the genitals until mutual orgasm, all without introduction of the penis into the vagina. Thus the hymen remains intact. The significance of petting lies in the achievement of mutual release of sexual tension without intercourse. The girl remains a virgin although in fact everything making up a marital sexual relationship occurs. These activities are harmless to health provided that ejaculation and orgasm take place. If not, a constantly unresolved sexual tension will lead to restlessness and nervousness and may cause other psychosomatic disorders.

Necking and petting are *forms of expression of premarital sex life*. They are a substitute for intercourse, used by those young persons who cannot have intercourse because of financial or moral taboos. But they are also an expression of sexual attraction and not to be despised, for they undoubtedly lead to a closer partner relationship than in a friendship without sexual exchanges. They are also an expression of the moral climate of our times, for if virginity were not so highly prized there would be no petting. Whether however they will disappear when more exact and reliable methods of contraception are available and the fear of premarital pregnancy is thus reduced seems doubtful, for they still represent a form of training for sexual experience. On the one hand this mutual and reciprocal stimulation leads the couple from the isolation of masturbation into an intense partner relationship. On the other hand it prepares them for actual sexual intercourse. This is not just a casual expression of intense feeling; in contrast to the purely sexual act, it is an expression of deeper love and a comprehensive relationship. Thus for many young people they represent a training ground, and it is not surprising that couples who have this closer relationship by necking and petting less frequently suffer from frigidity or impotence when they marry.

It should be added that in the progress towards full sexual maturity this training stage is not without risk if it persists for too long. Persistent petting may readily lead to a fixation on this form of release of tension and thus present difficulties for full sexual enjoyment. It should be abandoned at the latest when the initial satisfaction is followed by a feeling of dissatisfaction in one of the partners. This should be a signal for marriage so that full sexual intercourse can be begun in the security and safety of that institution. Premarital intercourse if undertaken with mutual respect, trust and responsibility and with the goal of prolonging the relationship, can no longer be described as a training period in the sense used above. It scarcely needs repeating that intercourse without any intention of maintaining a relationship has no training value but is an irresponsible isolation of sex.

Sexual Stimuli

We have seen that a healthy attitude to sexual intercourse can be gained only if it is recognized that the whole person is involved and not just a body conveniently placed around a genital organ one happens to want to use; the partner must be seen as another ego to be loved in its own individuality and on its own terms, for only out of this independence of egos and over a long-term relationship can a satisfying 'we' develop.

Sexual reactions
The nervous mechanism regulating events within the genital system and in sexual intercourse is extremely complicated. Because in recent years many biased, erroneous and mechanistic accounts have been given of this subject, an attempt will be made to look at the relationships so far as present scientific knowledge reaches.

The simplest type of human response is the reflex. This is the reaction of an organ, a part of an organ or an organ system to some stimulus from within or without which is specific for the organ and its receptor apparatus. Thus the ear responds to sound waves and not to light waves. The sense of touch responds only to touch and not to odours. The stimuli consist of changes in the existing situation (dark to light, quiet to noise, heat to cold), and it depends on the amount of change and also the initial state of the organ whether the change is actually perceived as a stimulus. (If for example anyone took an alarm clock into an engine room, the ear would cease to perceive its ticking, though it would be immediately obvious at night in a bedroom.) Perception of a stimulus also depends on preparedness to receive the stimulus. Anyone concentrating on playing or reading a book may fail to hear with the inner ear the summons to a meal although his ear has been reached by the sound waves. He is simply not tuned in. If however he is hungry and just passing the time in playing or reading he will hear the slightest trace of a call, or even imagine one. The point at which a stimulus becomes effective is called the threshold.

When the threshold has been crossed, simple stimuli are first recorded by the appropriate nerve endings. The recording passes through nerve paths to the spinal cord, and this is the simplest type of conduction (see fig. 34). The nerve paths end in nerve cells in a bulbous thickening on the posterior roots of the nerves just outside the spinal cord proper (see the swelling in fig. 34, on the right and above).

In the grey matter of the spinal cord the stimulus is then relayed to other nerve cells which will distribute it further. This distribution takes place both to the opposite side

FIG. 34 *Diagram of a spinal reflex arc (shown for one side only).*

The nerve paths from the organ have their cells in a (ganglion) node outside the spinal cord. They transmit the stimulus further to nerve cells, which either relay it to other centres in the cord or react back on the organ. The stimulus and response are not experienced, and cannot be influenced voluntarily with such a reflex arc.

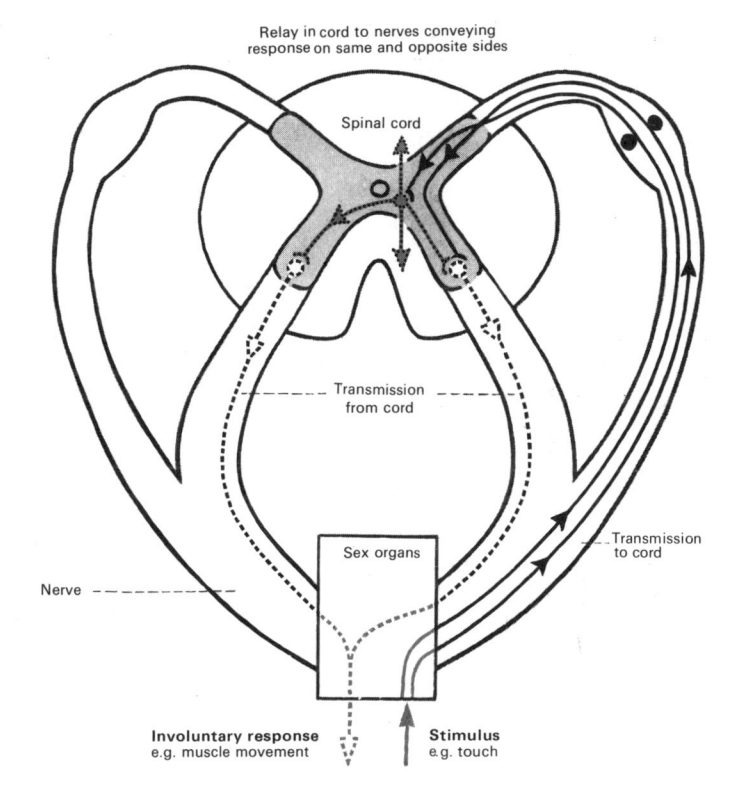

(from right to left and vice versa) and to points above and below. Moreover the stimulus is distributed to nerve cells connected with parts of the stimulated organ and is able to effect changes in the latter.

Thus the two relays of the stimulus in the spinal cord encounter nerve cells whose fibres run back again to the stimulated organ, or are distributed to other organs. These impulses leaving the spinal cord cause the organ to respond to the stimulus, in the form of a change of state appropriate to the latter (for example, a blow on a muscle sends a stimulus to the spinal cord, which is relayed in the cord and then conducted back to the muscle causing it to contract and move a joint). The whole process takes place without our cooperation or our will; it is involuntary and is called a 'reflex'.

Many such reflexes are related to the genitals. They function without any conscious effort, or learning, and because our bodies are constructed in this way. We know that they continue to function even if the section of the nervous system involved is cut off from the rest of the system, as can happen in certain severe illnesses affecting the spinal cord.

The genitals, which form an entire organ system, consisting in both sexes of various organ groups and glands, erectile bodies, receptors for stimuli of various sorts and muscles, are connected with a whole gamut of reflexes. These are interwoven in a most remarkable fashion through a variety of relay centres with nerve cells, some outside the cord, so that complicated processes (such as ejaculation of semen together with erection, or moistening and rhythmical movements of the female genitals) can go on reflexly, completely unconsciously and involuntarily.

Copulatory reflexes
The sum total of these reflexes associated with the genitals and their function are known as copulatory reflexes. They depend on the presence of certain amounts of pituitary hormones acting on the genital glands (gonadotropic hormones). This means that the reflexes first develop fully at puberty but are maintained until old age, even in the woman after her period of reproduction has ended at the climacteric.

The effectiveness of a stimulus is not limited to its capacity for starting a reflex. We have already noted that the stimulus may be distributed upwards, downwards, or across in the spinal cord and also through relay centres outside the cord. Distribution however is much wider, in that the stimulus can also be conducted up to those parts of the brain (see fig. 35) in which, as in the spinal cord, reflexes take place (though in a much more complicated way), and other responses which regulate either consciously or unconsciously the whole behaviour of the individual.

All human responses which only pass through the simple reflex arc in the spinal cord are called involuntary reactions, while all those which involve the brain are called voluntary reactions. This does not mean that the so-called voluntary reactions are necessarily consciously carried out. In the interests of clarity it should be pointed out that a distinction is made between the spinal cord and brain, the central nervous system, on the one hand, and the peripheral nervous system of nerves, nerve paths and other relay centres on the other. We also distinguish an autonomic or self-governing nervous system, mostly connected with viscera and regulating many involuntary primitive functions reflexly, such as the movements of muscles in the intestines, the digestive glands, and even the heart.

The arrival of a stimulus in the brain is not always experienced consciously and not always in the same manner; frequently the only sensation is indeterminate, generalized or perhaps referred to the organ system. Thus if the glans penis or the clitoris (figs. 6 and 17) is touched, a first reflex is set off causing the erectile tissues of the male or female genitals to swell. This swelling and further contact leads to a primary pleasurable irritation which seeks further gratification. The reflex process is thus reinforced to eliminate the stimulus. The latter is however possible only when the increased blood flow into the erectile tissues and thus the excitement have subsided. Hence this reflex, which is reinforced by reactions regulated by the brain, finally leads to orgasm (see p. 148 ff.). The reflex has now reached its peak and gradually subsides. A similar stimulus immediately after orgasm induces no new reflex process because the threshold for stimulation of the organs has been greatly raised through exhaustion. A new stimulus at this time will be experienced as painful and not pleasurable.

Setting aside the question of pain and pleasure, it is clear that the events described above represent a voluntarily influenced reflex process (since the brain has been involved) but also a process which is to a large extent reflex; in other words, it takes place unconsciously without thought and without involvement of other brain elements such as feeling and recollection. This elementary process of sexual response is common to all highly organized animals. In animals the process depends on the presence of a certain quantity of oestrus hormone secreted in the season of 'heat' and this is why animals do not respond to otherwise appropriate stimuli outside this season.

In humans this hormone is always present, and therefore we have to regulate our sexual activity with the help of culturally imposed customs. In human beings another mechanism plays a decisive part in the sequence of sexual events. The experience yet to come or the indeterminate sensation is subject to control and supervision by memory and the material stored in it; the latter may be immediately accessible, or inaccessible because it is in the unconscious but nevertheless just as effective. These recollections and experiences go back into early childhood besides including recent memories. In addition, impressions and experiences flow in, which are not all directly related to the presently affected sexual sphere; some may be remotely related, others less remotely. If all these factors are summarized under the heading of 'memories', it will be seen that the arrival of a stimulus may possibly be attended with both pleasant and unpleasant, pleasurable and displeasing, happy and anxious memories, both conscious and unconscious. There may indeed be simultaneous recall of emotionally opposed memories.

If the opposed memories are conscious ones it is possible to sort them out and give one preference. If however one of them lies in the unconscious it is not easy to make this decision, because unconscious recollections are usually stronger, so that they may overshadow the 'conscious' will to action and the person may have a feeling that he no longer understands himself. We have already encountered such happenings in connection with frigidity and impotence. If most recollections have a pleasant, sensuous and happy element, the result will be to reinforce the reflexes aiming at a peak of sexual experience; if however unpleasant or anxious recollections predominate they may completely interrupt the reflex, even in its simplest spinal form, so that in spite of all conscious efforts of will no reaction follows. It is impossible to set out all the various elements of these significant recollections, and we will therefore limit discussion to a few of importance because they interfere with reflexes.

It has already been pointed out that disparagement of sexuality and the genitals beginning in early childhood and perhaps continuing into puberty, together with disparagement of the associated sensations of pleasure, may lead to inhibition of reflexes so great as to

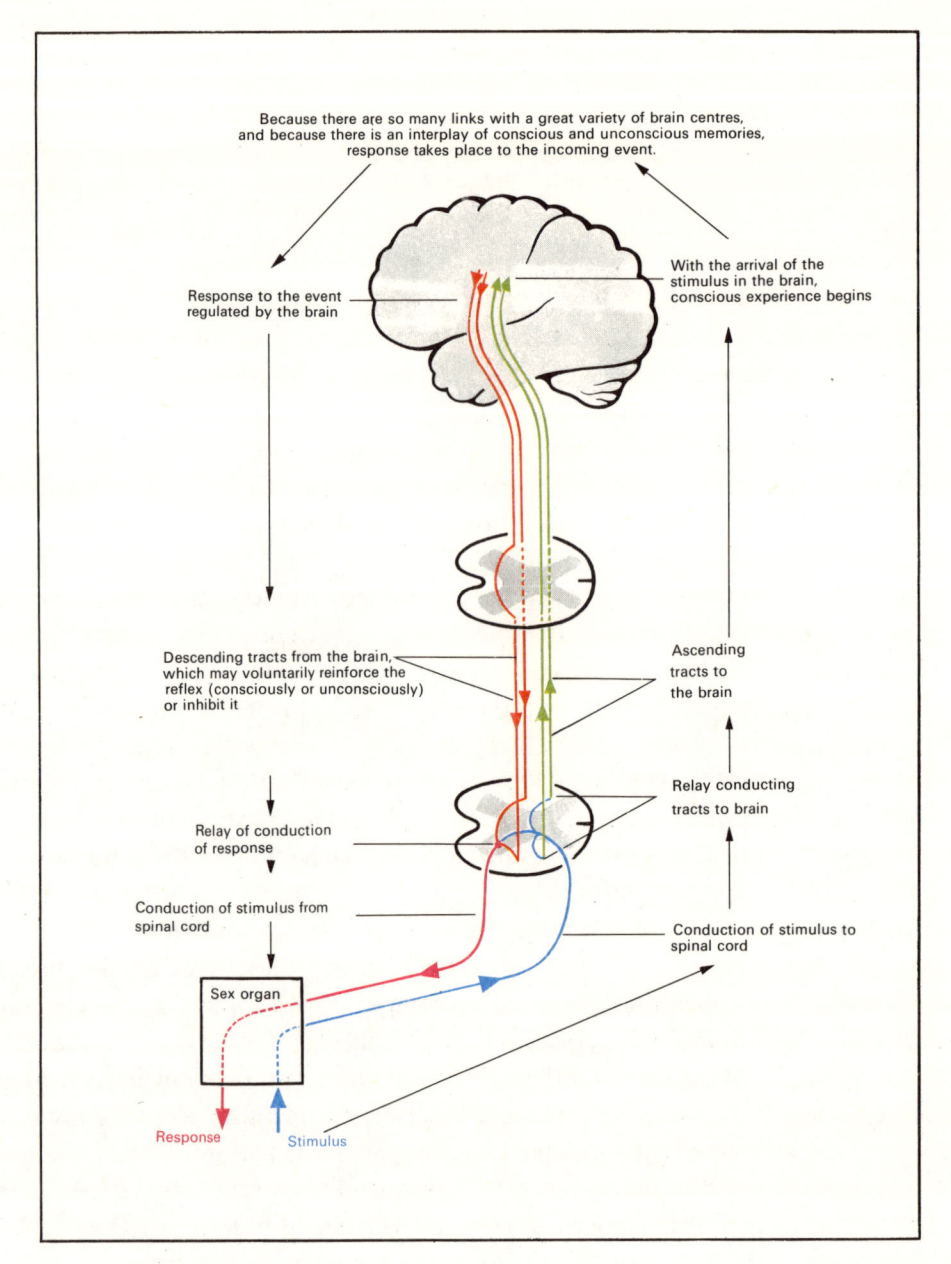

FIG. 35 *Diagram of response to a stimulus.*

The descending conduction paths from the brain (red) which influence the event via spinal cord centres, cross over in the upper part of the cord. Response may occur: 1. involuntarily (entirely through the nervous reflex arc in the spinal cord); 2. voluntarily (as a result of events in the brain), with both conscious and unconscious factors.

create impotence or frigidity. Disturbances of this sort may also be related to unconscious remains of childish associations of the boy with his mother and the girl with her father. If such an association is later transferred to the sexual partner, the adult is inhibited from giving himself sexually, for simultaneously with the association there is a transfer of the knowledge that there must be no sexual intercourse with the partner, i.e. the father or mother. Rape and other sexual experiences which may upset the emotional state of the victim have a similar action. Unfortunately lay circles often underestimate the effect of another type of memory immediately related to the person of the sexual partner or to the expectations entertained of him (or her) and of the sex act in general. A woman or even a younger girl is particularly receptive to such memories or wishes because she is much more closely wrapped up in the sex act than a man. The most important genital organs of the woman lie inside her, and she takes the penis and semen into her. Emotionally also she loves more from within than from without. The male genital organs, on the other hand, lie outside the man, and their action is away from him; emotionally, the man at first loves externally and towards the outside before he learns to love within.

The general mood in respect of the partner and the situation is decisive. The partner who knows that he is taken by the other only because he is a living object with suitable genital organs and not because he is loved in his entirety with all his mistakes and weaknesses, or indeed in spite of these, cannot abandon himself without inhibition to the sensations aroused, and will often stick at the stage of the physical act. If sexual activity persists at this level, which many people think to be sufficient, a well worn track of experience at this level is created from which it is hard to escape. It is exactly like driving along a track with ruts, which get deeper each time they are driven through so that eventually even if the driver knows he is on the wrong road he cannot get the wheels out of these ruts without help. Physical functions carried out without mental or emotional participation can readily turn into the ruts of incorrectly learned reflexes. They can become as much a habit as cleaning the teeth in a morning to get rid of the nasty taste in the mouth, but with more serious consequences. It is harmless to exchange a toothbrush when it is worn out. To exchange a sexual object just because attraction has waned and it no longer excites or gives pleasure is to injure the other person's sense of dignity after invading his privacy, learning his most intimate behaviour and promising him love. To achieve emotional harmony the sexual encounter must be incorporated in mutual trust, respect, care and responsibility for the partner, far beyond the mere physical exercise of the genital organs.

This shows how hopeless the illusion is that people must try each other out to see if they are suited. So elastic and adaptable are the genitals of both man and woman that theoretically any man could have intercourse with any woman and vice versa. The nerve paths and their relay stations are so arranged in every man and woman that they can conduct all the appropriate stimuli, sensations and pleasures and respond to them.

There is a reason why man and woman must strive after trust, care and respect, mutual responsibility and understanding beyond mere infatuation, so as to create a mental and emotional unit; only such a love can raise sexual communion above the physical, and make it a unique expression of man and woman as one flesh.

Orgasm is certainly associated with a reflex process as described above, and is certainly a special type of brain function, but the details are a mystery and will probably always remain so. One can only summarize by saying that orgasm more than all other physical functions is an expression of the psychosomatic unity of man and requires this as a prerequisite. Sexual pleasure and ejaculation of semen, rhythmical movements of the uterus, sexual tension and relaxation do not constitute orgasm, although the latter is not possible without them.

Orgasm presupposes an internal readiness to give oneself entirely to the partner, but the will to this is less significant than the unconscious attitude. The attitude of wanting the partner for oneself, and of wanting to experience a peak of sensation with him and through him (expressed as 'I *want* to find happiness with you') may be as disastrous to orgasm as the almost challenging attitude: 'You *must* be happy with (and through) me, I *will* make you happy'.

It is better to adopt the attitude: '*I am ready to serve you actively with all my human sexuality*'. Almost every word in this sentence is of significance. '*I*' means my whole consciousness and not just some drive in me or some dark id in my unknown soul. '*I am ready*' means that I am not requesting anything from you for me but I am waiting with my reaction for your reaction. But '*I am ready . . . with all my human sexuality*', not only my sex organs, means that not only do I make the latter available to you but also I offer all my male or female nature with its strength and weaknesses, its pleasures and joys; I offer my body to stimulate you and I focus on you my caresses, my skin and my touch, my voice and my odour, my eyes and ears, indeed all the senses and fibres of my being, as well as all my thoughts. This presupposes that the individual can love himself as he is, can affirm his own personality without reserve and is an integrated self-assured person ('I *can* live without you, but it is nicer to live with you'—Margarete Seiff).

'I am ready to serve *you*' means that I will enjoy orgasm with you and nobody else, because you and I enjoy each other's trust, respect, care, responsibility and understanding; you are neither unknown nor strange to me. 'I am ready to serve you *actively*' means that I am not just passive, self-sacrificing because you need me, but also myself involved in the production of happiness, rejoicing in myself and my ecstasy as much as yours and seeking to promote it for both our sakes. 'I am ready *to serve* you' means that I am only for you in this encounter; I am ready to offer you my whole existence not as your slave but because it pleases me. It is my happiness that you should be happy with me and because of me.

Complete abandon in sexual intercourse is possible through such an attitude and only through it. For a matter of seconds the two existences fuse into one; each has the sensation of being powerless over his own body and momentarily losing himself in an extreme of pleasurable unconsciousness. Man and woman give themselves entirely and achieve what each alone cannot reach, a unique experience of joy involving body, mind and spirit for a few seconds. At the peak of experience, at orgasm, the facial expression is not one of unalloyed pleasure. The experience lies between the death of the ego and the life of a new unity, between egoistical pain at abandonment of one's own personality and the joy of gaining an entirely different ego in the new unity. Thus the facial expression is torn between joy and pain, between life and death.

We have mentioned the copulatory reflexes which all converge on orgasm; we should now add that all organs and systems converge on this unity. At this moment body and soul attempt to mingle entirely at peace, and all the sense organs are aimed at this. The environment and indeed the whole world passes away. The breathing deepens as though the partners were trying to liberate themselves from oppression, the hearts may beat as one and the muscle movements also strike a uniform rhythm. It is only in the brief moment of orgasm that union becomes physical and induces an otherwise unattainable pleasure; for in a marvellous manner the partners are aware of every physical element involved, in spite of the tremendous finale to the sexual act.

Orgasm is the culmination of sexual tension and simultaneously the release; the latter takes place relatively slowly and is associated with single rhythmical bursts of excitation. Tension gives place to relaxation with a feeling of well-being, permeated with a sense of thankfulness towards the partner.

Not every act of intercourse ends in orgasm. To seek it constantly may give it too much prominence, so that orgasm may be regarded as a performance conveying the maximum of pleasure. Sexual activity then becomes a matter of prestige, with psychosomatic harmony dependent on orgasm. The result is to put it beyond one's reach, though it is accessible to patient mutual perseverance. This is the whole aim of preparation for marriage and training during marriage itself.

These facts should be known to the couple and they must practise tactfully towards this end. Mutual orgasm is rare at the first act of intercourse because the tension directed at oneself is much too great. Husband and wife gradually learn to obtain orgasm together provided they love themselves and their partner. Experience with partners other than the true one is useless, for one partner is different from another and wants intercourse in another way. It is therefore of no consequence for success with one partner that orgasm has been reached with another, since the decisive point is personal readiness to give oneself. Experience of abandon of self in orgasm is something quite different from the reflex release of tension in intercourse. The situation is similar to that in sexual dreams or masturbation, for these are expressions of incomplete orgasm or preludes to the latter. This is not a question of difference of degree. The abandonment of the body is so complete and so permeates the whole person that it cannot be repeated with anyone else. The exclusiveness of this experience strengthens the tie between the partners, leads to fidelity and makes possible the next orgasm.

Excitation graphs
A much discussed problem refers to the relationship between the speeds with which male and female reach orgasm, for the latter and also the amount of pleasure obtained from the copulatory reflex is more intense if both partners achieve orgasm simultaneously. However the graphs of excitation in male and female deviate greatly.

The male reaches orgasm rapidly after a relatively steep climb of excitation, and excitement then falls off rapidly (a). The woman gets excited more slowly but remains for a while at each level of excitement before climbing to the next level. Her excitement falls off more slowly and the curve is a wave (b). In general, the male reaches orgasm about five times as fast as the female and is sexually aroused about three times as often as his partner. These figures represent approximations for the initial situation in the two sexes. If the two curves are superimposed from start to finish of male excitement, the result shows roughly the situation when a couple first have intercourse together (c). The male has reached orgasm long before his partner, who now, because the man's excitement has subsided and his interest wanes, experiences an interruption of her own rising excitement and remains unsatisfied. Such disappointment almost always occurs during the first acts of intercourse between a couple.

Even today there are men who have not noticed all their lives that their wife never has an orgasm; there are also women who are unaware that they can reach a peak of pleasure in orgasm. It is only through loving and tactful management of each other that both partners learn to adjust their curves of excitation so that they coincide and permit simultaneous orgasm. This situation is shown in curves (d) and (e); the husband has reached orgasm either together with his wife (d) or immediately afterwards (e).

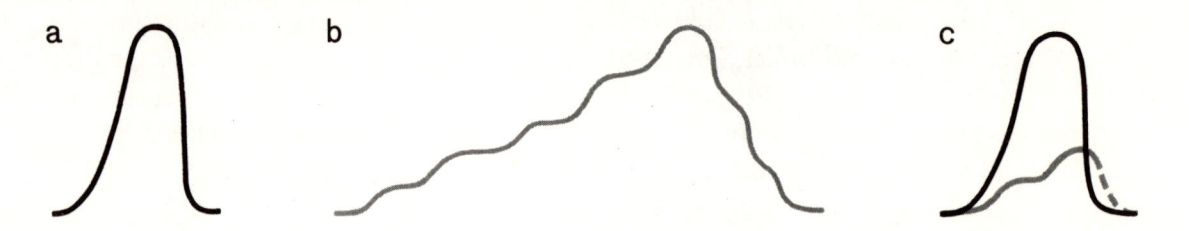

If all these graphs are compared it will be seen that the essential change has been in the

d   e

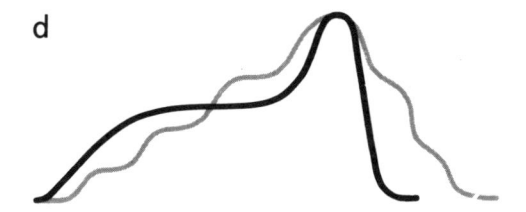

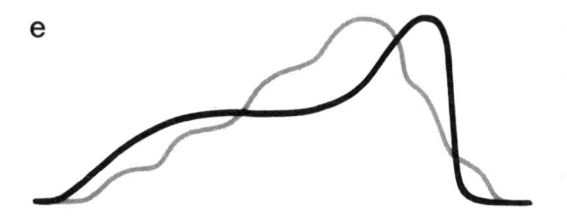

male. This is perhaps not quite accurate, for a wife who is handled lovingly by her husband can achieve orgasm more quickly. The significant point is the man's behaviour. If he is interested only in his own pleasure he will hardly be likely to help his partner to orgasm, and they will never experience simultaneous orgasm. By turning his attention to his partner and forgetting about himself he will succeed in holding back his excitement at an intermediate level, sufficiently high to continue to stimulate his partner but sufficiently low to check his own orgasm until his partner has made it quite clear through her own activity that she has reached an irreversible point in her own climax. (Irreversibility of the male copulatory reflex begins with the sucking out and expulsion of the sperm cells from the seminal duct into the urethra: see p. 94 ff.)

Mutual devotion
Sexual intercourse should not be an event separated off from the rest of marital life. 'Sleeping together' is an expression which accents the fact that the couple should stay together afterwards. The use of 'living together' as an euphemism also makes the point that one cannot have intercourse to the fullest extent without living together. Sexual intercourse belongs within the framework of living and sleeping, within the four walls where a couple can be undisturbed. Both these expressions make it clear that sexual intercourse should not be separate from the rest of conjugal life. The inclination of husband and wife towards each other is not restricted to intercourse, but affects all aspects of everyday life. If the latter is disturbed, it is not surprising that complete sexual union is also disturbed or shaky. The prerequisite for success in intercourse is not direct contact of the genitals or erogenous zones but mutual aid and comfort in the little things of ordinary living.

In sexual intercourse there is also more than stimulation and excitation of genitals. In discussing necking and petting (p. 140 ff.) we noted that mutual caresses form a necessary preparation for coitus. It is therefore an essential part of erotic intimacy that husband and wife should both pay some attention to preliminary love play in preparation for intercourse. This activity does not necessarily fall entirely to the husband, although he is likely to play the leading part, especially at the beginning of sexual union. His attentions should not be limited to those we have described as relevant during the act itself. They should include the whole personality of his partner and be transmitted to her as an all-embracing tenderness. On the other hand, the wife should also not shrink from expressing her tender emotions.

Expressions of intimacy between man and woman can be very varied. In the foreground lies consideration, but there is a never-ending scale embodying all possible active media of communication from the loving word to the understanding and contented look and beyond to the fondling and caressing of the whole body, from the transitory but meaningful touch to the powerful embrace and so on. The expression of togetherness can often be clearer in love play with its hundreds of variations than in the final stages of the copulatory reflex. Moreover all these attentions are a necessary forerunner of orgasm. The love play accompanying sexual activity is a prelude of delicate tuning-in for the subsequent act and makes the union of the genital parts particularly stimulating because it has attuned the woman and started the rise in her level of excitement before the act proper. She is ready to open herself to the man if he has first stimulated her by his general attention and contact.

In his approach the husband will initially concentrate especially on those zones in his wife which particularly excite him. Here a great variety of individual variations appear as regards the areas of the woman's body which most stimulate the male and the order in which their contact arouses him more. Independently of this, each woman will also have her scales of values for the exciting effect of touch of one part or another of her body. Each woman has a different response to her partner's body and his touch, and this is equally true of the man. It may be that a contact which excites the woman disturbs the man; conversely, a certain contact which the man finds stimulating may upset the woman rather than excite her.

As a marriage goes on, understanding of this should be achieved. If both partners are really ready to regard the happiness of the other as their aim, they can work out within certain limits a gradual adjustment to each other. The continued wooing of each by the other, which should not stop after marriage, can make an essential contribution.

The sort of contact which can stimulate both the active partner and the recipient varies greatly. Hands and mouth are the principal means of contact. But these offer all kinds of variation from a tender fleeting touch with the fingertips to a firm pressure of the hands, from a scarcely perceptible brush of the lips to a firm kiss. The mode of reception of the contact can also vary from shy withdrawal to energetic reciprocity, from passive acceptance to active participation.

Not only hands and mouth, but any contact of skin with skin, can have a stimulating effect, the sensation not always confined to the general erogenous areas. With increasing excitement the desire for more intense and energetic contact usually grows and finally leads to involuntary and intense orgasm. While recalling that the entire skin area in human beings is receptive to erotic stimuli, we may enumerate some particularly sensitive areas of skin and body, the so-called erogenous zones; this list should however be taken with some reserve and not be considered as a scale of values or a recipe for a sequence of areas to be contacted before and during sexual activity.

Erogenous zones in the woman
As regards love play and petting in general, the male would be well advised to begin his expressions of tenderness by touching first those erogenous areas which are furthest removed from the genital organs. The *palm of the hand* is an area of the body which is not only a donor but also a receptor of erotic stimuli, particularly by rhythmic stroking, pressure and kisses. Even more excitable are the *bend of the elbow* (walking arm in arm) and the *outer side of the thigh* (walking close together). The *inner side of the upper arm* and the *hair line* (especially on the back of the neck) are also excitable areas which can involve the whole of the woman's body in response. The *lobe of the ear* is less excitable than the *dimple behind the ear*. This is the reason for applying perfume there to attract the male to this spot. The *neck*, and the *upper part of the back* from the nape of the neck to between the shoulder blades, are areas of even stronger response to erotic stimuli.

Apart from the genitals, the *breasts*, including the areola and nipple particularly, are most responsive in the majority of women. However, many women find touching the breasts or playing with them unpleasant if their partner begins too soon or too roughly. As love play and petting advance, the *waist, hips and lower part of the back* including the sacral area respond to stronger stimuli. The *buttocks*, formerly as greatly emphasized by fashion as the breasts are now, usually require stronger stimuli but are receptive to delicate stimuli at the transition zones to the back and inner sides of the thigh. Touching the delicate skin on the *inner side of the thigh* has a powerful effect on a woman whose excitement has already begun and, provided the touch is gentle and not too premature, it will make her all the readier to open herself to her partner. Direct stimulation of the *genitals* embraces the whole pudendal region with variations from almost casual stroking through playful rhythmic touch to intense and continued contact. The lips (labia), the vestibule of the vagina and the clitoris should all be involved in this play. When the woman shows by her behaviour that she is ready the man should proceed to union, not forgetting to continue his love play.

A woman who has been led to orgasm learns to develop her own activity and to communicate similarly with her partner. She can thus become more active and display a whole gamut of possible ways to excite, stimulate, challenge, and request so that she becomes the determining partner in intercourse. Finally, a woman who has learned to recognize and appreciate orgasm will have more depths of experience than her partner. Because she is a woman, she will experience the transforming and satisfying unity of love more deeply and will later experience it more often than the man, who will often remain at the stage of simple enjoyment of the copulatory reflex. At this point his wife can by her tactful collaboration bring him to full orgasm.

Erogenous areas in the man
These are in general more sparse than in the woman. Whereas the woman's whole body is readily excitable, response to stimuli in the man is confined to his genitals. It is usually more important to him to feel a response in the woman to his efforts at arousing her, as an encouragement to him to proceed further. When his wife shows him by gently stroking his hands, his head, his lips and his hair, his arms and legs that she has recognized his efforts, his own excitement will also increase. Gentle or firm grasping of his erect penis and gentle stroking of his scrotum may arouse him greatly. However both man and woman should remember that all this may bring his excitement to a peak surprisingly rapidly and cause him to ejaculate, especially if he is inexperienced or has difficulty in holding back for his wife's sake. A wife experienced in love will almost always have a desire to touch the penis and grasp it, and many men find this exciting. However every woman at first feels shy about touching the penis, and there are many men who do not like to be touched there. This is a matter for mutual understanding of the partners, and there is no general rule.

In summary, we can only repeat once more that all knowledge and technique in intimate encounters is superficial and therefore incomplete unless it is based on a deep mutual attraction, respect and admiration and reinforced outside the sexual side by expression of this in mutual readiness to collaborate and care for each other and in the tenderness of everyday life.

Intercourse: frequency, forms, duration
We have seen that there is a wide range of possibilities in the game of love. In any individual partnership recognition and communication will teach the partners what is appreciated and what not; a basic type of approach will emerge with several variations around it, and in the course of time one or other variation will come into prominence. All this depends on mutual understanding. In this relationship as in others unchastity means treating one's partner as merely an object of one's will or ill-will. Chastity means therefore that intercourse should proceed with mutual comprehension and with respect for the personal needs and wishes of the partner.

This is also true for frequency of intercourse and its form. In every partnership of husband and wife there develops a specific rhythm of intercourse, for which no general rule can be laid down, and which will from time to time be changed to suit the wish of one or other of the partners; in general however, after the partners have achieved mutual adjustment, the rhythm will remain constant for years and the frequency of intercourse will first fall off in old age, though even then intercourse may not cease altogether (see p. 156 ff.).

Much the same situation holds good as regards positions adopted in coitus. There are all sorts of possibilities as regards position of the two bodies while the genitals are in contact. In general, forms in which the partners are face to face are to be preferred, because they allow visual contact and thus permit the partners to see each other's facial expression. Whether the wife lies, sits or kneels on the husband, or the husband lies on his wife, kneels in front of her raised pelvis or stands, or both lie facing on their sides in relatively close physical contact, or finally the wife turns her back and buttocks to her husband, is a question of agility of the partners, their ability to tolerate extra physical stress and finally and most important their mutual wishes. In rare cases, the physical position may depend on adaptation of the two physical conformations and sizes; in others the governing factor will be the type of contact between the genitals desired during the act. In yet other cases the position adopted will depend on the weightbearing ability of one or other, as in pregnancy. After an initial period, during which the partners will have allowed free rein to each other in experimentation (a situation which should continue into later years), they usually settle down to a basic pattern enjoyable to both. This basic pattern will of course have a number of variations, at least in the earlier years. No generally valid recommendations can be laid down.

The duration of individual sexual acts also varies greatly. But living together would miss its point if coitus consisted merely of lightning thrusts or surprise attacks, although an occasional encounter of this sort is not without its charm. It is usually the untried and inexperienced male who is responsible in the early days of marriage, when he has not acquired self-control and consideration for his wife, for such quick and fleeting episodes. The more practice he has in the skills already discussed, the easier it will be to make physical intimacy into real togetherness. With a practised and mutually considerate couple, the act of love including the preliminaries should last on an average about 15 to 25 minutes (a quick encounter only about 5 minutes). It may be prolonged into hours but is then likely to be followed by serious fatigue lasting up to a week.

The beneficial relaxation after orgasm gradually turns into sleep, which should be accompanied by a grateful tenderness. An old proverb has it that one kiss after orgasm is of more value than a thousand beforehand. The gratitude of the partners, as they retreat from the peak of unity into their separate selves, is an expression of their belonging to each other and already forms a basis for the next encounter.

It must be repeated that real intimacy is scarcely possible unless the partners live together physically. Readiness for repeated intimacies grows out of living together in space and time in one's own private dwelling place. Hence marriages accompanied by major separations in time and space, such as 'weekend marriages' of students or commercial travellers, are more easily upset in their intimacies, even if there is the continuing stimulus of beginning again. The tension of expectation accumulating during the separation is more likely to lead to fading of the stimulus than to orgasm.

In this chapter we have traced the arc from simple reflexes in the sex act to orgasm, and from there on to the many variations in the game of love and in the form, duration and expression of intimate encounters. It has become clear that the decisive factor in the achievement of a happy sex life depends on the inner attitude to sexuality and in particular to the partner. There is no area in human life where the unity of body, mind and soul is so clearly demonstrated as in its highest fulfilment in physical intercourse. This unique union is more than a mere event affecting the sex organs; it is an eminently mental and emotional act; the partners retreat from their unity to their separate ego situation. The memory remains as a stimulus to a fresh beginning. Repeated experience of union is only possible from the distance and integrity of the individual 'I' and 'thou'. It is therefore always rewarding to start afresh with mutual consideration as a deliberate preparation for the next time.

Sexuality in Later Life

It has already been said that the male remains capable of producing sperm cells into old age while the female becomes infertile with the onset of the climacteric (see pp. 101 and 127, 136 and 175). This biological distinction used to play an important part in the emotional field as well, for in the former climate of moral opinion sexuality was mainly related to reproduction and recognised as licit only in this respect. Once she could produce no more children, a woman looked upon herself as sexually useless. We now acknowledge that capacity for orgasm has nothing to do with reproduction and that completion of intercourse without desire to reproduce has its own rights; so that the sexual consequences of the climacteric have diminished. Women now 60 years old, i.e. 10 years after the menopause, have almost all been influenced by an education which played down a woman's sexual activity. Nevertheless, many during their lives have found the way to orgasm and they do not want to give it up just because of the climacteric. On the other hand, there are younger women aged between 35 and 50 who more and more frequently say that they look forward to their menopause as a time when they will be freed from the anxiety of pregnancy and able to give themselves up to sexual enjoyment as experienced persons; this is something their mothers would never even have dared to think. The change in concept of sexuality thus lags behind actual behaviour. The decisive effect of extinction of gonadotropic hormone function is not the end of the fertile period of life but the end of cyclical rhythm. The woman is liberated from the emotional swings due to her hormones, which she had to come to terms with, and now achieves an intense but smooth and level pattern of life. This not only affects her general life and professional activity, something which incidentally should be developed more for women of this age group, but also has a stabilizing influence on her sex life.

The switch from a cyclical and rhythmical emotional state to a stabilized one is the problem of the climacteric in modern women. The woman thus finds herself in a totally different situation from that of the man, for at the age of fifty she has to learn to deal with a new situation and not to mourn the one she had got used to. Yet this is a source of strength in comparison with the male. If she succeeds in changing she can begin to create for herself a new life with a new purpose. The complaints of the climacteric are grounded in this crisis. They are organic and functional expressions of a failure to master this change. The climacteric is not an illness, even if transitional endocrine stages with their transient failures of control may lead to severe hot flushes and similar manifestations. A woman with a positive approach to the transformation will not suffer. However, wherever there are relatively unconscious disturbances of emotional attitude they will make themselves felt as psychoneuroses, the ageing organs often forming a welcome focus for the disorder. It is quite clear that there are no differences regarding the married and single, the women with children and the childless as regards experience of climacteric symptoms and their conquest. Overcoming the climacteric is not a matter of exercise of sexuality or not, or of confirmed or unconfirmed fertility, but of the individual's attitude to these facts.

Men are free from these problems of hormonally conditioned changes. They remain fertile even in old age; the production of male sex hormone continues even if the amount diminishes, and their capacity to have intercourse in old age, though less frequently, has never been doubted. However men do encounter occasionally, over a much greater span of years (sometimes as early as 35 or as late as 55–60 years), symptoms similar to those in menopausal women, so that some doctors have been led to describe a male climacteric. Once again, normal ageing changes in body organs are exaggerated into signs of illness, while emotional conflict situations may also occur. Men may suffer from neurotic symptoms as well as women. The trigger mechanism for these symptoms of the so-called 'male menopause' is in most cases a recognition of waning function in competition with youth and in comparison with their powers of adaptation. If sexual activity is measured in terms of the number of orgasms—a scale of values which sets the man in imaginary competition with himself—the biological and natural decrease in this capacity with age must lead to a severe emotional shock which can then be unconsciously excused on the grounds of 'illness'.

Men who do not suffer from this disability are not necessarily more virile but simply those who have not rebelled against growing old. They have a positive attitude to the plateau and later decline of physical capacity, finding compensation in intellectual development. As numerous examples have shown, the latter increases with the years. There is no point in increasing intellectual work beyond the amount appropriate to the age group, although experience of life together with the sum total of knowledge acquired may lead to a higher level of judgement and wisdom than in youth. In addition the mature intellectual can accept his waning physical powers, neither bemoaning their loss nor finding life boring. This is equally true of men and women.

Marital intercourse becomes less frequent in later years though no guidelines can be laid down for this; frequency depends entirely on the tastes of the partners. Manifestations of tenderness are no longer so stormy but they are often deeper. The union of married couples, at first experienced only as fleeting episodes of mutual surrender, becomes increasingly an expression of mutuality apart from sex. With experience of life the unimportant appears small and the important big. Hence older people are often more tolerant and far-seeing than the young.

Modern statistical study of sex has shown that, on an average, sexual intercourse is desired by married couples up to the age of about 60 as frequently as at the age of 45. Between 60 and 75 years there is a definite decline in frequency. But even beyond 75 years intercourse need not cease completely.

This period however can be difficult if the partners do not communicate freely about their problems because of lack of mutual trust, or if a considerable difference in age (10 years or more) creates a biological difference in vitality which cannot be bridged. Even more difficult are those marriages in which the husband thinks he can no longer satisfy his wife and therefore neglects her, while she feels that she has lost some of her first bloom. Even now, about half the married women over 50 are sexually deserted by their husbands and suffer greatly from this, sometimes seeking alternative sexual outlets. The same men may dream of being sexually stimulated and therefore more potent with a younger girl or woman, only to find that such liaisons add nothing to their self-esteem. They may have engaged on a false hunt after prestige and thus have departed from their proper path of taking the ageing process seriously and facing it together with their wives. Ageing cannot be avoided. It is best dealt with by accepting it, and recognizing dreams of eternal youth for the sham they are and abandoning them.

Ageing, a biological process of degeneration of organs and cells, runs counter to intellectual maturity. It is therefore a poor service to mankind if the natural fear of death is enhanced and the biological processes of intellectual maturation are impeded by a vain attempt to maintain physical youth as long as possible. It is of course the task of modern medicine and biochemistry to preserve ageing persons from illness and keep them healthy. But health in old age does not mean maintenance of the physical capacities of youth; it means maintenance of performance in accord with organic regression. A small child does not possess the capacity and style of living of a 30-year-old although it is organically younger and more elastic, because it has not yet achieved control over expenditure of its energies; similarly, an older man can no longer with impunity maintain the style of a younger one, although he knows how to employ his mental capacity better and more economically. Whoever takes away from a man the possibility of maturing intellectually and offers him instead the illusion of eternal youth with the help of pills and tablets, also takes away the possibility of recognizing the challenge of ageing and of ending one's life with dignity.

Inheritance

In the last chapter we described the area of sexual relations between man and woman. During the fertile period of a woman's life, completion of intercourse is always associated with the possibility of fusion of spermatozoon and ovum and thus with production of a new life, the child of the couple. Before we discuss in subsequent chapters the physical and emotional processes of conception, pregnancy and labour, we will say something about inheritance and its mechanisms.

Germ Cell Maturation and Inheritance

Children resemble their parents to varying degrees, sometimes being as alike as two peas, sometimes very different, and sometimes resembling other relations such as an uncle, aunt or grandparents. On occasions some peculiarity or other of the father reappears in feminine form in his daughter, or conversely a characteristic of the mother reappears in masculine counterpart in her son. If we exclude the fact that many external nuances of behaviour appear to arise through imitation (for example, the gait, the way of crossing the legs or carrying the head, moving the eyebrows and many other movements) and the fact that many other forms of attitude and behaviour are also transmitted during development from one or other parent (for example, courage and anxiety, frankness and withdrawal, extraversion and timidity), there still remain many characteristics and modes of behaviour which are not acquired simply by living together with the parents or other people. These characteristics are transmitted from father and mother by specific physical vectors. This is the true process of inheritance; acquisition of characters through close contact with relatives is 'social inheritance'.

Man and woman form germ cells (spermatozoon and ovum) in their genital glands.

Through fusion of these a new life arises (see figs. 40–48), modelled on internal blueprints transmitted to it, with the addition early in life of factors depending on the mother and her feeding (see figs. 46, 47, 48, 72) and later with additional influences from both parents in accordance with the identification processes described in the opening chapter. After the fusion of spermatozoon and ovum, the new living organism receives nothing more of paternal or maternal substance (apart from physical and later mental and emotional 'nourishment') which can affect the inheritance of physical characters. Physical inheritance in contrast to emotional acquisitions must therefore be contained in the sperm and the ovum.

Chromosomes

Research has shown that the hereditary substance is associated with the nuclei of the spermatozoon and ovum, and in fact with certain carriers of hereditary characters known as chromosomes (a word meaning 'coloured bodies', because they are rendered visible by staining with dyes). These carriers are present in every cell, or rather every cell nucleus, and not only in the reproductive cells.

The number of chromosomes is the same in every human being, amounting to 23 pairs or 46 single pieces. One of these pairs (two carriers) determines the sex of the individual, so that we can say that a human being has 44 carriers of characters plus the two sex chromosomes. If every mature spermatozoon and every mature ovum contains 46 chromosomes, fusion of two such cells would mean that the child had 92 chromosomes, its progeny would have 184 and so on. Since this is not the case but the number of chromosomes remains constant, there must be a reduction in their number somewhere during maturation of the spermatozoon and the ovum. This reduction takes place in a peculiar manner during cell divisions occurring while they mature.

Genes

Before describing in detail the processes of maturation divisions (meiosis), let us take a look at the structure of the carriers of hereditary characters and their mode of action. A chromosome looks like a ribbon of varying length, formed of a number of bands which are stuck together in a certain order (see fig. 36). These bands or discs contain the real carriers of the hereditary substance, the genes. It is however not true that one gene is responsible for transmission of one definite character and no more. One external physical character is not determined by a single gene but in certain circumstances by several genes and by the way these genes are placed and linked with other genes in the same chromosome or in other chromo-

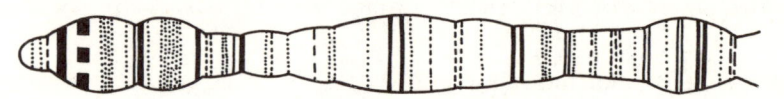

FIG. 36 *Chromosome threads.*

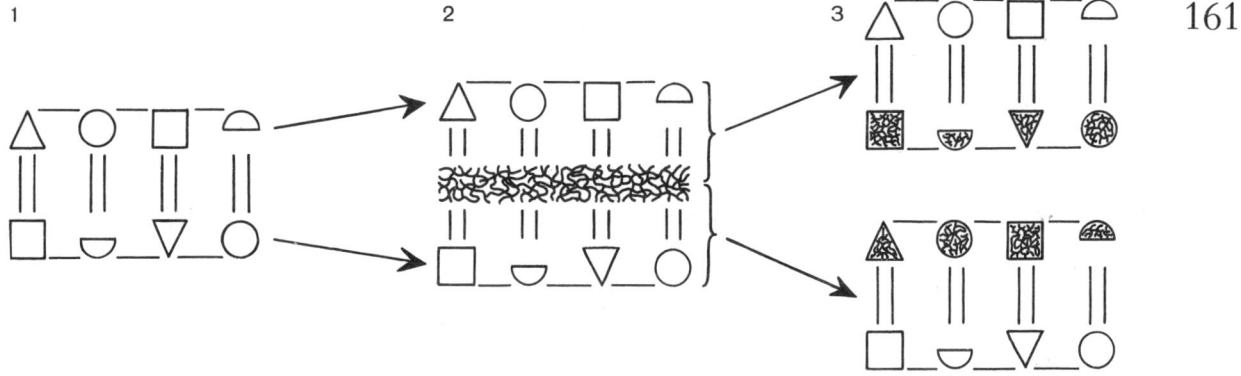

FIG. 37 *Increase in hereditary substance: simultaneous duplication (identical reduplication) of the substance.*

1 A double chain (greatly shortened in the diagram)   2 Split double chain with nutrient protein (relatively unformed) in between   3 Two double chains, of which a part has been formed out of the nutrient protein

somes. Thus it happens that although the same genes are present in parents and children, children may have other physical characters because the relevant gene occupies a different place in the chromosome. Moreover, genes do not always act directly on the cell in which they are present and thus determine what will happen to that cell. They may intervene in physical structure through chemical intermediate products (so-called gene hormones and gene enzymes).

The above does not exhaust our present knowledge of structure and mode of action of carriers of hereditary traits. The genes can be looked upon as a double chain of building bricks of protein (molecules) arranged in a certain fixed order; their special arrangement represents the code or building blueprint. This double chain of protein building bricks (made of so-called deoxyribonucleic acid or DNA) is responsible for the capacity of the body to reproduce itself with the aid of other protein substances (nutritional) and thus to double itself (identical reduplication, see fig. 37), and also for the capacity to act as a code for a clear text, or in other words to cause other nutrient proteins to arrange themselves in a definite and persisting order (see fig. 38). In these protein units therefore lies the secret of what we call life, at the lowest scale of development, that is, the ability to use other substances to multiply and grow.

Maturation division
How are these blueprints transmitted from father and mother to the children? For simplicity's sake, we will keep to the larger unit, the chromosome, leaving aside for the moment the particular significance of the sex chromosomes.

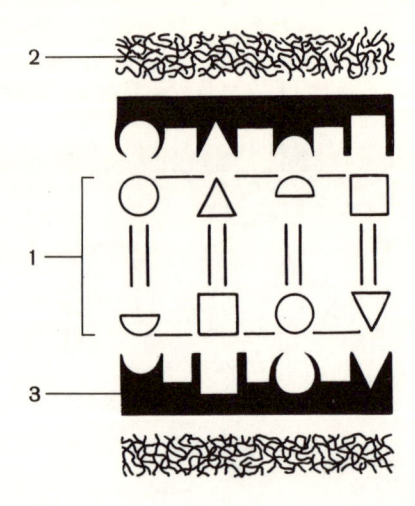

FIG. 38 *Construction of body substance (effect of double chain on matrix composed of nutrient protein).*

The structure of the protein molecules, united in the double strands as genes, contains the plan which governs the future organism.

1 Double chain as coded formula for laying down body substance
2 Relatively unstructured nutrient protein
3 Constructed body protein (decoded protein formula)

We have learned that human beings have a total of 46, i.e. 23 pairs of, chromosomes. Of these one chromosome out of each pair comes from the father and one from the mother. To keep the matter in proportion we will look at these chromosomes undergoing maturation division, which takes the same course during maturation of the primary oocyte to the ovum and of the primary spermatocyte to the spermatozoon. In the diagram (fig. 39) the chromosomes coming from the mother are coloured red and those from the father blue. At the beginning of the first maturation division, the corresponding chromosomes lie close together. This is termed chromosome conjugation or pairing. During this apposition, there may be an exchange between parts of the chromosome from the father and corresponding parts of the chromosome from the mother. This exchange of hereditary factors (genetic material) is called crossing over. The result is that, within one chromosome, genes from the father are combined with those from the mother. (In our example we have, for the sake of simplicity, shown crossing over in only one pair of chromosomes.)

The pair of chromosomes then separate again, divide once more lengthwise and thus end up with 4 instead of 2 chromosomes lying together; the latter also shorten and thicken (tetrad formation). The cell then divides (primary spermatocyte into two secondary spermatocytes; primary oocyte into one secondary oocyte plus one polar body). The nuclear capsule is lost. In the cell substance a spindle appears, whose threads serve to draw the chromosome into the new cell. The cell walls separate off from each other, and a new nucleus arises in each cell.

At this division, it is not preordained which chromosome will go into which cell. All that is laid down is that every new cell will contain the same set of chromosomes. If at this division the chromosomes are not equally distributed in full complement to the two new cells, malformations will arise. In the subsequent second maturation division (with a fresh

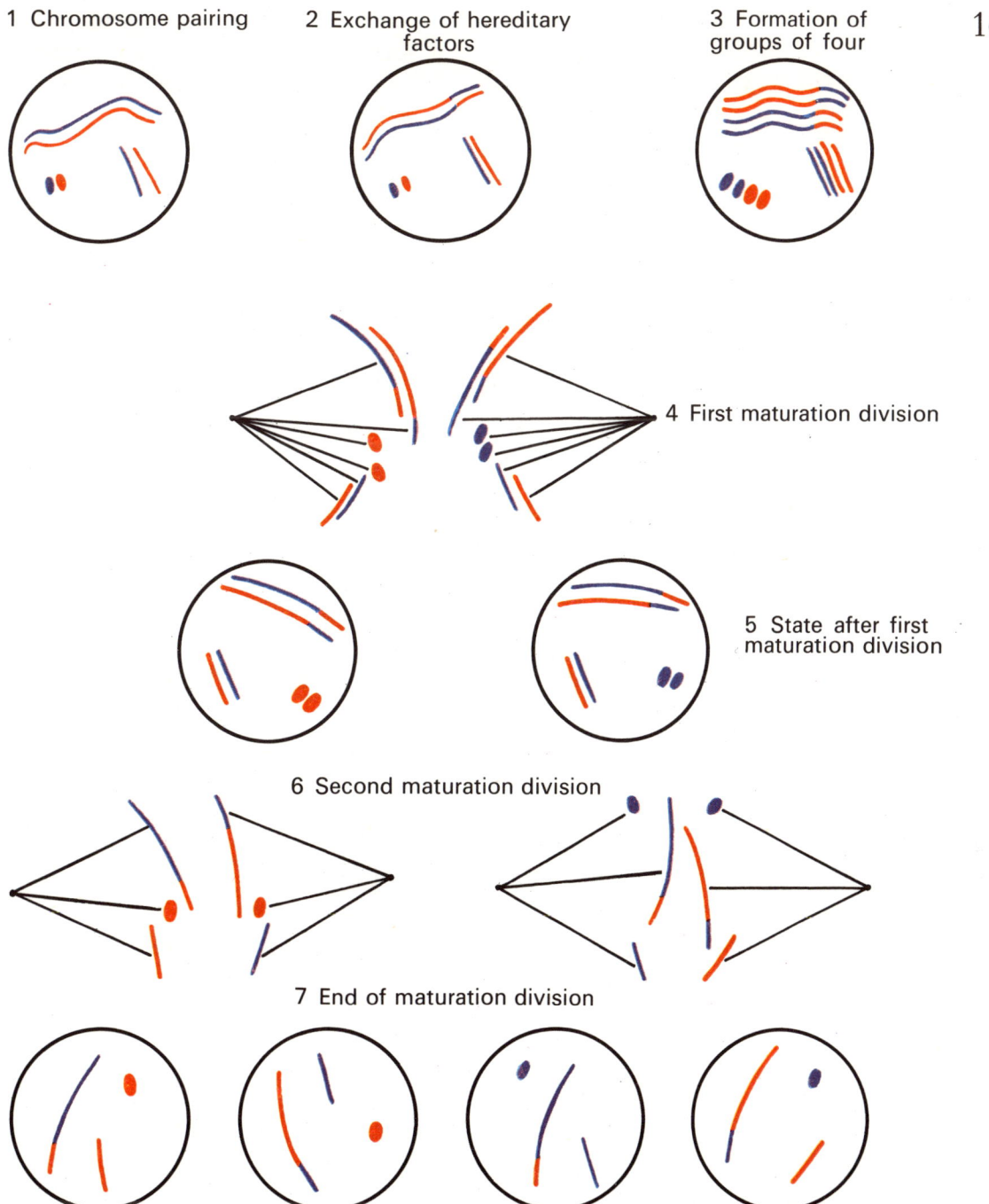

1 Chromosome pairing
2 Exchange of hereditary factors
3 Formation of groups of four
4 First maturation division
5 State after first maturation division
6 Second maturation division
7 End of maturation division

FIG. 39 *Diagram of maturation divisions of ovum and spermatozoon.*

spindle) the chromosomes are distributed among the progeny cells without further doubling. (From two secondary spermatocytes four spermatids arise and develop into sperm cells, and from the secondary oocyte with one polar body an ovum plus three polar bodies.)

The example shows clearly how, in mature spermatozoa or ova, the paternal and maternal 'characters' are differently distributed. If there were no crossing over, the child would possess only the characters of his grandparents. Crossing over serves to mix up the characters in the hereditary substance of father and mother. The characters the father has inherited from his parents, or the mother from her parents, take effect as a result of the mixing of chromosomes and thus determine physical components of the child.

The above clearly indicates also that the composition of the hereditary material in the spermatozoa or the ova is independent of the physical properties of the father or mother; these physical characters are expressed only after total mixing. This is the explanation of the poor degree of resemblance between some children and their parents.

The rest of the cell, the plasma, is not without significance for the appearance of characters. A given character inherited in the chromosomes will be differently expressed in different plasma environments. Since the spermatozoon contributes hardly any plasma in the fusion process (the sperm head consists almost exclusively of nuclear substance), this plasma factor in human subjects is contributed only by the ovum. Thus, hereditary factors associated with paternal and maternal nuclei in sperm and ovum, as well as factors associated with the substance of the ovum, affect each other mutually and together determine the hereditary process.

Social inheritance
At the beginning of this chapter, we pointed out that as well as the inheritance determined by the chromosomes there is a social inheritance. This social inheritance in its widest sense has a say in which parts of the hereditary matrix will develop later in life. An example will make this clear. If peas of pure strain are sown and exposed to different conditions of nutrition, weather and sunshine, many of those harvested will be much smaller or much larger than the ones sown, although the majority will resemble the original ones. Hence a great variety of environmental influences affect the development of the hereditary matrix, yet the latter determines the extent of variation in size between the smallest and largest. The expression of physical characteristics and other properties may vary within these limits as a result of such environmental variations as those of nutrition, education, milieu and so on. This also means that education can be effective only within these limits. We have already shown how far-reaching and decisive educational influences can be in relation to character, attitudes, response to life challenges and relations with partners. The fact mentioned in the introduction that all human life is either male or female needs some further explanation.

Asexual reproduction

A superficial look at the living world around us suggests that sexual life, with male and female examples, is universal, but this is not absolutely true. Lower forms of life which may be regarded as the forerunners in the evolutionary story of more highly organized life, may reproduce asexually for thousands of generations by simple cell division. A single cell retains the capacity to divide indefinitely and thus to produce progeny without itself dying unless it is killed by external circumstances, as for example by being eaten. Under favourable conditions these cells appear immortal. When external conditions of life get worse and there is a danger that the entire species will die out, we observe something new—the fusion of two cells which seem exactly like all the other cells. The new cell they jointly produce is, in comparison with other cells, more resistant to external circumstances and can (sometimes by resting for a prolonged period) withstand unfavourable conditions of dryness, cold, pressure, lack of oxygen and so on. When the environment is again favourable such a cell grows, divides and reproduces itself asexually indefinitely until hard times once more threaten its existence. The fusion of two cells to form a new and more resistant organism is the simplest form of sexual life. It does not yet serve the cause of reproduction but only that of maintenance of the species. It is still not known whether the fused cells can be distinguished as 'male' or 'female'. They appear rather to be bisexual, with possibilities in both directions. The above is mainly true of single-celled organisms. Organisms consisting of several cells living together in union, in which at first there is little differentiation of cell function but later a more marked distribution of work in the cell state, are at first more susceptible to external influences. Hence maintenance of the species becomes more difficult. Although such organisms can still reproduce by division, there is a growing trend for certain cells to be the only ones able to fuse with a similar cell from another organism of the same species to produce a more resistant cell, out of which an entire organism of the species can develop.

Sexual reproduction

With the appearance of such highly developed forms of life as cell complexes (with increasing distribution of function between different cells within the complex) the organism becomes more susceptible to external disturbances and it therefore becomes necessary to make the innate capacity of every cell to preserve the species more specialized. At first these organisms and their sexual cells cannot be distinguished as male and female externally. Increased development of life on this planet has led first to differentiation of sex cells and later to difference in the entire organism. It should be noted that the presence of water, even a few drops of moisture, is essential for the union of the different sex cells in the entire animal world. Whereas in lower forms of life the sex cells simply leave the rest and then find each other (by chance or by chemical attraction), in more organized creatures the sex cells are associated with special organs. Union takes place because the sex cell of one organism

166

Mother

Father

44 chromosomes each
xx = female
xy = male

First maturation division

Second maturation division

Germ cells ripe for fertilization

22 ♀ x

22 x   22 y   22 x   22 y

Possibilities for fertilization

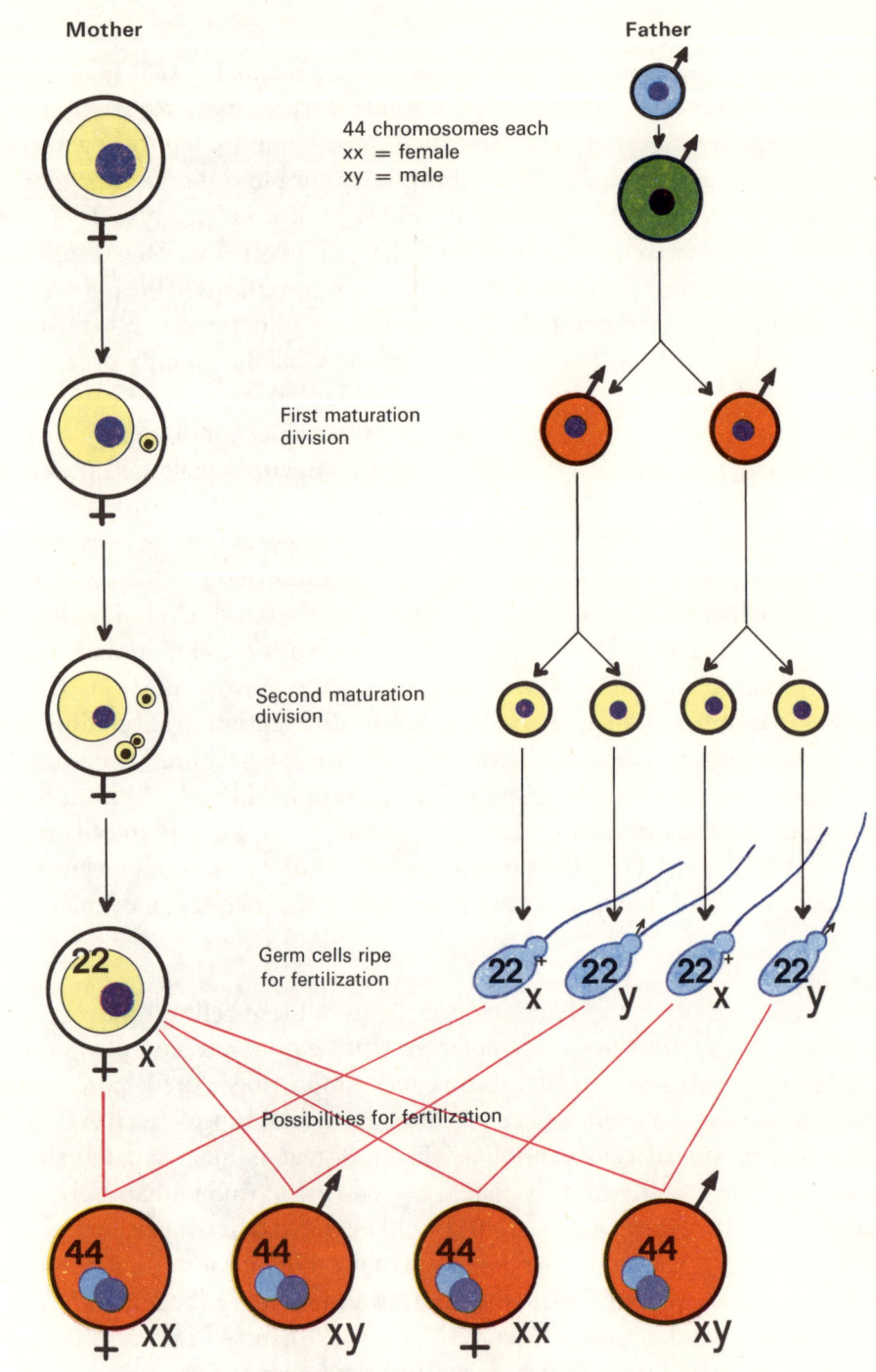

44 ♀ xx   44 xy   44 ♀ xx   44 xy

FIG. 40 *Boy or girl? The decision is made by the spermatozoa.*

is brought to the sex cell of the other through particular organs, the sex organs or genitals. The cell which awaits the other is known as the female, and the cell which comes to the other as the male. Fusion of male and female cells is called fertilization, and the male and female cells are the parent cells.

In humans as in other highly developed animals, the further development of the new organism takes place within the organs of the female, because ever greater specialization makes the newcomer particularly sensitive to disturbances during the first months of life. It is set free into the world (birth) only after it has attained a certain degree of independence, and the woman is then delivered of her fruit. The child however remains, especially in the human race, dependent on the help of its parents after birth.

Boy or girl?
How is it that after union of male and female sex cells either a boy or a girl is formed? We have seen that the characteristics of a new living organism are associated with the reproduction of certain carriers in the cell nuclei of sperm and ovum. The forerunners of the spermatozoon have a special chromosome pair (containing an x and a y chromosome). In the forerunner of the ovum there is also a special pair but they are not different—they are both x chromosomes. Hence the chromosome schema for the sex cells of male and female is as follows:

Male: 44 somatic chromosomes and one pair of sex chromosomes xy

Female: 44 somatic chromosomes and one pair of sex chromosomes xx

This shows that the y chromosome determines maleness and the x femaleness. During the maturation divisions of sperm and ovum cells, the chromosomes are distributed as shown in Figure 40. Thus within the sperm cells there are both female-determining x and male-determining y spermatozoa while the ovum is always a female-determining cell. Whether a boy or a girl is born is dependent therefore on which of the father's spermatozoa fertilizes the ovum.

In theory therefore, equal numbers of boys and girls ought to be born, but in fact there are 106 male births for every 100 female births. If premature births and abortions are included, there is a further shift in favour of the male sex, so that immediately after conception there are actually only 100 females to 135–150 males. Hence many more male foetuses are produced than female, but male foetuses die much more commonly within the womb than do female ones, often within a few days of conception, so that the only sign is a somewhat heavier loss of blood. The extra bleeding is not a true menstrual period but a very early abortion, which can be proved medically. How is it that more male embryos than female are produced?

It has been shown that the male-determining sperm cells with a y chromosome are somewhat smaller than those carrying the female x chromosome alone, and more resistant in the milieu of the female sex organs. There is therefore a higher probability that a male-determining spermatozoon will fertilize an ovum. The actual reasons why such a spermatozoon is more resistant than a female-determining one remain unknown, as do those for the lower resistance of male embryos in the uterus. The peculiar increase in male births during times of war and afterwards, as well as in times of hardship and oppression, has not been sufficiently studied, although there is no lack of attempted explanations.

Hermaphrodites
Apart from the sex-determining factors in the chromosomes (XX—female, XY—male), a second group of hitherto unknown factors also affects the sexual development of the child and may give rise to disturbances. There may also be disturbances during maturation division, giving rise to incorrect distribution of the X and Y chromosomes in sperms and ova, and therefore to abnormal circumstances when the two meet. The products are true and false hermaphrodites (2–3 per thousand pregnancies). In all true hermaphrodites there are *both* male and female sex organs. These children are sterile and self-fertilization is impossible. False hermaphrodites possess sex organs of only one sex (either male or female) but show considerable disturbance in the development of external and internal genitals, so that with male sex organs the external genitals usually appear female or vice versa. Certain forms of hermaphrodite also suffer from other malformations.

Since the external genitals determine which sex will be entered in the official register, it can happen that a mistake is made because the external genitals do not correspond to the sex glands present in false hermaphrodites, and the sex of the child may be incorrectly registered. If for example a boy has a very small penis which looks like a clitoris and the two halves of the scrotum have not adhered together, while the testes have not descended into the latter, the external impression may be one of a female. Conversely, if the girl's clitoris looks as big as a penis and nobody notices that the urethral opening lies below the organ, while the labia look like the two halves of a scrotum and the vaginal opening is closed, she may be taken for a boy. Such a decision determines the upbringing of the child, beginning with its clothing and continuing with gender assignment as regards its role in the family and later in the world. The fact that the individual is a false hermaphrodite may often not be discovered until long after he or she has been established emotionally in a female or male sex role. Discovery may take place at puberty, when the alleged boy under the influence of his ovaries develops breasts or the alleged girl under the influence of her testes grows a beard, develops a deep voice and takes on male bodily conformation; the error may even not be discovered until the 'girl' wants to marry. This leads to considerable mental shock because the 'sexual' life style so far allowed is shown to be biologically false, even if it was an involuntary deception for which the individual was not responsible. With the hormonal activity of puberty this has been unconsciously indicated, but there now arise serious problems of future living. The role that has been inculcated and learned, for example, to behave, think and feel like a man, must be abandoned and a new role, that of a woman, learned and performed; all through his former life the individual has had no preparation for the part. If we recall that the essentials of character and behaviour have been implanted by the end of the sixth year, the burden of having to change one's life basically later on will be obvious. Whether the person is helped to overcome these problems by postpubertal operative transformation of the external genitals into a state corresponding to that of the internal sex organs (sex change of a 'false' male into a 'true' female, and vice versa), together with appropriate hormonal treatment, remains undecided. Every effort should therefore be made to unmask false hermaphrodites at birth—by comparison between external genitals and results of sex chromosome examinations—so that operation can be undertaken early and the child can be reared in accordance with its true sex.

Mutations and Injury to Hereditary Material

General mutations, radiation injury, healthy inheritance
The effects of radioactivity of all sorts on the genes is now well established. Radiations consist of small particles which penetrate the body without our noticing it, as for example in radiography or radioscopy. (The differences in density of body tissues, for instance, between bones and soft parts, cause different amounts of braking on the particles as they pass through. These particles show up the internal structure if allowed to leave the body again and visualised in various ways, as on an X-ray film or a radioscopy screen.) If radiation particles as they pass through the body with a given energy and in given numbers meet a gene they may injure the protein molecular structure of the latter. Since the effectiveness of a gene depends on its protein molecular structure, the effect of the gene is therefore altered, and with it the character it determined. Such a change in a character due to change in a gene is called a *mutation*.

Mutations are not only caused by radiation and are not always limited to one gene but may affect either a segment of a chromosome, the number of chromosomes or the entire set of chromosomes. They may also affect crossing over. Certain mutations leading to so-called hereditary diseases are related to the age of the parents, such as mongolism which is related to the age (of the germ cells) of the mother while another malformation of cartilage and bone with dwarfism is related to the age of the father (and his sperm cells). It would take us too far to discuss other hereditary diseases in detail. (To avoid misunderstanding it should be said that mongolism, now better known as Down's disease, may also arise independently of the mother's age and as a result of incorrect attachment of one chromosome to another during maturation division, so-called chromosome translocation.)

Mutations are not necessarily disadvantageous to the germ cells or the later progeny, or the body cells of the organism. Because there is a complicated exchange of genes during the maturation divisions which precede every fertilization, and also because mankind has always been exposed to cosmic radiation long before the era of x-rays and atom splitting, these effects on hereditary material have occurred and will continue to occur. Thus there have always been mutations or changes in inherited characters due to changes in the genetic material, and this will go on. They explain the changes in hereditary background during the course of human and world history. Since the changes in genetic substance due to mutations are usually further inherited, benign mutations will lead to better adaptation of a people to external environment, while life-disturbing mutations will threaten the life of the individual and his reproduction and may in fact prevent it. Such mutations may appear out of the blue in previously genetically 'healthy' families; what is regarded as genetically healthy depends of course on what the current society expects of its members as regards appearance, performance and adaptation. For example, the present average body size of the white race would have appeared gigantic in the Middle Ages. We may designate as genetically healthy those genes whose effect is harmoniously adapted to the manifestations of life as a whole and does not disturb the balance of characteristics. Thus with healthy genes there is a greater probability of survival and reproduction of their carrier.

In recent decades however, many more pathological mutations, i.e. those disturbing the balance of characters, have been observed; the massive radioactivity associated with nuclear fission has a greater effect than X-rays in causing disorder and destruction of genes. For this reason, all measures protecting human beings from excessive X-ray and atomic radiation deserve support.

Ever since it has been known that aimed irradiation can also lead to mutations favourable to life, at least in animals, there has been a continuous clamour in favour of positively altering the genetic material of man, or at least of a definite race or group. But this is a scientific utopia, for such 'aimed' irradiation must have a side-effect leading to extensive damage to neighbouring genes it was not intended to hit.

There has also been speculation on the possibility of cleansing an entire population genetically from all those members who carry 'bad' genes. This idea is also in the realm of utopia, however attractive it has seemed to certain scientists, simply because of mutation. Because mutations can occur without any artificial intervention, because undesired hereditary characters may be transmitted undetected for generations, and because hereditary diseases often appear only if the genes transmitted from father and mother are arranged in a certain way, theoretically any member of a population might be the cause of undesired characteristics. To get a genetically healthy population one would have to exclude all possibilities and therefore to prevent all members of the population from reproduction. Pure hereditary material exists only in theory, never in practice.

Quite apart from scientific discussion of such questions, there is also an ethical angle to consider, for such interference with human heredity is an affront to the personal dignity of man.

This warning against interference with human genes should not be confused with the demand that husband and wife be aware of their responsibility as future parents for the hereditary make-up of any children they produce. Where hereditary disease has been demonstrated in the blood relations of a partner, it may be better to abstain from marriage; the mutual love of the partners does not necessarily mean that they will love a child with hereditary disease, nor does their mutual love help the diseased child to overcome its handicap. It might be added that proof or exclusion of hereditary disease now depends in part on examinations conducted in the chromosome laboratories.

Marriage with relatives
I should perhaps make here a few remarks about marriage with relatives. Probability statistics show that in a marriage between first cousins the chance that both partners will have inherited the same disease-evoking gene in their make-up is 7·6 times greater than with unrelated partners. If the two disease-evoking factors unite when sperm and ovum fuse, certain diseases may appear although the two partners have been and remain healthy. However, for this to happen it is essential that the two hereditary factors be present in the particular sperm and the particular ovum which unite. Thus we see that the risk to the children in marriages between relatives is not very great if the couple are themselves apparently healthy. When first cousins marry and reproduce, however, there are more than the normal number of malformations and deaths in childhood.

The risk attached to marriages of relatives diminishes rapidly as the degree of relationship becomes more distant. First-cousin marriages and those between uncle and niece represent a small but notable risk. With second cousins, the risk of malformed children is no greater than the general risk in the population. Blood relationships between grandparents and even earlier are of no significance for the health of the progeny of a marriage.

Effects of alcohol
Constant abuse of alcohol may also damage the germ material in both male (forerunners of sperm) and female (forerunners of the ovum). But is there any risk of hereditary injury to a child conceived after intercourse following a single drinking bout? It has been shown that alcohol is very quickly found in the sex organs in the same concentration as in the blood. Even alcohol concentrations in the blood of one in a thousand damage the substance of the spermatozoa (causing rolled up spermatozoal tails, broken off heads, and distended middle pieces), and interfere with their motility (paralysis, oscillations instead of forward progression, reverse movements). It is known that spermatozoa so damaged are infertile because

172 they cannot penetrate into the ovum. It is also supposed, but without proof, that fully developed spermatozoa or ova cannot undergo injury to their genes as a result of a single dose of alcohol; such a dose may however damage the genes during maturation of the sperm cells in the tubules of the testis and the head of the epididymis, or the maturation divisions of the ovum in the ovary. All this has not been definitely proved, and it will be difficult to establish. It should simply be borne in mind that an inclination to alcohol abuse by one partner may at least have certain relations to defects of character. Even if the latter are not hereditary, they will represent a disadvantage for the environment in which the child grows up. In the choice of partner this deserves consideration in the context of future responsible parenthood.

Conception and Contraception

Impregnation and Conception

At the peak of sexual excitement in the male, his orgasm, the seminal fluid containing spermatozoa from the male sex glands, is ejaculated from the urethra. The involuntary spasmodic movements of the lower abdomen during this event drive the penis deeply into the vagina, so that ejaculation of semen takes place immediately next to the cervix. If the ejaculation leads to fertilization of the ovum, the event is called *impregnation* or *insemination*. Without fertilization the event is merely copulation.

The spermatozoa first reach the vagina, whose fluid is mildly acid as a result of certain bacterial and chemical reactions. This property causes the spermatozoa to migrate, and since the mucus plug in the cervix offers them better living conditions, they swim in this direction, impelled by chemical attraction. They move about as fast, in comparison with their length, as a world record swimmer would, swimming their own length in one second. They keep this speed up later within the uterus and tubes.

The cervical canal with its mucus plug is the real receptor organ for the spermatozoa (see fig. 41). If intercourse has taken place at a time when the fallopian tube contains a fertilizable ovum, the mucus plug is particularly watery and sticky. Protruding from the cervical canal, it advances a little towards the sperm and facilitates their entry. A disturbance in the chemical composition of the mucus plug at the time of ovulation may represent a cause of diminished conception and therefore of infertility in marriage.

The rhythmical movements of the uterus when the woman has her orgasm, associated with rhythmical to and fro movements of the mucus plug, may assist the uptake of spermatozoa in the internal genitals. However, these movements are not necessary for penetration of the spermatozoa and for fertilization; a woman can conceive without orgasm. Conception is in fact possible if the semen merely wets the external genitals; spermatozoa are capable of wandering through the vagina to the cervix. This can also happen during petting if the hands deposit semen on the external genitals. This is why the so-called coitus interruptus

174 (see p. 181 ff.) is not a safe method of avoiding conception. Methods which mechanically or chemically prevent penetration of the cervical canal by the spermatozoa are safer; these include the intact rubber condom over the penis, mechanical closure of the cervical os, or chemical injury to and disturbance of movement of the sperm by substances introduced into the vagina before intercourse (see p. 183 ff.).

In the *mucus plug of the cervical canal* the spermatozoa undergo a chemical cleansing from foreign (i.e. male) proteins in the semen which might disturb the female organism. The mucus helps the spermatozoa to penetrate more deeply into the woman's internal organs. Penetration is hindered in the uterus by the stream of fluid outwards and in the tubes by the ciliary movements as well. There is no chemical attraction towards the ovum. The spermatozoa either meet an ovum by chance or they swim past it. The great number of spermatozoa is designed to ensure that if there is a living ovum around, at least some of the spermatozoa will meet it somewhere among the complicated mucosal folds of the tube. Many spermatozoa die on the way, others wander into the wrong tube, and many more miss the ovum or pass right through the tube into the free peritoneal cavity, where they perish among the coils of intestine and are dissolved.

The spermatozoon penetrates into the ovum (*insemination*), and fusion of spermatozoal nucleus and ovum takes place a little later (*fertilization*). The latter process begins pregnancy, and the further events will be described in the next chapter. Insemination of the ovum takes place in the funnel-shaped beginning of the tube, and the ovum then takes about five days to pass into the uterus, aided by the cilia and the fluid stream in the tube.

Timing of conception
Experience has shown that conception is commonest when intercourse has occurred 22 to

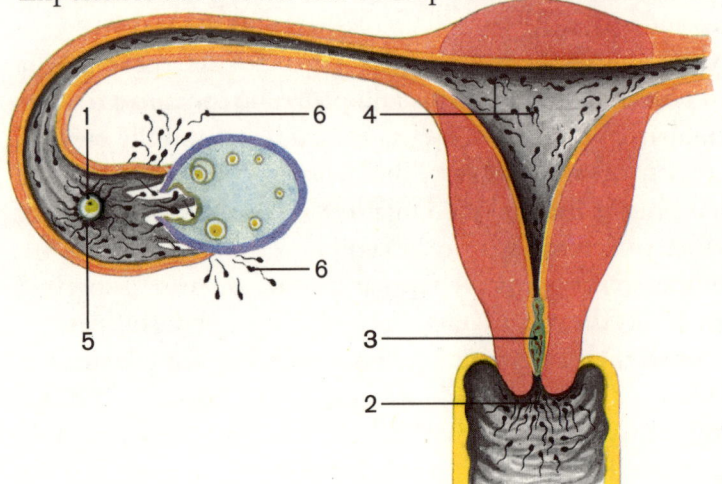

FIG. 41 *Insemination.*

1 *Ovum in funnel-shaped end of tube*
2 *Spermatozoa just outside os*
3 *Spermatozoa in mucus plug*
4 *Spermatozoa sorting themselves out for entry into tubes*
5 *Spermatozoa meeting the ovum*
6 *Spermatozoa issuing from tube into peritoneal cavity*

13 days before the next menstrual period. If only the length of survival of the germ cells were taken into account, this period would be much shorter.

The spermatozoa after deposition outside the cervix remain fertile for at most 2 complete days or 48 hours. Thus they may find themselves in the tube two days after intercourse and there meet an ovum which is just leaving the ovary. Provided they are still alive, they may lie in wait for an ovum just about to leave.

If the ovum is not fertilized it will die a few hours after leaving the ovary. The favourable time for conception amounts to only about 2 to $2\frac{1}{2}$ days. However, the time of ovulation cannot be determined accurately beforehand and may be influenced by many factors. The follicle may rupture earlier under a variety of stimuli—intense sexual excitement, direct stimulation of the cervix during intercourse and especially frequent intercourse within a short period or an increase in secretion of gonadotropic hormone from the pituitary due to intense emotional and sexual stimulation. There is thus a possibility that a fertilizable ovum may leave the ovary at a time when it would not have done so without these stimuli. Equally well, maturation of a follicle in the ovary and its rupture may be delayed, for reasons not sufficiently known.

In practice, it has been found that conception may take place at any time between two menstrual periods. However, with a regular menstrual cycle there is only slight probability that conception will occur during menstruation and in the week before the period is expected. The probability of conception after intercourse is greatest 22 to 13 days before the next period. For calculation of the time of the next period, see p. 178 ff.

Although in general it is true that when menstruation ceases pregnancy is no longer possible because no more ova mature, pregnancy has been known to occur after the menopause. The record is so far held by a woman of 63, who had her seventh child after a gap of thirteen years, and some eleven years after the menopause. Another 59-year-old gave birth to her first child nine years after her last period.

Statistics from several big cities and countries show that the probability, or in other words the risk, that a woman over 50 years old will become pregnant is extremely small. According to a variety of statistics, it lies between 1·75 and 79 per million live births. Because women in the first year of their menopause predominate in these figures, it is suggested that the usual contraceptive measures be continued for one year after the last menstrual period. Obviously it is impossible to calculate fertile days during this year.

The Bases of Contraception

Responsibility and sexual intercourse
Sexual intercourse should be based on a sense of responsibility to God, the partner and the

children; because of this, consciously practised contraception is included among the intimate relations of husband and wife. It is therefore necessary for both husband and wife to inform themselves properly about the means available, and to reach a mutual decision on this point. One of the unavoidable responsibilities of married couples today, lying beyond desire, love of pleasure and convenience, is to plan their parenthood on humane, social, economic and financial bases, and with due consideration to the circumstances of the couple, the upbringing of the children and the ability to support a family.

Responsibility for children begins with the choice of partner, for this decides the environment into which children will be born. It also decides what kind of a home will be offered to children and to what extent the father and mother can provide an appropriate and secure milieu. Children born before marriage often upset the latter not only financially but also emotionally, so that the child not uncommonly finds itself in an environment which has undergone disruption on its account. Apart from this, husband and wife after marriage need some time to accustom themselves to each other, and too early a birth may disturb this. The child needs an intact marriage for its well-being, and it is wrong to imagine that a child can heal the rift in a marriage. For this reason experienced marriage counsellors always recommend that the first child should be born two years after marriage if possible. The most favourable interval between children for both mother and children is about two years. The number of children born to a couple should depend both on their social circumstances and their state of health and emotional state.

Abortion and sterilization

Since a new life begins with the fusion of ovum and spermatozoon, contraception implies prevention of this fusion for as long as the couple feel unable to take responsibility for parenthood of the first child or other children.

Killing an existing new human being (abortion) as a method of family planning cannot be justified ethically and is also not without risk to the physical and mental health of the mother. The introduction into the uterus of devices (IUCD, see p. 185) and the use of tablets after intercourse, designed to destroy the uterine bed before the ovum gets into the uterus, probably produce continuous abortion. We should also reject definitive organic prevention of the encounter of sperm and ovum (sterilization) because it makes almost impossible any later desired pregnancy.

According to Protestant thinking, the *medical indications for abortion or sterilization* are justified only if there is a present or future risk of substantial damage to the physical or mental health of the woman and there are no other medical means of dealing with this, or if the means available are insufficient to make her cure probable. Since medicine should deal with the whole person, not only physical disease and hereditary disorders should be considered but also all the personal and social circumstances of the woman, her marriage and her family in coming to a decision. In the Catholic view, of course, such medical indications are inadmissible.

Social disorders can be combated just as little by abortion as by sterilization. This is true not only for the individual marriage and family but also in greater measure for society. Social disorders and grievances must be overcome by other methods than these.

The concept of 'responsible marriage and parenthood' includes:

1. *Responsibility for marriage.* This begins with choice of partner and continues with an appropriate preparation for marriage as the basis for a favourable atmosphere in the home into which the child will be born and in which it will grow up.
2. *Responsibility for securing parental care for the child.* This includes the maintenance in both parents of vitality and capacity for love, with due respect for the individual physical and mental capacities of the parents. It also includes the assurance that the child will receive the attention it needs from its mother (not its aunts or its grandmother) during the first six years of its life, and especially the first two years. Husband and wife must already have found fulfilment in their marriage before they are in an emotional state to receive one or more children into their circle. Otherwise, there is a risk that the child may be used as a substitute for this fulfilment, or regarded as a nuisance and therefore impeded in its development. For this reason, the time of the first conception and the intervals between babies should be chosen voluntarily and with responsibility.
3. *Responsibility for personal and social development of the child* in accordance with the prevailing cultural norms and degree of civilization of the society. This signifies responsibilities to the individual child and also as regards the number of children.
4. *Responsibility for assuring the necessary means of satisfying the legitimate social demands* of the couple.
5. *Responsibility for development of the personality of the child,* for its education and guidance on the way to maturity.

Responsible parenthood with voluntary family planning is ethically justified. A decision about the necessary methods and measures to regulate conception must always be in the hands of the partners themselves. All methods demand of both partners a conscientious application of the rules. This is possible only when both partners study the matter, discuss it together and take joint responsibility. They must behave chastely to each other, in that each abstains from making the other the object of his or her will. Chastity is not related to the life style and behaviour of one individual, but refers to the partnership. Chastity is no virtue in itself but only in a relationship. It is a part of chastity for the partners to talk about their intimacies, to decide together on the methods of family planning and to collaborate in their conscientious application.

The doctor or family planning clinic should be available to advise on suitable methods. The doctor's task in practice and in marriage counselling with regard to contraception includes reminding the couple of their responsibilities and helping them to work through their inhibitions and conflicts. The actual technical advice, recommendation or prescription of methods, and supervision of their effects is only secondary; without a general assumption of their responsibilities and without a wholehearted acceptance of the need for family planning, all these methods will fail, even if many of them appear safe in theory.

Methods of Family Planning

Abstention from intercourse

Abstention from intercourse is obviously the safest method of avoiding conception. In many marriages there are times at which, with mutual consent and respect, abstention is employed not only as a necessity, for example five weeks before and five weeks after a delivery, in illness or absence of a partner, but also as a means of strengthening the inner bonds of marriage. However, abstention cannot be recommended or justified as the sole method of family planning, because it prevents the union of husband and wife for prolonged periods and hinders that intimacy in marriage which is an end in itself. Abstention as a means of contraception disturbs a marriage, because it must be employed continuously for long periods, even for years. Intellectual workers may succeed in sublimating or transferring their sexual drives into mental energies and performance, but this is a road open to few. One should not lightly consider oneself an exception among men. The demand for abstention often slights the other partner. Such a demand is unchaste because it reduces the other partner to an object of one's decision for inaction. Thus abstinence from intercourse cannot be regarded as a contraceptive method of greater merit than others; on the contrary, it is problematical whether it is as good, for it is ethically inconsistent.

The safe period

The safe period, based on calculation of the fertile and infertile days in a marriage, requires exact calculation. Not only must the menstrual cycle of the wife be taken into account (see p. 127) but also the viability of the husband's spermatozoa (see p. 174). For these reasons, and since the wife cannot be fertilized without semen, it is better to talk about the safe period of the marriage rather than of the wife. The calculations must be respected by both partners, and are made as follows: from the menstrual calendar of the last twelve months, the shortest (s) and the longest (L) cycles are abstracted and inserted in the formula: $(s-22)-(L-13)$. The figures so obtained cover those days in the cycle within which the probability of conception is greatest. This formula takes account of the so-called safe days, but it must be emphasized again that it offers no absolute guarantee. For example: Shortest (s) and longest (L) cycles in the last 12 months.

Mrs A., aged 24: s = 21 days, L = 26 days
(s − 22) = 21 − 22, i.e. less than zero
(L − 13) = 26 − 13 = 13

This means that for Mrs A. from the first day after menstruation begins until the thirteenth day of the cycle, there is a greater probability of conception than on other days of the cycle.

Mrs B., aged 38: s = 26 days, L = 32 days
(s − 22) = 26 − 22 = 4
(L − 13) = 32 − 13 = 19

For Mrs B. from the fourth day after menstruation begins until the nineteenth day of the cycle, there is a greater probability of conception than on other days of the cycle.

It is therefore clear that any pronouncement about the possible fertile days of a woman and her marriage must be based on her own dates and not on those of any other woman. It would be erroneous to base such calculations on an 'average' length of cycle derived from statistics. Anyone who relies on these will soon discover this fact, often confirmed in the practice of marriage counselling. The important prerequisite for calculation of fertile days is regular, continued and conscientious keeping of a menstrual diary (see fig. 30). Calculation must be based on the observations and entries for the previous 12 months. This is emphasized in the section on menstruation.

It might be added that maturation of the ovum is exposed to psychological influences via a regulating centre in the hypothalamus (see fig. 32). Ovulation may be either expedited or delayed by joy, for example at a reunion with a loved partner after long separation, so that fertilization becomes possible outside the previously calculated days (see p. 175). Similarly, delay may be due to fear (for example, of pregnancy after rape or in an alarming situation such as a general upheaval in society), with complete suppression of ovulation (and of menstruation, maybe for years). Other mental stresses or changes in emotional atmosphere may cause considerable and irregular deviation in ovulation and hence uncertainty in calculation (trips, severe illnesses, accidents, operations, or admission to communal dwelling places or institutes), especially if the situation makes personal privacy impossible. Every delivery is also followed for a while by very irregular menstrual cycles. Breast-feeding itself offers no guarantee of safety from conception, even if it is accompanied by no menstrual periods. In practice, conception is possible almost immediately after a delivery.

Calculation is also rendered difficult if not impossible in the climacteric with its frequently irregular variations in menstruation (for pregnancy after the climacteric, see p. 175). However, as long as menstruation continues a woman can become pregnant. It must also be recalled that in the early years after the onset of menstruation (menarche) irregular cycles are common enough to hamper exact calculation. During a woman's reproductive life her ovulation time may also vary and affect the length of her cycle. All this shows that the reasonably exact calculation of infertile days is possible only with an orderly marriage free from mental stress, provided that the wife is not too young or too old and has no obvious irregularities of her menstrual cycle due to other causes. Because cycles are indeed often irregular, the method is of limited value in practice.

Another drawback is that this method often demands abstention from intercourse precisely on the days when many women feel their greatest need and their greatest readiness for sexual intimacy; moreover, it calls for periodic abstinence and compels both partners to undergo considerable limitation on their needs for marital union.

Basal temperature measurement

This method (see p. 132 ff.) depends on the fact that one to two days after ovulation a woman's body temperature rises, though by only a few tenths of a degree. Basal temperature is measured as follows. Every morning, immediately after awaking and while still lying quietly in bed before eating or drinking, the woman must take her body temperature for five minutes (with the thermometer in the mouth or rectum; axillary temperature is unreliable), and plot it on a special chart which she can construct herself. (Temperature measured after prolonged rest without bodily activity or digestive activity is known as the basal temperature.) The curve of basal temperature in ideal cases is described on page 132.

If the chart is to be used for contraception, the essential point is to establish the rise in temperature one or two days after ovulation. Since the ovum can live only for one day, there is no further possibility of conception when the temperature has risen.

This method seems at first glance attractive, but there are many cases, if not a majority, in which a chart showing a sudden rise in temperature cannot be plotted in spite of careful measurements. This does not mean that ovulation has not taken place. In about 10% of women the curve is individual and irregular because of some personal peculiarity, and therefore of no use for this purpose. Moreover, it may change because of mental stress, disorder, disturbance, or illness, and may be affected by quite simple infections such as a cold, a septic finger (even if the latter is painless), a tooth infection or mild neck pain, i.e. by minimal illness for which one normally does not take one's temperature or go to a doctor. Basal temperature may also rise after major physical exertion, such as a climbing holiday or a spring clean. Since every woman is exposed to infections and exertions such as these, the method is fairly unreliable in practice. If it is to be used, the method demands a certain expenditure of time each day, year in year out, and therefore has disadvantages even for a responsible household. Will the children be contented if mother does not appear at once when they feel poorly? Or will mother allow herself five minutes extra in bed if the telephone or doorbell rings, or if she has overslept, or she simply wants to leap out of bed for pure joy on a nice day? The possibilities of interference with conscientious temperature-taking (essential if the method is to be even approximately reliable) are too numerous, whether objective or subjective, for it to have won many adherents. Marriages in which everything is carefully arranged, particularly those between obsessional partners, are probably best suited to this technique.

In spite of all their limitations the two methods discussed above have one advantage. With both there is a period before the next menstruation in which intercourse can be indulged in freely without use of any other measures. This is the reason why these 'safe period' techniques have obtained a slow but steady increase in followers from various classes of society. We will return to discussion of a combined technique later.

Petting

In circles where marriage must be postponed for social and educational reasons (see p.140 ff.) the practice of petting, not because of moral objections to direct premarital intercourse but because of fear of premarital pregnancy, carries the danger that it will be continued after marriage as a method of contraception, especially in younger people who have practised it for fairly long periods before marriage. The practice is more likely if the couple object to other methods. It has obvious disadvantages, for it prevents maturation in lovemaking in general and it is relatively unsafe. I have encountered several cases in which a virgin has unintentionally become pregnant through insemination by the hand during petting. Hence petting, even if it relieves sexual tension, cannot be recommended as a method of contraception in marriage, on account of its uncertainty as well as on psychological grounds.

Interrupted sexual intercourse

Interruption of intercourse, technically called coitus interruptus, is a widespread method of contraception. The husband concentrates his attention on his impending orgasm, so that he can at the decisive point, not too soon and not too late, withdraw his penis from the vagina and empty his semen outside the female genitals.

Reliability is not very great (failure rate up to 60%), for a little semen with a few spermatozoa may be unconsciously expelled early in intercourse. Moreover if after interruption the semen is not ejaculated far enough from the vaginal entrance, but near it or directly in front of the opening, sufficient spermatozoa may get into the vagina and the uterus to reach the ovum. In practice this is not really an interrupted but rather an unfinished type of intercourse (coitus abruptus), since there can be no reunion after ejaculation because the penile swelling subsides.

It is no particular credit to the husband if he denies his wife that part of intercourse in which she can share physically, at the acme of male excitement and experience, the joy of being fulfilled, both in the literal and metaphorical senses. In many cases, or even in a majority, the husband cannot contain his orgasm until his wife has also had hers. He is of course frequently exhorted to try to hold back until his wife has been satisfied, or at least if he cannot hold out that long to use his hand to bring his wife to orgasm.

In any case, rupture of intimate contact is always a shock to the wife which sets her excitement back; after ejaculation the husband is not in any mood to carry out intensive petting, and may even find it annoying that his wife is so slow to achieve orgasm. Usually a man is able to take part in delicate love play only if he wants intercourse as well and has not reached his own orgasm. Love play after ejaculation will be less sophisticated, rougher and only undertaken as an obligation; many women experience such activities as a nuisance rather than a delight after so short an intimate contact.

If coitus interruptus or abruptus is constantly used as the sole method of family planning, friction in a marriage is common. A woman cannot love if not fulfilled. She avoids intercourse and substitutes the household mending. Her built-up tension shows itself by day as irritation, or else she is always tired. The husband, who has had his tension relieved, cannot understand her; she finds his advances a torment, and he does not know why. If husbands who complain that their wives are uninterested in sex or reject it only realized that their own behaviour has often contributed, they would abandon the method and show more understanding for their partner. Incidentally, husbands may also find continued coitus interruptus emotionally disturbing.

Carezza
Carezza refers to the prolongation of coitus, even up to hours, without a male orgasm; after a while, perhaps a couple of hours, excitement subsides through exhaustion and the penis becomes soft. The woman does not have a really full orgasm with its sensation of temporary death, but a series of minor orgasms punctuating a persistently high level of excitement. The technique arose as a form of so-called higher erotic art, with emphasis on the erotic (magnetic) heightening of union rather than on release of tension through orgasm. Connoisseurs of the technique always stress that the subsequent feeling of exhaustion is much less than with 'normal' intercourse. Carezza, also known as the magnetic method, does not appear to cause emotional disturbances. From the standpoint of Christian ethics, the method is dubious if it leads to a sort of religious cult.

In one sect the method has been used with success for contraception, but it cannot be recommended for this purpose; the unreliability is related as in coitus interruptus to the possibility of failure on the part of the husband (especially if he is inexperienced) and that of unconsciously depositing semen during the act.

Other unsuitable methods
Unreliability is also the hallmark of some other methods, briefly mentioned below. They must be discussed because they are used in a desperate attempt to achieve safety by the ignorant who fear other techniques, and may be irresponsibly propagated, sometimes secretly by word of mouth.

'Spanish intercourse' means deposition of semen in the outer part of the vagina with subsequent douching; this is both unsafe and inconvenient (see p. 186 on douching). In another technique the wife is supposed to squeeze the hind end of the penis with her hands at an appropriate time to make the semen flow backwards into the man's urinary bladder. This technique is not only painful but also unsafe. The various positions adopted for intercourse are of minor importance for contraception. In some positions the semen is deposited only in the lower part of the vagina or into a vagina sloping downwards so that outflow is assisted. None of these methods is at all safe, and it would be irresponsible to recommend the use of a particular position as a method of contraception.

At best, certain positions may be recommended for the reverse purpose, if a wife has difficulty in conceiving and wants children. For this aim, all positions are suitable in which the top of the vagina and the uterus lie lower than the vulva, so that after orgasm the semen gravitates towards the cervical os. The best thing is for the woman to lie on her back with her pelvis raised by a cushion underneath.

The Apparatus of Contraception

The condom or sheath
The modern condom is made out of heat-vulcanized thin rubber and covers the erect penis down to its root (tips or caps which only cover the glans are not recommended since they are liable to slip). Before putting on a condom the foreskin should be peeled back. At the tip of the penis a space of half an inch or so should be left, to take up the semen, otherwise the condom may tear here. It must be remembered that after ejaculation the penis goes soft relatively quickly and no longer fills the condom. If therefore the husband keeps his penis in the vagina for a while, semen may trickle out between sheath and penis. As a result, fertile spermatozoa may enter the vagina and reach the uterus long after intercourse is over.

Most modern condoms are now provided with a lubricant powder which inside the vagina forms a thin mucous layer and makes it unnecessary to wet the sheath. It may occasionally be necessary to reduce friction between the penis and a rather dry vagina by using an extra lubricant. For this purpose, the industry now provides 'moist' condoms in various styles. Condoms made by firms with a reputation for conscientious work represent the safest contraceptive means, provided the instructions are followed and the rubber is not allowed to become brittle through long or inappropriate storage. In contrast to popular opinion, a sheath does not reduce sensitivity appreciably, provided not too much lubricant is used.

Special 'stimulating' condoms should also be mentioned, whose outer surface is modified to produce greater stimulation of the female genitals. These are either scaly or fitted with harder bits of rubber in the form of a ring or comb, or with softer hollow protrusions in the form of fingers or combs. The idea is to increase stimulation of the clitoris, labia or posterior wall of the vagina, depending on the site of the elevations, and thus bring the woman to an earlier orgasm. Many (if not a majority of) women regard the use of such condoms as a personal insult, for they suggest that the husband is not satisfied with his wife's responses. As with other stimuli to skin and mucous membranes, such as application of heat or drinking hot liquids, the body acquires tolerance to extraordinary stimulation, so that the desired effect of employing these condoms may be defeated by habit formation. Their use also means a sacrifice of sensitivity for the man, since they tend to be thicker and thus to transmit stimuli less easily.

We have seen that genital excitability in both man and woman is not only closely related to emotional capacity for love and readiness for giving, but indeed directly dependent on them. Hence, greater stimulation of the woman can scarcely be attained by mechanical means; in a healthy marriage it requires intensive application on the part of the husband, and in cases where capacity for love has been pathologically disturbed some suitable psychotherapy. One might add that many women do not find these special condoms stimulating but downright painful. Their employment cannot be recommended either for their original purpose or for contraception. They should not be condemned however as 'unnatural', for the intention to help the wife to orgasm is laudable even if the means are inappropriate.

The pessary
Solid pessaries are worn by the woman to prevent entry of spermatozoa into the uterus. Advice, examination and instruction from a gynaecologist are needed, while the wearer must be examined at intervals determined by her doctor. This is because the wearer cannot really tell whether her pessary is correctly sited and of the right size, or whether it is causing undesirable pressure or other rarer changes in the vagina and cervix. The woman must be shown by her doctor how to insert the pessary, how to take it out and how to clean it. Most wearers of pessaries need a medical check up after every menstrual period, but this appears to us the lesser evil in face of undesired pregnancies or attempts at abortion, especially if the husband is careless and has no sympathy with his wife.

Although some pessaries afford a great deal of security if correctly employed, they are much less popular than sheaths, because most women, young or old, dislike having their genitals touched and examined by strangers. Others are of course unaware of the possibility of using this method. In family planning clinics pessaries are usually prescribed only if husband or wife rejects the condom and is unwilling to try other methods.

The general term 'pessary' includes a number of different articles offering different degrees of security from pregnancy. Before describing them, we should repeat that whenever a mechanical device is used by the wife its use must be supervised by the doctor.

Caps
These are usually made of plastic, and fit over that part of the cervix which protrudes into the vagina (the portio), remaining in place by mechanical suction or adhesion. Obviously they can remain from one menstrual period to the next only if there is no vaginal discharge.

Diaphragms
These consist of a thin layer of rubber stretched across the vagina by means of a spring ring (usually made of rubber-covered annular spiral springs) and separating the greater and anterior part of the vagina from a small posterior part, closed off to prevent entry of spermatozoa into the uterus. Before the diaphragm is removed, which should be about 6 to 8 hours after intercourse and not earlier, the vagina may be douched out to remove any semen if a spermicidal jelly has not been used (see p. 186). For douching, the apparatus must not deliver fluid at a greater pressure than a height of two feet of water (length of the tube from an irrigator hung up above the woman), otherwise water or douche fluid may get into the uterus and thence into the fallopian tubes and peritoneal cavity, where it may set up highly dangerous inflammation. A doctor should prescribe the apparatus to be used and the composition of the douche fluid. (The old-fashioned vaginal douche with a cuff to close off the cavity is unsuitable and dangerous.)

Unsuitable, unsafe and dangerous means
Because of official reticence over these things and their propagation by highly effective whispering campaigns, these techniques deserve a mention here.

Intrauterine pessaries are mechanical agents partly or totally introduced into the uterus or cervix. They used to be made of plastic, silk or metal (sometimes precious metals) and they were condemned by leading gynaecologists in the 1930's. One danger is of causing an ascending infection with subsequent adhesions within the fallopian tubes (and thus infertility), or even a lethal general infection not responding to modern medical measures.

In recent years a new form of intrauterine pessary has been developed. This is (usually) a plastic ring, loop or spiral introduced into the uterus and commonly known as an intrauterine contraceptive device (IUCD). As far as one can tell from collective experience abroad, such devices do not prevent migration of spermatozoa and therefore conception but mechanically disturb implantation of the fertilized ovum in the uterus, or else interrupt the pregnancy at a very early stage. The apparatus is therefore not a contraceptive one but a means of procuring continuous abortion. It has been stated to cause symptoms in 20 to 44% of cases (menstrual disturbances, cramp, pain, discharge, bleeding, suppuration, fever, injury to the uterine wall, peritoneal infections and so on). In 1 to 4% the method fails, or in other words the woman becomes pregnant in spite of the presence of her device. Some more failures may be due to expulsion of the IUCD with the menstrual flow. Because of the by no means inconsiderable risks, though these are played down by some authors, these modern IUCDs cannot be recommended here.

Vaginal douching alone, even immediately after intercourse, is obviously unsafe since enough spermatozoa may have been taken up into the uterus during the act. Apart from this, douching disturbs the gradual relaxation which should follow orgasm.

Sponges and tampons were known to the ancients, but even if they are soaked in suitable liquids they are unsafe and may have unpleasant side-effects. Lastly, we may summarize by stressing once more the need to get medical advice, especially in cases of doubt and uncertainty.

Chemical agents: tablets, suppositories, jellies, foaming preparations
These have to be used by the woman, and depend for their action on the introduction into the vagina before intercourse of one of a variety of substances killing or paralysing spermatozoa. The substance is distributed in the vagina and penetrates on to the posterior vaginal wall and the cervix. The time before intercourse at which the substance must be introduced varies with its nature. Effectiveness and tolerance depend not only on the chemical compound but also on the way it is used and the sensitivity of the vaginal mucosa. Unfortunately there are no universal standards established for effectiveness, tolerance and harmlessness of these chemical contraceptives, so that married couples will have to obtain advice from their doctor.

Modern preparations are put up as tablets, pessaries, jellies and foaming preparations, and exact instructions are supplied with the packing. All these agents must be introduced as deeply as possible into the vagina.

Tablets dissolve in the normal vaginal moisture with foam formation, but may have to be moistened.

Pessaries distribute their effective substance, after solution due to bodily warmth, as a thin fatty or creamy film over the vagina and cervix.

Jellies permit distribution of the finely divided effective substance in the vagina.

Foaming preparations. The effective substance is rapidly and evenly distributed in a thick white foam over the vault of the vagina and adheres well to the moist mucosa.

Since the material introduced will always be expelled (together with the semen) again, there is increase in discharge from the vagina after intercourse, so that the toilet (washing, use of sanitary towels or tampons to avoid soiling of underwear) must be more careful than usual. The increase in moisture in the vagina when any of the above preparations is used (due to foam, fatty substance, or jelly) will diminish the friction between male and female skin; some couples find this a nuisance because it blunts sensation. Occasional intolerance (for example, burning of the affected mucosae) can be neglected in comparison with the favourable general assessment of these agents. However their effectiveness and safety can be guaranteed only if they are conscientiously used in accordance with instructions. Occasional complaints about their unreliability are usually due to obvious errors of employment.

Combinations of several methods and agents
As we have seen, reliance solely on calculations prevents union of the couple, just at the times between menstrual periods when desire for sexual intercourse is generally greatest. Outside these fertile days in a marriage, there is theoretically no need to use any agent. It is of value therefore to combine careful calculation of the fertile days with the use of another method *only during these days*. If the woman's cycle is regular, calculation is not hard. If there is doubt about the result of the calculation, it is best to refer this at once to a doctor experienced in the method.

Apart from this combination of the safe period with an agent used at other times, it is possible to combine agents to increase safety. If caps or diaphragms are used, it is very advisable to combine them with use of a sperm-killing jelly, and there is then no need to douche; when condoms are used there is generally no need for additional safeguards. A jelly may be used simply as a lubricant, but the small amount so used will not be enough to guarantee contraception.

Because the mechanical pressure of a condom applied by a sexually inexperienced man may lead to such powerful stimulation that he quickly ejaculates (possibly even before introducing his penis into the vagina), this method of contraception is often rejected at the beginning of a marriage. In addition the newly-wed man has to learn how to control his ejaculation until his wife has reached her climax, and he therefore needs to avoid any means of increasing his excitement prematurely. (The necessary experience, with tactful cooperation between the couple, may take up to two years.) For these reasons chemical agents (especially jellies) are often given preference at the beginning of a marriage, since they lower the stimulating friction between penis and vagina and make it easier for the husband to delay his ejaculation. The wife at the beginning of her love life rarely finds the increased moistness of the vagina due to the jelly a hindrance to her excitation. As the marriage progresses and the partners have more experience in their responses to intercourse, it will become easier to use a condom.

Hormones for prevention of ovular maturation
The effect of the contraceptive pill depends on inhibition of maturation of the ovum through hormones, and therefore prevention of ovulation. As a result no ovum gets into the fallopian tube, and the woman is rendered infertile for as long as she takes the pill. The hormone effect of the pills is not due to direct action on the ovary itself but on the pituitary

hormone which regulates ovarian function. Thus previous experience has suggested that a direct injury to the ovaries can be excluded, for during pregnancy much greater doses of hormone than the tablets contain are excreted via the pituitary to prevent any further ovulation. We also know that in the days when many women had one pregnancy after another, and therefore had their ovulation suppressed for most of their fertile life, they suffered no ill-effects. These preparations simply produce a pregnancy-like hormonal situation at a lower level with corresponding effects on ovary and genital mucous membranes.

If the tablets are taken continuously, the woman does not menstruate. The endometrium will swell up in a different manner, and occasionally at irregular intervals break away, with bleeding resembling a menstrual period. This irregularity upsets some women because they believe that regular menstruation is a necessary expression of their health and welfare. Moreover, the appearance of a period on time is a guarantee that they are not pregnant.

For these reasons, the classical pill is taken from the fifth to the twenty-fourth or twenty-fifth day (inclusive) of the menstrual cycle. Two to four days after the drug is stopped, that is around the twenty-sixth to twenty-eighth day of the cycle, there will be a 'withdrawal' bleeding resembling a menstrual period. The loss is usually somewhat less, but occasionally is more than a normal period. The commonest type of pill is used as follows.

The woman waits until a menstrual period. She then counts from the first day of bleeding and starts her tablets on the fifth day, regardless of the length of her period, taking one each evening from then on. This continues for twenty or twenty-one days, according to the number in the packet. If she forgets one evening, she should on the next day take the overdue tablet in the morning and the proper one in the evening, i.e. two on that day. The 20 or 21 tablets in the packet will thus bring her to the twenty-fourth or twenty-fifth day of the cycle. Two to four days later she will have a withdrawal bleeding. The day this begins is counted as the first day of the next cycle, and on the fifth day of this she will start her tablets again. She must realize that 'the pill' is *not* taken just before intercourse; doing this will give her no protection against pregnancy.

When a woman starts on the tablets, she may not bleed on the twenty-sixth or twenty-eighth day. This does not matter if she has taken her tablets regularly. She must simply wait for seven days after taking her last tablet and then start with a new pack, thus imitating the usual interval. If by any chance she is pregnant, and this can only happen if she has been careless with her tablets, there is no need to fear that continued intake of hormone will injure the embryo, for the tablets usually contain the hormones present in even greater doses in the body during a normal pregnancy.

All commercial preparations of these pills are accompanied by exact directions for use, among which is one advising the woman that if she does not have a withdrawal bleeding or experiences any other unusual symptoms, she should consult her doctor. She can make the doctor's task easier if she keeps a careful menstrual calendar. Two contraindications to use of these tablets are the presence of liver damage and the existence of inflamed leg veins or other diseases likely to be associated with thromboses (clots).

Side-effects may include increase in weight and (early in the story) headache, irritability, stomach and bowel disturbances, or tension in the breasts; there is also diminished readiness for intercourse in about 6% of cases and increased readiness in about 38% of cases.

It is still not entirely clear how many of these side-effects are emotionally conditioned. It is possible that an unconscious resistance to the agent may lead to symptoms or enhance existing symptoms. On the other hand, freedom from fear of pregnancy can increase desire for intercourse.

The relationship between hormone secretion and the woman's emotional life has already been mentioned (see p. 133 ff.). If the pill is taken for a long time, there is a decrease in pituitary hormone secretion and thus a decrease in sexual sensibility. The peaks and troughs of a woman's emotional life are also flattened out. The result is a dominance of the basic emotional attitude to sexuality, which may have an adverse effect on the approach to intercourse (see p. 135 ff.).

Disturbances with menstruation-like bleeding are not uncommon in the first months on the pill (in up to 35% of cases). These disorders disappear with persistent use of the tablets (as do side-effects, see above) in most cases; in others the type of tablet may be changed. It is exceptional to find that they continue enough to warrant abandoning this type of contraception.

Tablets are *not recommended* under the age of 21, because the internal sex organs are still developing up to that age; nor in the immediate period after delivery. It is best to wait for two or three normal menstrual periods after a delivery before starting the tablets again.

If two or three normal periods have elapsed after a delivery, suckling the baby is no contraindication; the climacteric is also not a contraindication, for these preparations seem to be of advantage at this time of life as a protection against disorders and irregularities of menstruation. They can also be used temporarily by women who would like more children later on. Experience so far has shown that after the pill is discontinued the rested ovaries seem to work better than usually, so that pregnancy is earlier and easier to achieve.

Injury to the resting ova in the ovaries during prolonged administration of the tablets has not so far been observed; nor would it be expected theoretically, since the effects are not direct on the ovaries but indirect on the pituitary. Because the preparations are reliable if used correctly, there is also no need to worry about possible malformations if an ovum is fertilized. Observation periods are still insufficient for us to say with certainty or with near certainty that there are *no* undesirable late effects. Whether the pill exercises a promoting or an inhibiting effect on specific cancers must remain undecided until we know more about the exact causes of cancer. However, our present knowledge would suggest that the possibility that these agents actually promote cancer is remote.

In summary, present medical research and experience suggest the following. Use of oral hormones for contraception represents a new technique in responsible family planning. At the moment there are limits to their use. These limits will be clarified in the light of further developments and observations, as well as through the development of new preparations with other modes of action and fewer side-effects. However, there will always be some limits to their employment. At present and probably in the future these agents will need medical supervision and prescription.

Development of a pill for men with a direct effect on male germ cells is still in its infancy. This is also true of agents which can be taken by the woman some time after intercourse and still used to prevent pregnancy (see p. 196).

Pregnancy

Responsible sexual intercourse by no means excludes pregnancy. On the contrary, it accepts conception, pregnancy and the birth of a child as an expression of the conjugal will to parenthood. This chapter therefore deals with the physical and emotional processes in pregnancy and labour.

Fertilization and the Early Stages of Embryonal Development

Penetration of the ovum by spermatozoa.
Those spermatozoa which after copulation reach the ovum via the fallopian tube attempt to penetrate it (see fig. 42). This can only happen however when the corona around the ovum has been so far loosened by the secretions of the tubal mucosa that there exists a gap in it, through which the spermatozoa can reach the surface of the ovum proper unhindered.

Out of the 120 to 540 million sperm cells ejaculated, a few reach the ovum, but there is no chemical attraction between the sperm cells and the latter. A few hit their target by chance while other spermatozoa swim past it. Those which do hit the ovum usually stick to it and arrange themselves perpendicularly to its surface. Finally, the whole surface of the ovum is covered with spermatozoa which rotate on their own long axis, move their tails powerfully and regularly, and try to get through the surface by boring and with the aid of a special chemical substance present in their head. The ovum is often rotated on its own axis by their movements. This activity may last for 20 to 30 hours. Finally, a few spermatozoa enter the ovum simultaneously or shortly after one another.

The ovum takes no active part in this process. It shows no preference for any of the candidates nor does it close its walls to the others when the first has entered. The intruders swim with short and spasmodic but less frantic movements through the egg yolk and the rest of the

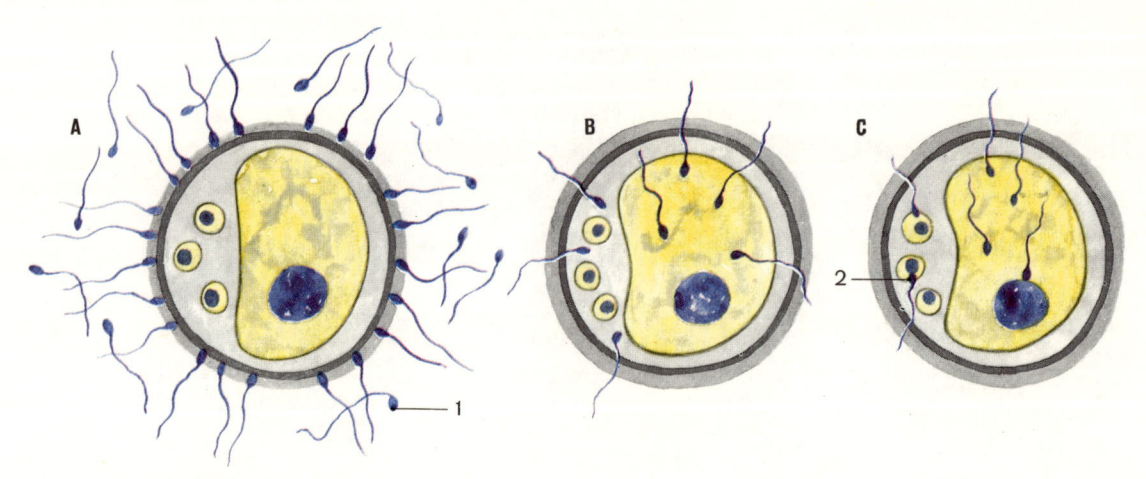

FIG. 42 *Fertilization*.

A Ovum surrounded by spermatozoa seeking entry; other spermatozoa (1) have missed the ovum and are swimming past
B Penetration of several spermatozoa, including tail, into the ovum
C Contact between ovum nucleus and a spermatozoal nucleus; impregnation of a polar body (2)

cell substance and seek out the cell nucleus. Since polar bodies are also present at this time, a spermatozoon may make contact with one of these and fertilize it (a possible cause of a disordered multiple pregnancy or a malformation). Although several sperms may reach the nucleus, only one unites with the latter to fertilize the ovum. The lucky sperm is the first to reach the nucleus.

Union of spermatozoa and ovular nuclei
After one of the spermatozoa has reached the nucleus of the ovum and either come in contact with it or arrived very near it, the nucleus of the male cell (head of cell) assumes a rounded shape almost the same size as the nucleus of the ovum (see figs. 42 and 43). The other sperms within the cell perish. The polar bodies also disintegrate, usually including those which may have achieved fertilization.

First cell division
After about 30 hours the fertilized ovum has already divided once (two-cell stage). Ten to twenty hours later (i.e. after a total of 40 to 50 hours) it has already reached the four-cell stage. At this stage the daughter cells may separate and each may develop independently into a whole individual; in other words, at this early stage of life each cell has an unrestricted capacity for forming an entire body (the cause of uniovular twin pregnancies). This capacity is soon lost, and from then on the cells can form only a part of the body. They have a

specialized role within the body and lose their universality in favour of further specialization 193
or organization.

The peculiarity of being able to separate off at the two to four cell stage seems to be inherent in the ovum and inherited through this, for it has been observed in some families that uniovular twins are relatively common in females (great-grandmother, grandmother, mother, daughter). About 72 hours after the first encounter between spermatozoon and ovum, a cell state of 32 cells has arisen, which looks like a mulberry (hence its Latin name, morula). Division continues with formation of a cavity open on one side and the embryo enters the blastocyst stage (small bladder embryo), starting at about 96 hours after fertilization and ending after about 120 to 140 hours. The cell layer lying nearest the outside will

Fertilization   After 30 hours

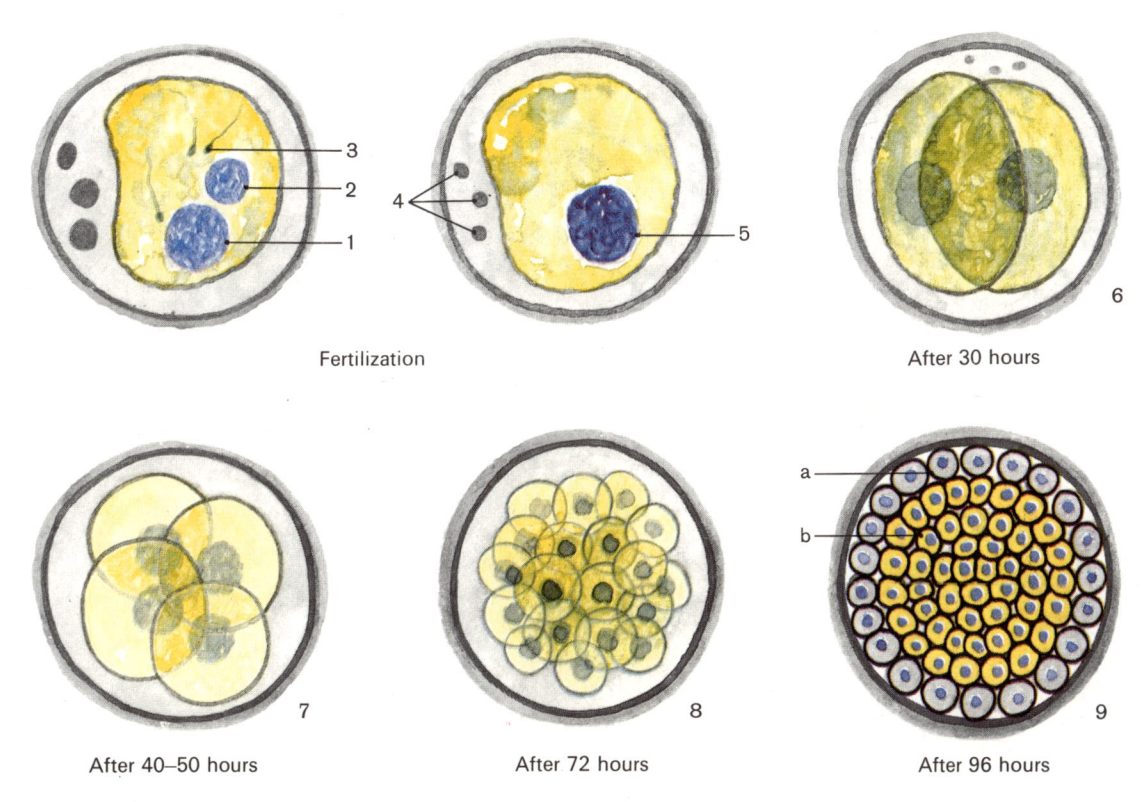

After 40–50 hours   After 72 hours   After 96 hours

FIG. 43 *Fertilization and early cell division.*

1 Nucleus of ovum
2 Swollen nucleus of spermatozoon (sperm head)
3 Other disintegrating spermatozoa
4 Disintegrating polar bodies
5 Fusion of male and female cell nuclei

6 First cell division (two-cell stage—uniovular twins)
7 Four-cell stage (—uniovular quadruplets/triplets)
8 Morula
9 Blastocyst with (a) early embryonic trophoblast (nutritive tissue); (b) remaining embryonic tissue

assume at the somewhat later stage of implantation the role of supplier of nourishment to the embryo. By the time this happens, about 5 or 6 days have gone by and the embryo has not grown in size because it has received no nourishment. Hence, development has taken place entirely within the still intact external cell membrane.

Embedding or implantation of the embryo
While the embryo has been going through the above stages of development, it is being swept towards the uterus by the tubal cilia and the stream of fluid; it arrives in the uterus on the fifth or sixth day as a blastocyst and embeds itself in the mucosa. The endometrium or uterine mucosa, which is full of nutrients, then takes over its task, and is therefore maintained and not shed. The corpus luteum, which has formed in the abandoned bed of the ovum in the ovary, does not disintegrate but grows (at the end of pregnancy it is about the size of the end phalanx of a thumb). It is responsible for seeing that the uterine mucosa fulfils its multiple functions in maintaining the embryo (see fig. 44).

On its arrival in the uterus, the embryo destroys the superficial layer of endometrium and penetrates with its nutritive tissue into the deeper parts of the latter. The preparations undertaken by embryo and endometrium are complementary and harmonize; at and from this moment, the new being begins to acquire its own living space, digging actively into the tissues of the mother and changing them. There can be no doubt that this undifferentiated being already represents a human life even if it cannot maintain its privileges without help and support.

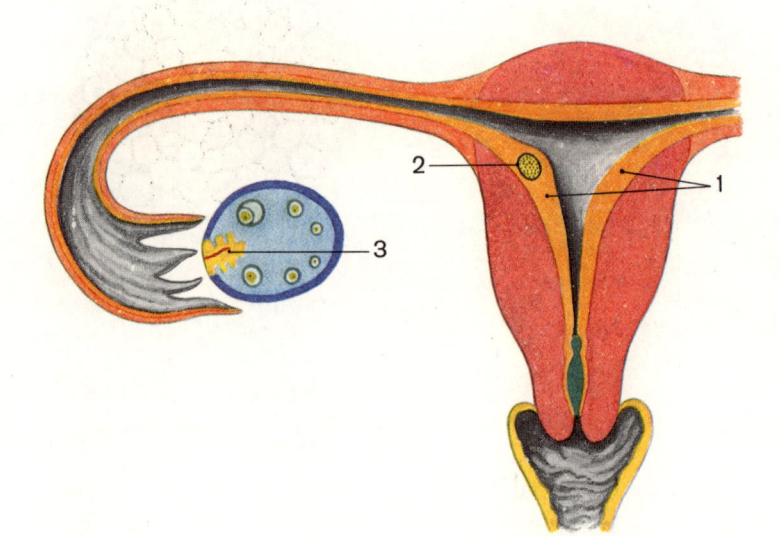

FIG. 44 *Beginning of pregnancy.*

1 Prepared endometrium
2 Implanted embryo
3 Corpus luteum of pregnancy

Ovarian Function and Pregnancy

The corpus luteum or yellow body in the ovary is responsible for the proliferation of nutrient material in the endometrium, intended to maintain the embryo. After implantation of the embryo in the endometrium so prepared, the embryo's own nutritive tissue produces a hormone similar to that made in the pituitary and acting on the corpus luteum. Through this pregnancy hormone, the embryo acts on its maternal organism to ensure that the corpus luteum does not perish (as it does in menstruation) but remains in being. Under its influence, the corpus luteum grows and soon occupies a large part (about one third) of the ovary, so that the latter increases somewhat in size. The increased secretion of luteal hormone ensures that the endometrium does not collapse, but persists, together with the implanted embryo. The next menstrual period does not appear, and the embryo can develop further (see fig. 45).

If the hormone secretions are disturbed, abortion takes place but may be prevented by medical intervention with administration of the appropriate hormone. The very large

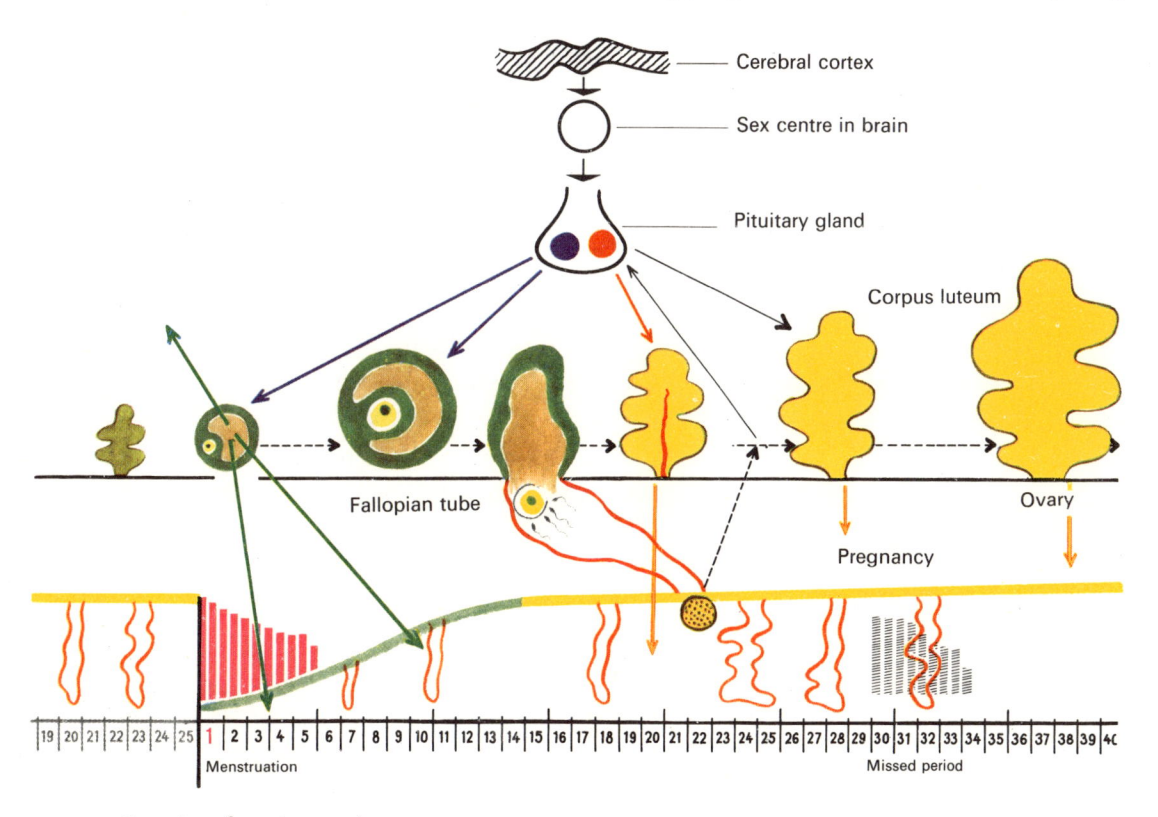

FIG. 45 *Ovarian function and pregnancy.*

amount of pregnancy hormone formed in the nutritive part of the embryo also acts directly on the pituitary gland and indirectly on the increased secretion of corpus luteum hormone, so that no more ova mature and no more fertilizable ova leave the ovary. Hence no new pregnancy can begin during an existing one. It is important to know this, because further sexual intercourse will likely take place at the beginning of a pregnancy, at a time when the couple do not know that the woman is pregnant and perhaps think that menstruation is simply delayed.

Sexual intercourse is possible throughout pregnancy and is in many instances also desired by the wife. These intimacies during a pregnancy do no harm. It is only in the last five weeks before the woman comes to term that intercourse should be avoided, since her tissues are now loosened up in readiness for her delivery, and damage to her pregnancy is then possible.

The effects of pregnancy and corpus luteum hormones on the female body go still further. Both hormones have effects on the maternal tissues and organs such that the latter can undergo the enormous changes due to growth of the foetus and then cope with the mechanism of delivery (see p. 217 ff.).

The excess of pregnancy hormone formed is excreted in the maternal urine and its presence in the latter can be demonstrated. Tests for early recognition of pregnancy depend on this fact. A positive pregnancy test can be obtained as early as 6 to 8 days after conception, and therefore 2 or 3 days after the ovum has been implanted in the endometrium. The test is usually carried out on frogs and reverts to negative eight days after delivery.

Maturation Stages of the Embryo

Seventh to ninth day
The first developmental processes in the human embryo as it lies in the endometrium, with an age of 7 to 11 days (see fig. 46a), are still not clear, for results of studies of early stages in other mammalian embryos cannot be transferred to human embryos with certainty. The embryo wanders for about five days through the tube and implants itself in the endometrium on the sixth day. This process of implantation can be taken as complete when close relations exist between maternal and embryonic organisms for the nutritional supply of the foetus. The nutritive tissue (trophoblast) of the embryo burrows into the cell layers of the endometrium, lays open the blood spaces and begins to take over the supply of nutrients to the embryo.

In certain illnesses or artificially produced changes in the endometrium, the embryo cannot implant itself and its trophoblast cannot function but dies off. This process is the basis of effectiveness of the IUCD (see p. 185) and of some contraceptive tablets taken after intercourse. These techniques for upsetting the maternal bed really cause a very early abortion.

At this point (seventh to ninth days) the embryo shows the following structures: a germ or embryonic disc and two tiny cavities lined with cells, the amniotic cavity and the primary yolk sac. The human body is developed by a complicated process from the germ disc, while the rest of the embryo forms the protective coverings of the foetus and its nutritive and excretory systems in the womb.

After three weeks

Three weeks after conception, development has gone considerably further (fig. 46b). At one point the trophoblast has differentiated itself, sending finger-like processes (villi) into the endometrial tissue and thus increasing and intensifying the surface of exchange between mother and child. Another part has turned into a jelly-like mass, within which the amniotic cavity extends more and more to eventually envelop the whole embryo. One part of the trophoblast remains in close association with the foetus as the body stalk. From this the umbilical cord arises, which is still gelatinous at birth. Clumps of cells also grow out of the trophoblast into the germ disc, so that the human embryo comes to consist of essentially three layers, the ingrowing cells forming the middle of these. Blood vessels also form in the trophoblast; and finally the heart (at first in the shape of a pulsating tube) appears in the middle layer or mesoblast.

A groove forms in the inner layer of the embryo, and begins to close into a tube at either end to form the beginnings of the gut, with a canal into the body stalk along which the blood vessels of the umbilical cord will later develop.

The yolk sac (now related to the primitive gut as the so-called secondary yolk sac) gradually shrinks, for in man it has not the significance which it possesses in birds, in which it is responsible for nourishing the foetus with yolk material. Finally, all that remains of it is a little canal forming a part of the umbilical cord and at last disappearing entirely.

The outer layer of cells thickens to form the forerunner of the central nervous system, at first a flattened plate; the embryo thus rises above its supporting yolk sac (in fig. 46b this is particularly obvious at the head end) and grows well beyond the latter. Because it grows so rapidly and the yolk sac shrinks and fuses with the body stalk, the latter shifts from its early site at the hind end of the embryo and comes to lie on its abdominal side.

Thus in early stages (at the end of the third week of life) the human embryo consists of outer, middle and inner layers of true embryo, covered by an amnion with its cavity containing fluid and by some nutritional tissue, the chorion. Embryo proper and nutritional tissue meet at the body stalk, but everything has originated from cells formed by repeated division of the fertilized ovum. Through displacements, migrations, foldings and formations of fissures or cavities, distinct forms and functions of cell groups can be recognized even this early. At this stage (as we have long known from comparative studies of less organized animals such as sea urchins or lancet fish) the cells are no longer interchangeable. Their

FIG. 46 *Maturation stages of embryo.*

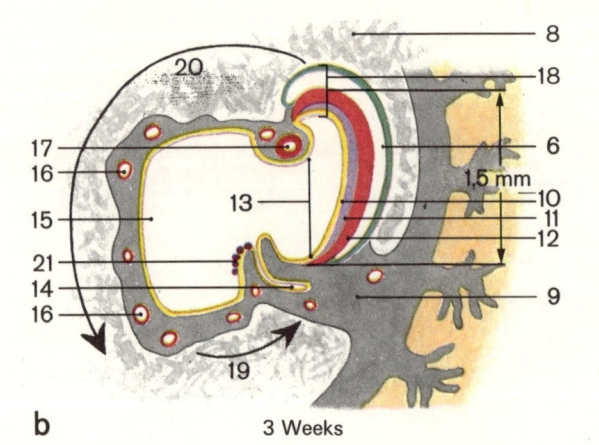

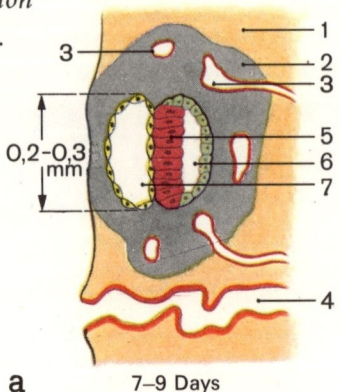

a   7–9 Days

b   3 Weeks

1 *Endometrial surface*
2 *Trophoblast (nutritive tissue) of embryo*
3 *Maternal blood vessels opened up*
4 *Maternal mucosal gland*
5 *Embryonic (germ) disc*
6 *Amniotic cavity*
7 *Primary yolk sac*
8 *Gelatinous mass of nutritive tissue*
9 *Body stalk*
10 *Internal germinal layer (endoderm)*
11 *Middle germinal layer (mesoderm)*
12 *External germinal layer (ectoderm)*
13 *Intestinal groove*
14 *Prolongation of intestinal groove into body stalk*
15 *Secondary yolk sac*
16 *Foetal blood vessels*
17 *Heart*

peculiarities and their position have already destined them for a certain course of development. This lack of interchangeability is notably present at an even earlier stage, and this is certainly true of some cell groups at the end of the fourth day. Hence cells are organized quite early, although we have no idea where the organizer is. It is however clear that at later stages, from about the seventh day on, the organization of one cell group (itself within an undifferentiated larger group) has an organizing effect on neighbouring groups so that the latter become committed to one course and no other. Life, cell multiplication after fertilization and cell organization all follow a remarkable innate blueprint, which will still seem remarkable when research has uncovered all the underlying mechanisms.

All later organs are the result of a complicated interaction and association of individual 'primitive' organizing systems, which in the end combine to form one functional unit.

The following is a somewhat simplified scheme of development of the various organs from the three germinal layers:

External germinal layer (ectoderm): Brain, spinal cord, nervous system, sense organs, skin and accessory organs such as hair, sweat glands and nails.

Middle germinal layer (mesoderm): Bones, tendons, ligaments and joints, blood vascular system, heart and blood, urinary and sex organs.

c 4 Weeks   d 6 Weeks   e 8 Weeks

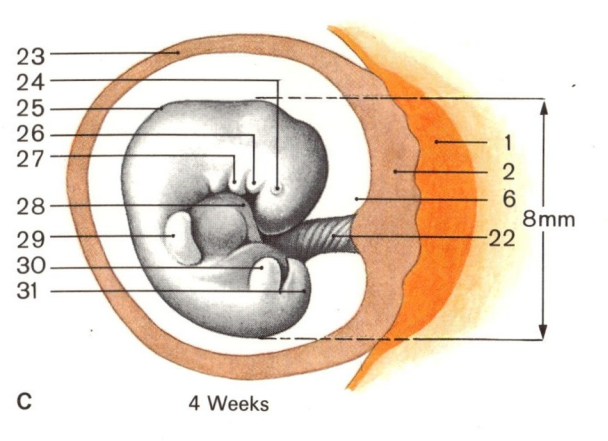

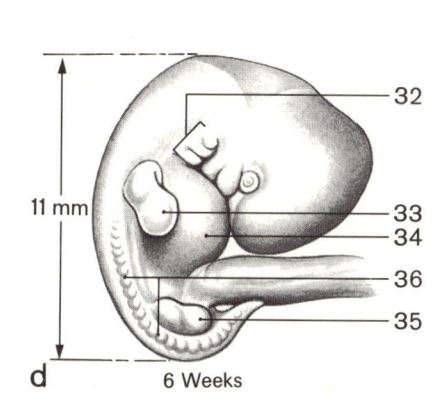

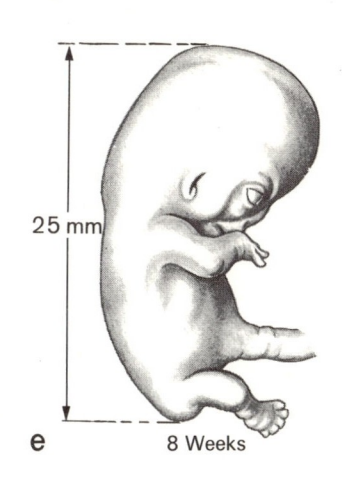

18 Head (cephalic) end
19 Direction of displacement of yolk sac
20 Direction of rotation of embryo on body stalk
21 Primitive germ cells
22 Umbilical cord
23 Amnion and chorion (membranes of embryo)
24 Primitive eye
25 Bend of neck
26 Primitive upper jaw
27 Primitive lower jaw
28 Primitive heart
29 Primitive arm
30 Primitive leg
31 Tail (caudal) end of embryo
32 Primitive ear
33 Hand plate
34 Heart and liver site
35 Foot plate
36 Primitive muscles

Internal germinal layer (endoderm): Organs of digestion and respiration with all their accessories (stomach, intestine, liver, pancreas, respiratory tract, lungs).

The precursors of male and female sex cells pursue a special path of development. They are very early separated off from the other specializing cells and maintained unaltered as germ cells, with the capacity to continue reproduction if united with corresponding cells of the opposite sex. The sex organs serve equally for their storage and multiplication, and they wait in these areas until the body reaches maturity and allows them to perform their task. These primitive germ cells can already be demonstrated in a three-week-old human embryo (between the secondary yolk sac and the appendages of the primitive gut). They migrate into the precursors of the genital glands and can be seen there from the end of the fourth month of pregnancy.

From the fourth to the eighth week

The external appearance of the human embryo depends on the development of its organs and systems, and this in turn is determined by the value of their functions in embryonic life. Those organ systems with a particularly complicated fine structure are most marked at first (see figs. 46c to 46e).

The organs of nutrition are dominant at first, while the embryo proper occupies a less prominent place. The vascular system, with the heart, is already in action by the fourth week of life, first as a yolk sac circulation, later as a circulation in the trophoblast and finally as a body circulation. Behind lie the forerunners of the nervous system, beneath which are those of the skeletal system, while the digestive system lies internally and abdominally. In the body wall, large muscle masses appear near to the primitive nervous system, and these project externally at first.

The appearance of a primitive nervous system, together with the excessive early development of the head in relation to other organs, leads to a marked bend in the back, and a curve in the neck. The huge mass of the primitive brain, together with the eyes, jaws and ears, is prominent. The part of the head containing brain long dominates in size the smaller facial part. The heart develops fast and bulges forward, as does the liver, which is the most important source of blood cells in the embryo (the bone marrow takes over this function only after birth). Both heart and liver cause the abdominal region of the early embryo to protrude and gradually compensate for the curve of the back. Pelvic and tail (caudal) areas are at first backward in development, so that the intestines have no room inside the body and are temporarily housed in the umbilical cord.

The limbs first appear as buds on a 3 to 4 mm. long embryo, the primitive arms somewhat earlier than the legs. These develop into stalks with furrows corresponding to the future elbow and knee and with end-plates for hands and feet, out of which fingers and toes bud off. The limbs at first lie at the sides of the body with their surfaces directed backwards and forwards. As the heart–liver complex grows, the arms rotate into their adult position. Later as pelvic and lower abdominal organs develop, the caudal part of the embryo is taken up into the body and the lower limbs are separated off from the umbilical cord. Meanwhile the umbilicus moves from the hind end of the body towards the middle of the abdomen.

In the third month of embryonic development the first hair appears on the eyebrows. In the fourth to fifth months, a delicate hairy covering is obvious everywhere.

Independent though initially very simple movements of the embryo are possible as early as the second month and become more refined as soon as the muscle masses, which at first lay at the back, grow into the abdominal wall and later into the limbs. At the end of the second month, the embryo already looks like a human being, and this resemblance becomes steadily more marked.

The sex of the child

The sex of the child is determined from the moment of fusion of spermatozoon and ovum. The external genitals of the boy or girl can be distinguished with some certainty from the middle of the third month of pregnancy. People have always been interested in the question whether a pregnant woman is carrying a boy or a girl, and a number of attempts have been made (some verging on superstition) to penetrate this secret, though no result has stood up to statistical examination. It is now possible, by measuring the hormone excretions from the foetus into the liquor amnii (fluid contained in the amniotic cavity), to determine the sex of the child towards the end of a pregnancy. The intervention needed for this (puncture with a needle through the abdominal wall, the uterus and the amnion) is not without risk, so that parents would be well advised to continue to await the delivery to find out whether it is a boy or girl.

Development of the embryo

The size of a human embryo depends on its age, but there are considerable variations, especially at the beginning. Since the moment when life begins (union of spermatozoon and ovum) cannot be accurately assessed in individual cases, it has been agreed to date the embryo in terms of its mother's menstrual cycle, from the first day of the last menstrual period. Pregnancy amounts on an average to 282 days from the first day of the last period, i.e. about ten lunar months, each of 28 days. This figure is about 10 to 18 days too long, because rupture of a follicle takes place between two periods and not when the new menstrual cycle begins.

The table on p. 202 gives an approximate timetable for development of the embryo.

At the turn of the century, the average length of Europeans at birth was about 20 inches, but it has now reached 22 inches in accordance with the general increase in height. The cause is not altogether clear, though it has been suggested that this increase is due to the balanced and varied diet our generation enjoys.

At the end of the second month of pregnancy the average weight of the embryo is a little more than 4 grams (about one eighth of an ounce); by the end of pregnancy it averages 3500 to 4000 grams (approx. $7\frac{1}{2}$ to 9 lb.).

If the speed of growth in length and weight before birth is compared with that afterwards, the enormous rate of development within the uterus will be appreciated. This is clearly shown by the table below. The column 'multiplication factor' shows the factor by which the figure in the preceding column must be multiplied each time to obtain the figure for the next stage of development.

	Length	Multiplication factor	Weight	Multiplication factor
Fertilized ovum	about 0·1 mm.	250	about 2 mg?	2000 (?)
Two month embryo	about 2·5 cm.	20–22	4·5 g.	800
Newborn child	50–55 cm.	3–3·5	3·5–4 kg.	20
Twenty-year-old	165–180 cm.		about 70 kg.	

Age of embryo in days or months of pregnancy	Overall length	Organs Laid down	Organs Functioning
5 days; still in tube	about 0·1 mm.	Nutrient tissue	
6–7 days; implantation			
9 days	0·2–0·3 mm.	Germ disc, amniotic cavity	Nutrient tissue
21 days	1·5 mm.	Intestinal groove	Heart and blood vessels
1 month	about 5 mm.		
31–35 days	about 8 mm.	Eye, upper and lower jaws, limb buds. Beginning lung development	Heart and body circulation, liver
Towards end of 2nd month	25 mm.	Eye, ocular fissure, upper & lower arm, rudimentary hand, elbow, knee, foot, finger, toe; body shape grossly present	First movements in response to external stimuli, i.e. muscle and nerve response
3rd month	9 cm.	Eyebrows, first hair	First gastric juice and urine produced
4th month	16 cm.	Sex organs distinguishable	Movements felt by mother
5th month	25 cm.		
6th month	31 cm.	Ossification of bone centres	
7th month	37 cm.	From 35 cm. the foetus is viable outside the uterus. (Incubator, special care)	
8th month	43 cm.		
9th month	49 cm.		
10th month	55 cm.		

Up to the moment of birth, the fertilized ovum has increased its length 5000 to 5500-fold, and its weight 1·75 to 2 millionfold. This shows what enormous energy must be available to the fertilized ovum, and what a prodigious performance is involved up to birth. Increases in length and weight after birth are in comparison quite small. Small children cannot believe that they have grown so enormously, and if they are shown pictures of themselves as babies cannot believe that they were once so small. (This of course also has some connection with the fact that young children have much less interest in the past than in the future, in comparison with older children and adults.)

Relation between mother and unborn child
The question whether an unborn child has a soul or not, and if so, when it acquires one, has been much discussed. It is of no medical interest and equally fruitless theologically, because with the fusion of sperm and ovum God has created this and no other human life and given it his blessing. The other question, of the human relation between a child and its mother, is psychologically interesting. In the first thirty years of our century it was assumed that these relationships were at first merely exchangeable object relations like reflexes, and that personal relationships arose only at the end of the first three months after birth. We now have an increasing number of studies which suggest that this is wrong, and that entirely personal and irreplaceable relations between child and mother or father can be formed from birth; with premature birth, therefore, these are formed even sooner than with children born at term. The human being lives through his relationships and his dialogue with others; he is approached and responds, not only with words. It might therefore be expected that a baby would from the beginning be able to respond, even if not in the way that adults respond as a result of their sophistication, but in a primitive 'speech' which the mother recognizes and understands.

The relation between mother and child is promoted during pregnancy by her sensation of her child's movements. The child moves as early as the end of the second month of pregnancy, but the mother cannot feel these movements as yet. In her first pregnancy she feels the movements through her abdominal wall during the fifth month. Women who have already borne children can usually detect faint signals about four weeks earlier. The relationship between a child and its unborn brothers and sisters is helped if the mother allows it to place its hand gently on her abdomen and feel the movements of the foetus. An explanation that the child itself was formerly in mother's abdomen and kicked around there helps the child to identify with the newcomer, and also to experience some of this primitive security for itself. The knowledge gives a better understanding of the relations between reproduction and birth, associated with the origin of children, and helps acceptance of the newcomer.

When a mother feels her child's movements, she will choose a name for it, if she has not already done so, with the collaboration of the future father. Frequently the likely names will already have been discussed, considered and perhaps decided upon. Naming the unborn child is not only the outcome of necessary deliberations, since the child must have a name anyway, but also an extraordinarily significant act of human relations. Naming the child means incorporating a hitherto foreign fact into one's personal system of relationships, feelings and thoughts. It contains an acknowledgement which, in addition to other phenomena such as the foetal movements, forms a basis for a relationship and expresses it. With the naming of the child, it becomes a person and enters into a unique personal relationship with others.

Supplying the Foetus with Food

Development of an embryo in the uterus is possible only if its food supply is ensured. Figures 46a and b already show a clear demarcation of the future nutrient tissues or trophoblast from the rest of the embryo. In Figure 46a the former outweighs the rest, and Figure 46b, which is simply a section, demonstrates the enormous development of this nutritive tissue. Bodily development of the embryo can begin only when the tools and the transport agencies for the supply and conveyance of nutrients and building materials, as well as the excretion and removal of wastes, are functioning.

Whereas the fertilized ovum on its way down the tube has been supplied with material from the yolk of its own cell, immediately it has been implanted it begins to take up nutrients from the prepared endometrium and to transfer them from cell to cell. Very soon the first embryonic blood circulation forms for this purpose (see fig. 46b). In the meanwhile, the outer part of the nutritive tissue, supported by new growth of embryonic tissue and blood vessels into the endometrium, makes close contact with the maternal uterine mucosa. It puts forth around the embryo a series of finger-like processes called villi into the maternal tissue; later, most of these will regress leaving active only those on the side of the embryo facing the mucosa (see fig. 47).

When the growing embryo has become so big that it presses the surrounding capsule against the opposite mucosal wall, small amounts of mucosa may break off and cause bleeding, which the woman may take for a menstrual period. A misinterpretation of this nature may lead to a false calculation of the date of delivery.

Placenta

The ingrowth of embryonic tissue into maternal tissue induces the latter in turn to change its structure, until finally a functional unit is created out of both embryonic and maternal tissue which ensures the nutrition of the foetus and the removal of wastes. This functional unit is called the placenta (see fig. 48). The foetus is attached to the placenta by the umbilical cord. Two blood vessels (umbilical arteries) lead from the foetus through the cord to the placenta and divide again and again in that part of the organ formed of embryonic material until the vessels enter the villi as very fine capillary loops. From these capillary loops the blood flows into larger and ever larger vessels and finally through a single vessel (the umbilical vein) into

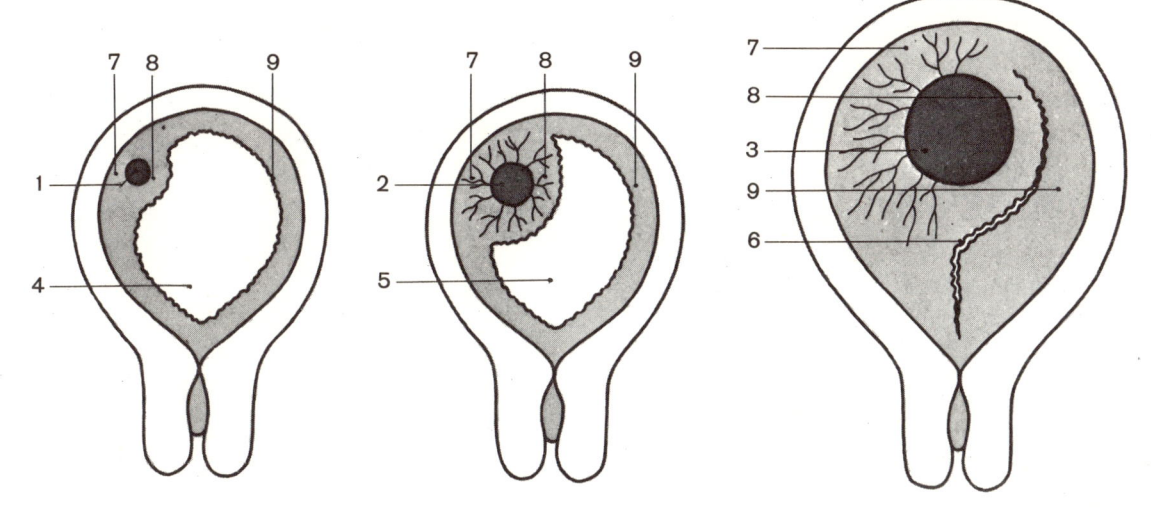

FIG. 47 *Development of nutritive tissue (placental formation) in uterus.*

1 *Completely implanted ovum lying under endometrial surface*
2 *Ovum with nutritive processes (villi) in all directions*
3 *Ovum with villi only on one side*
4 *Uterine cavity*
5 *Remains of uterine cavity*
6 *Cavity of uterus has disappeared*
7 *Basal endometrium*
8 *Capsular endometrium*
9 *Opposite endometrium*

the foetus. The villi dip into very small clefts in which maternal blood flows from a series of vessels. Other maternal vessels carry it away again. The entire placenta is stabilized by maternal septa as well as by adhesion of some embryonic villi to the maternal layer.

Maternal blood never flows into embryonic vessels or vice versa. However, maternal and embryonic blood are separated only by the vessel walls of the embryonic capillaries and a thin membrane covering the villi. This membrane consists of a thin cell layer in which individual cells send a large number of tiny prolongations into the maternal blood. This 'wall' between maternal and foetal blood in the mature placenta (at the end of a pregnancy) is only about 0·002–0·005 mm. thick, and serves for exchange of material between maternal and foetal organisms; exchange is in part governed by chemical and physical laws and in part due to active participation of the membrane itself. Nutrients from the maternal blood (oxygen molecules and units of sugar, protein and fat) cross this cell barrier to enter the foetal blood. Waste residues from the foetus (excretory products such as carbon dioxide molecules, urea, and many others) take the reverse road and are finally excreted through the mother's skin, lungs, kidneys and bowel.

It should be pointed out that transfer of nutrients means provision of building blocks for the foetal body. These are not parts of the maternal organism which the child takes over but

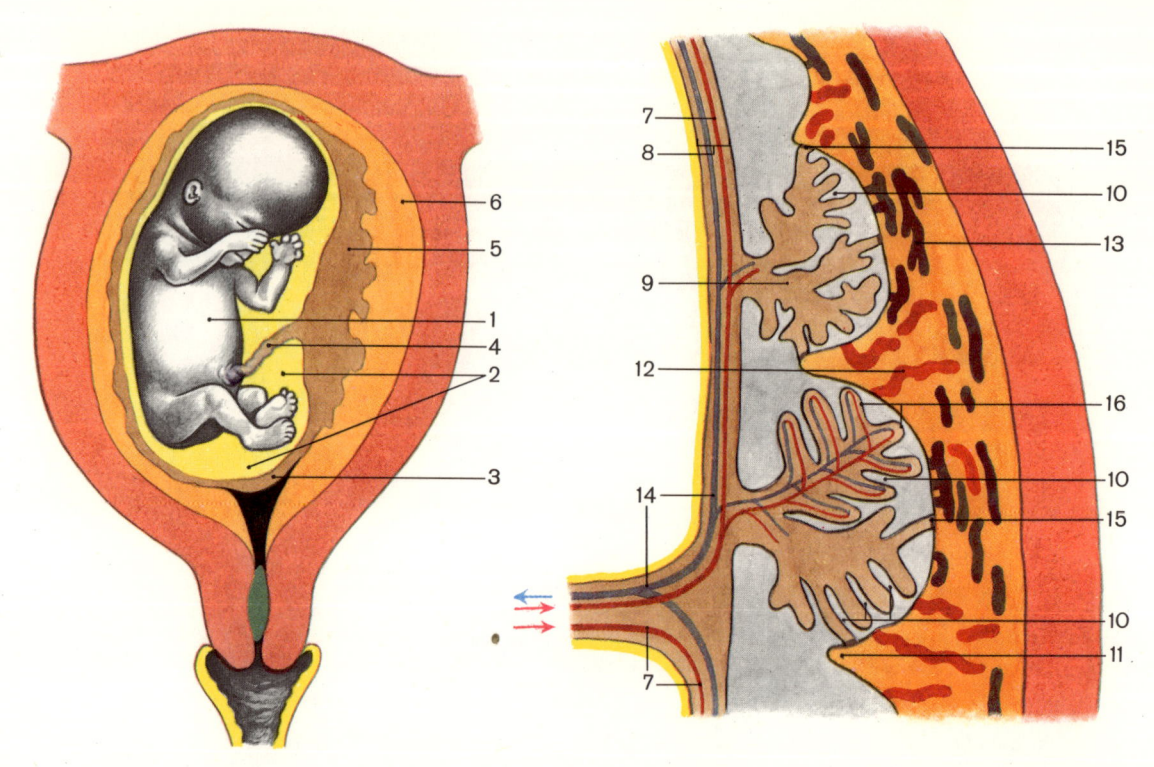

FIG. 48 *Foetal nutrition in the uterus (late stage). The placental barrier is only 2 to 5 micrometres thick.*

1 Embryo
2 Amniotic fluid
3 Amnion
4 Umbilical cord
5 Foetal part of placenta
6 Maternal part of placenta
7 Umbilical arteries (blood flows from foetus to mother carrying metabolic wastes)
8 Foetal capsule of placenta
9 Foetal villi containing blood vessels
10 Spaces containing maternal blood
11 Maternal supporting columns of placenta
12 Maternal arteries carrying maternal blood rich in nutrients to foetus
13 Maternal veins containing maternal blood carrying metabolic wastes from foetus
14 Foetal veins (flowing towards foetal heart with nutrients)
15 Boundary layer at point of contact between foetal and maternal tissue
16 Cell barrier across which exchange of materials between mother and foetus takes place (no blood flows either from mother to foetus or vice versa)

nutrient materials which have been broken down in the mother's organs, finally carried through the mother's bloodstream and transferred to the foetus for use in its own construction, for example, of protein which may differ from the maternal protein. Construction will be determined by the code in the foetal genes inherited from both mother and father, and therefore the end product will of necessity differ from that of the mother alone. If protein groupings occasionally correspond in mother and child, this is because the child has by chance inherited the same genetic formula as the mother.

Other materials also pass through the placenta from mother to child. Drugs given to the mother to relieve pain, or to help her to sleep, also make the foetus in the uterus sleepy. Alcohol and nicotine produce even greater effects on the foetus than on the mother. The organisms of infection and their poisons (toxins) may also be transmitted to the foetus. Not only can these produce the effects we are familiar with in adults but they may also have an adverse effect, especially in the earlier stages of foetal development, on those organs and groups of organs which are then at their most active phase of development. Hence infectious disease in the mother may cause malformation in the child.

An earnest plea must therefore be made for any woman who wants a child and thinks that she has missed a period, or any woman who knows she is pregnant, to abstain from all drugs (hypnotics, pain relievers and so on) unless the doctor specifically prescribes them, as well as from alcohol and tobacco.

The rhesus factor

A question which often arises is that of incompatibility of blood groups between mother and child, together with the possible consequences, treatment or prevention. Incompatibilities between maternal and foetal blood can affect any of the blood groups and factors. These groups and factors include the ABO system, the rhesus factors, the MN and ss systems, the factors P, Fy, Tj and so on. However at the moment, the most significant incompatibilities are those concerned with the rhesus factors, so-called because they were first observed in rhesus monkeys.

FIG. 49 *Simplified hereditary mechanism for rhesus factors.*

1 Hereditary characters of germ cells
2 Fusion of ovum and spermatozoon—pattern of inheritance
3 Properties of new individual

It is usual in cases of d/D inheritance to write Dd

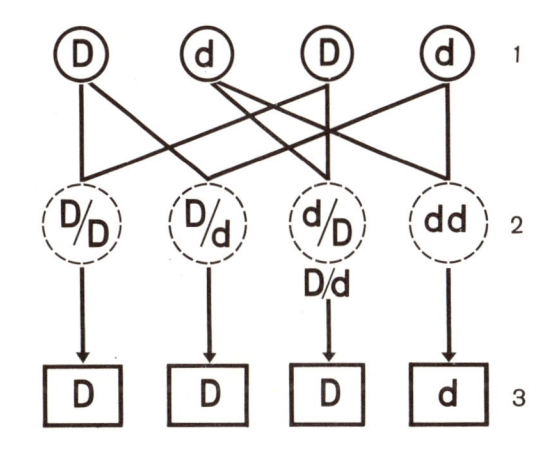

The prerequisite for the appearance of these incompatibilities is the passage of red cells belonging to the child into the maternal circulation, and the passage of maternal substances into the child. Both these can happen, although only to a very small extent; however, this is enough to produce an incompatibility reaction. Some explanation of the inheritance mechanisms and effects on symptoms is necessary. We will limit ourselves to only one of the Rh system factors, the so-called D-d factor, which in practice calls forth the commonest incompatibilities. The D factor was formerly known as the Rh-positive and the d factor as the Rh-negative one.

The blood character D or d is heritable. It is therefore not singly (through either sperm or ovum) determined but doubly so (from both). Thus spermatozoa or ova may have either the character D or d (after maturation divisions, see p. 161 ff. and fig. 39). Through the union of ovum and sperm the following combinations may arise—DD, Dd, dD and dd (see fig. 49). Since the character D is stronger than d, manifestations in the child, i.e. the actual composition of his blood cells, depend on the presence or absence of D. The inherited character d can appear only if D is absent. This means that a person showing the d character must have the formula dd. Persons with a pure inheritance of dd however will form antibodies against the character D (i.e. anti-D antibody), and this is the real cause of the incompatibility.

This is most obvious if there is a blood transfusion in which a person with the d character receives a comparatively small amount (relative to his whole blood volume) of blood with the character D. In such a case, the antibodies (anti-D) will damage the transfused blood, and instead of being a help the transfusion will be the reverse.

In pregnancy, matters are a little more complicated. The situation is only of significance if the mother is pure dd, carrying only the blood character d, and her child carries the D factor. If the child happens also to be dd, there will be no trouble. Nor will there be trouble if the mother is D and the child is dd or Dd, because as noted above, D does not form antibodies against d.

The diagram (fig. 50) shows all the possible and actual combinations and demonstrates how rarely incompatibility occurs in practice in comparison with the theoretical possibilities. Differences in Rh factors are found only in 11 to 13% of all marriages. Incompatibilities between maternal and foetal blood appear only in 2–6 per thousand marriages. This is because trouble arises only in 50% of all theoretically possible children born to a father with Dd and a mother with dd. In the children actually born, the combination leading to incompatibility may not however appear.

Incompatibility of red cells between mother and child does not immediately and directly lead to symptoms. When the foetal red cells carrying the character D enter the mother's (d) circulation, her organism must first learn to make antibodies. This takes a variable time, depending on the extent of the invasion with foetal cells and the individual response of the mother's immune apparatus. When finally antibodies are formed, these can

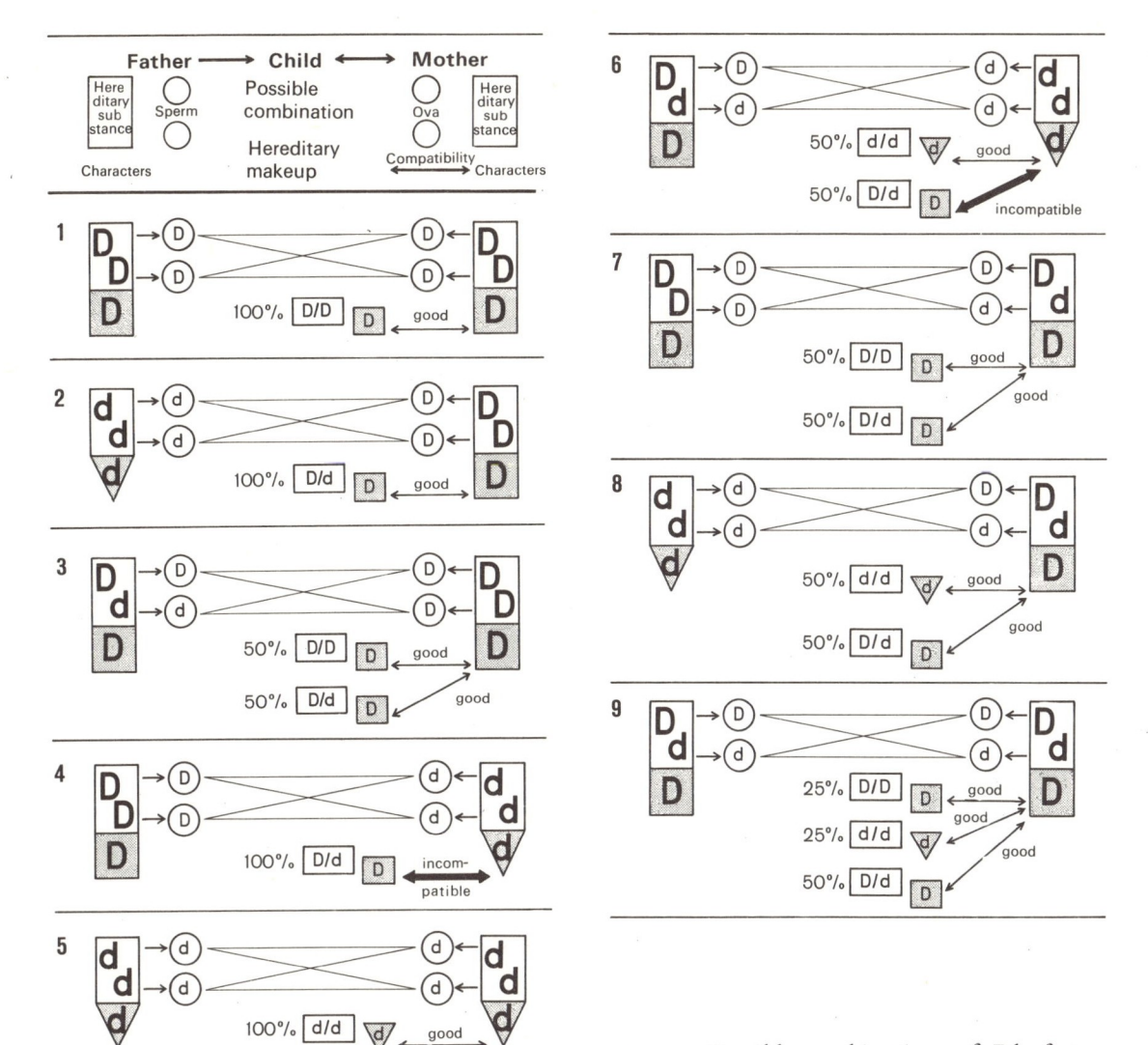

FIG. 50 *Possible combinations of Rh factors.*

of course make the foreign red cells harmless at once, but in order to get into the foetus they have to cross the placental barrier again. The latter varies in its resistance, so that it may be only at the end of a pregnancy that a small quantity of antibody leaks from the mother into the foetus, thus causing minimal damage (see fig. 51).

Example 6 in Figure 50 shows that several normal pregnancies may have preceded such damage, and several normal pregnancies may also follow the abnormal one. In example 4, however, a normal pregnancy is impossible. If a second pregnancy occurs with incom-

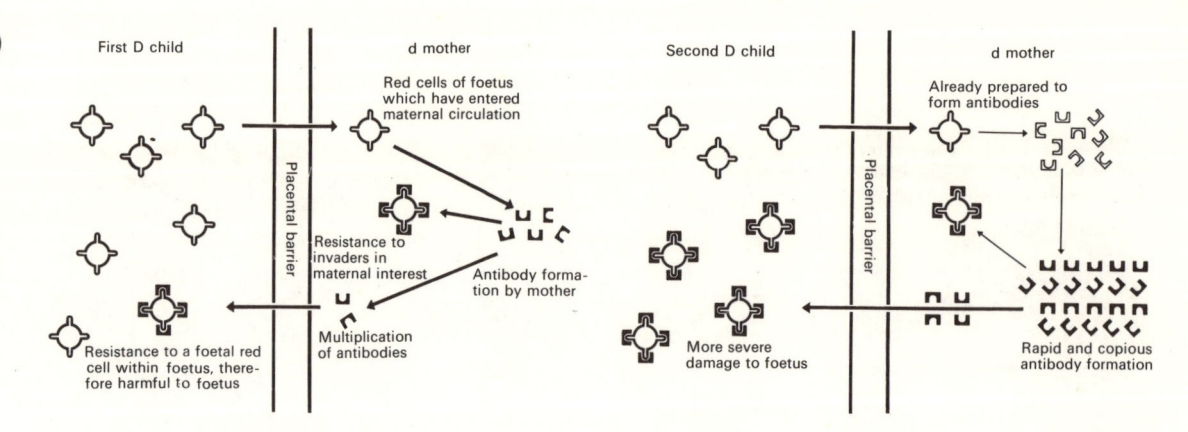

FIG. 51 *First formation of antibodies by mother, causing trivial damage to foetus.*

FIG. 52 *Formation of Rh antibodies by already sensitized mother; more severe damage to foetus.*

patibility of red cells, the maternal organism does not need to learn again how to make antibodies but gets on with the task forthwith. Hence they are made and can migrate into the foetal body much more quickly (see fig. 52). The consequences of damage to foetal red cells from maternal antibodies *may* be:

(a) anaemia of the newborn (in about 10 out of 100 cases of blood group incompatibility);

(b) severe jaundice of the newborn (in about 80 out of 100 cases of incompatibility) with the possibility of injury to the midbrain if treatment is not prompt;

(c) generalized severe swelling (oedema = retention of water) of the child's body, often with death in the uterus and stillbirth or with death a few hours after delivery (in about 5 out of 100 cases of incompatibility).

In cases (a) and (b) a so-called exchange transfusion may help; this means that the damaged blood in the child's body is pumped off a little at a time and replaced little by little with donor blood (of the same group but without the maternal antibodies). Obviously during this exchange there is a constant mixture of new blood and old, so that we have to introduce several times the total blood volume before all the sick foetal blood has been removed.

So that exchange transfusion immediately after the birth of the child can be arranged if needed, it has become customary to determine the blood group and blood factors in every woman who becomes pregnant. If she has the D factor, no further measures are needed, but if she has the d factor her husband must be examined. If he also has the d factor, nothing further needs to be done. Only if he has the D factor will the pregnancy need supervision with delivery in hospital, the child's blood group being determined immediately after birth (or even during delivery). All further steps depend on the outcome of this.

If an Rh incompatibility has already occurred, it may be necessary in some circumstances to interrupt the pregnancy by performing caesarean section between the thirty-seventh and fortieth weeks, and then to undertake immediate exchange transfusion on the child. This is done because the serious damage to the child occurs in the last weeks of pregnancy when the barrier between the maternal placental spaces and the foetal capillaries in the placenta becomes thinner and more permeable.

The suggestion that people in love should have their blood groups determined to see whether they ought to break off their relationship seems to go too far, though Rh incompatibility between a couple may mean a limitation of their family. New techniques will probably make it possible to prevent the harmful effects of an Rh incompatibility in certain (or indeed all) cases, by a procedure resembling protective immunization.

Independence and Dependence of the Foetus

We have shown that, apart from its nutrition in the uterus, the foetus leads a fairly independent life, even if it is dependent on its mother and her organs to a great extent.

False maternal claims
Enough has been said above to refute the statement of the romantic mother that her child 'is her own flesh and blood'. She may not know that she is wrong, but she says this in order to establish unconsciously some claim on the child. There are three possible aspects to such a statement. She may say: 'I must love my own flesh and blood', or 'I can do what I like with my own flesh and blood', or finally 'My own flesh and blood ought not to turn against me'. The first statement represents a defence against the fearful thought that she may in fact reject the child. Such a claim (culturally determined) to have to love the child at any price may be dangerous, because if she has thoughts of rejecting the child she will feel guilty, and since such feelings are as little permitted as those of rejection, they will remain beneath the surface. The consequence is all too often that the child is spoiled as an unconscious act of reparation for having such thoughts. This leads to a conflict when the child really has to be checked. At such a time her dammed-back feelings of rejection may burst through, and she may punish the child excessively and unjustifiably, a fact realized by the victim. If she knows why she has done this, she will then compensate by excessive spoiling. Children who have subconsciously seen through these rules of the game will be quick to take advantage of them when they want to be spoiled. They gladly risk the possibility of severe punishment which their conduct is provoking, for the sake of what comes after. Behaviour of this sort might not have such serious consequences if the emotionally plastic child did not learn a basic pattern of behaviour (great happiness must be preceded by self-induced punishment,

humiliation, suffering) without which it cannot be 'happy' later in life; the greatest happiness for such a child throughout life will lie in receiving personal attention.

In this modern age in which almost every woman works before and early in marriage, only to abandon her job when she is pregnant, these considerations seem significant to me. Giving up a job always means a loss of independence, self-esteem and self-respect, and this cannot be countered by the formula 'instead of that, I will now be a happy mother', even if the pregnancy and a family are desired.

The claim to love the child as one's own flesh and blood goes deeper, for it is really self-love. The child is not loved for itself alone but because it is a part of the mother. Much maternal pride is really pride in oneself. This is the cause for exaggerated affection for the child, and the tragedy is that the child will end up not as a separately developing creature but as part of the mother, and will feel happy only in dependence on her.

The first claim is closely related to the one that a mother can do what she likes with her own flesh and blood, and indeed the second is a consequence of the first. Here again the child remains a dependent but is not stifled in its emotional growth by excessive maternal tenderness; instead, it is openly manipulated, often right up to its adolescence. Even the choice of a profession and a partner may be determined by the mother. If the child tries to free itself from this emotional dependence, it must of necessity find itself running counter to the desires and wishes of its mother. The latter considers such behaviour as a personal insult and tries to bring the child back to order by entreaties and exhortations, by reproaches of ingratitude or even by a retreat into illness.

Perhaps the knowledge of how her child is nourished in the womb may help to show a mother that, even in the purely physical sphere, the child while to some extent dependent on its mother nevertheless builds for itself and develops independently. If the womb gives the foetus this freedom, the mother should surely realize that the child is not her property and never was, and that she not only brings it into the world but must also let it go out into the world. She can teach and accompany the child but she must not hold on to it. Cutting the umbilical cord at birth is not a separation of mother from child, but a separation of the child from its own organ which happens to be intimately associated with the maternal organism. It is true that the child may then suckle at the breast, but that is essentially a less intimate process.

False claims by the father
The father may also get a false idea of his property rights in the child and be misled into false attitudes and behaviour. When man discovered thousands of years ago that children grew in the woman because of his seed and not because of some mysterious power, and thus realized the connection between sexual intercourse and pregnancy, he began to take steps to ensure that he was in reality the father of his children. He acquired an interest in the

exclusivity of his intimate relations with a certain woman, and later in seeing to it that she had had no other men before him. He began to regard his seed (a term used for his progeny) as something of promise and also of care. This was the beginning of patriarchy and of female virginity before marriage, as well as of monogamy itself.

The man's claims related not only to his wife but also to his children. The meaning of the word 'virginity' changed; it used to mean that a woman was still free and belonged to no man, whether she had had intercourse or not, and it came to mean that she had not had intercourse either. However, the male reserved to himself the right to do what he liked with his sperm either before marriage or during marriage (double standard of morals). On the other hand, he felt obliged to marry any woman he had made pregnant before marriage, not for the sake of the woman but for the purpose of retaining his rights in the product of his sperm, the child. It is not surprising therefore to find modern men fighting for the possession of their children, even if they do not want to marry the mother or cannot do so.

The authority of a father over his children is based on a sort of copyright, and expressed in his claim to dispose of his own property. This was the basis of the traditional legal ruling that a father had the final say in the fate of the children.

Recognition of the part played by the semen in the production of a child led to common parental care of the latter (the mother also took pride in her infant), and to a common responsibility for its rearing, education, and preparation for life, out of which the concept of family grew. Yet even today some fathers pervert this idea to mean that they have absolute authority, that they can educate the child exclusively in accordance with their own beliefs, and that in short they can do what they think right with their own seed. This type of father is just as guilty of self-pride as the mother may be (although he asserts that he is proud of his children), and he also demands as much gratitude and unconditional obedience, surrender and dependence, as the mother may; the only difference is that he sometimes acts more rigorously.

It is not long since women became emancipated from male dominance, and we are now discovering that the child is also an independent person. However, in her demands for equal rights with the male, modern woman has perhaps gone a little far and imperilled all our cultural development. We may expect that the marriage pattern will continue to be monogamy and that the family will remain the bulwark of decent human behaviour as it has become in cultural evolution. But the circumstances will have changed. Modern woman is justified in taking heed of her own sexual needs but must also learn to take responsibility for them in the framework of human relations. The man must strive for the same goal. Both have to learn that their care of their child must no more interfere with its independent development than others may interfere with their own personal decisions. They must learn to accept the child as a gift and a challenge but must not prevent its progress towards independence by making false claims to possession or authority over it. This demands of modern parents a higher degree of individual thought than in the days when traditional social customs could be taken over without reflection, since things had always been that way.

This is not to say that earlier educational practices were wrong in their content, even if they were based on what we now know to be false principles. They were certainly well adapted to the then circumstances and led to fitness for life and to health. These practices are now ill-suited to the times, and if they are continued out of mental laziness they will lead to maladaptation and illness.

Uterine Muscles and Pregnancy

The uterus in labour functions for only a few hours, while its function as a container for the foetus goes on much longer. As the foetus grows, the uterus undergoes enormous enlargement (from about 3 inches to about a foot in length). It is only at the height of this enlargement that the services of the uterine muscles will be required to ensure delivery. After delivery, the uterus must once again get ready for a fresh pregnancy and must therefore return to its original size. This cycle is possible only because the muscles are arranged in a special way (see fig. 53).

Structure and changes in the uterine wall
All the muscles in the uterus form spirals which traverse the uterine wall, obliquely to its axis from outside to inside like springs in a watch whose coils lie in one plane (fig. 53B). As a result there exist (schematically simplified in fig. 53A) functional units of spiral muscle. Since there are two intertwining spiral systems whose angle of incidence increases as the tubes are reached i.e. over the body of the uterus, it is clear that the uterus can expand most in the area where implantation takes place and the ovum increases in size. Expansion of a hollow organ mostly takes place through stretching. If this were true of the uterus, the organ would sacrifice its muscular function in labour, for an overstretched and thus thin-walled organ cannot contract powerfully. Function is preserved in spite of great increase in size by letting the muscle spirals running between outer wall and cavity uncoil. The two ends of the spiral are displaced in opposite directions, so that the number of turns is diminished. The significant point is that the muscle fibres do not need to increase in length to increase the size of the uterus (figs. 53B and C). They simply grow somewhat thicker in order to retain the strength of the muscle wall (important for the development of force during delivery). Thus it is possible for the uterus to adapt itself effortlessly during pregnancy to the demands of the foetus for more room.

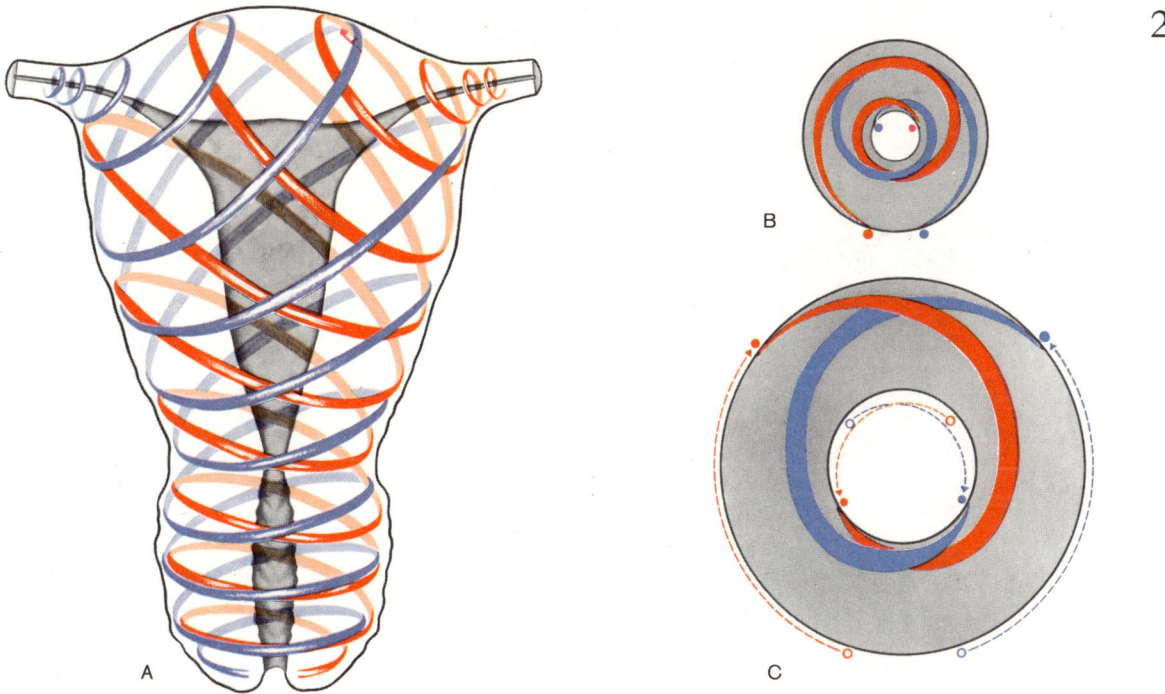

FIG. 53 *Structure of uterine musculature.*

A Three dimensional diagram of uterine musculature   B Uterine muscle fibre in resting phase: narrow lumen
C Uterine muscle fibre in pregnancy: increased lumen due to unwinding of coils. No increase in fibre length but increase in thickness

Changes in uterine size (fig. 54)
At the beginning of pregnancy, the uterus cannot be felt, for it is hidden behind the pubic bones. At the end of the fourth month of pregnancy (each month being reckoned as 28 days) it stands about two fingerbreadths above the pubis. By the end of the fifth month (twentieth week) it is about midway between pubis and navel. By the end of the sixth month (twenty-fourth week) it has reached the height of the navel. At the end of the seventh month (twenty-eighth week) it lies three fingerbreadths above the navel. At the end of the eighth month (thirty-two weeks) it is halfway between navel and breastbone. By the end of the ninth month (thirty-six weeks) it has reached the lower limits of the rib cage.

During the last month the uterus sinks a little, because it rounds itself off and because the foetal head has already descended into the pelvis. Moreover, the abdominal wall has become slacker and lets the uterus sag. Hence at the end of the tenth month (forty weeks), the uterus reaches only to about one fingerbreadth below the breastbone. The descent of the

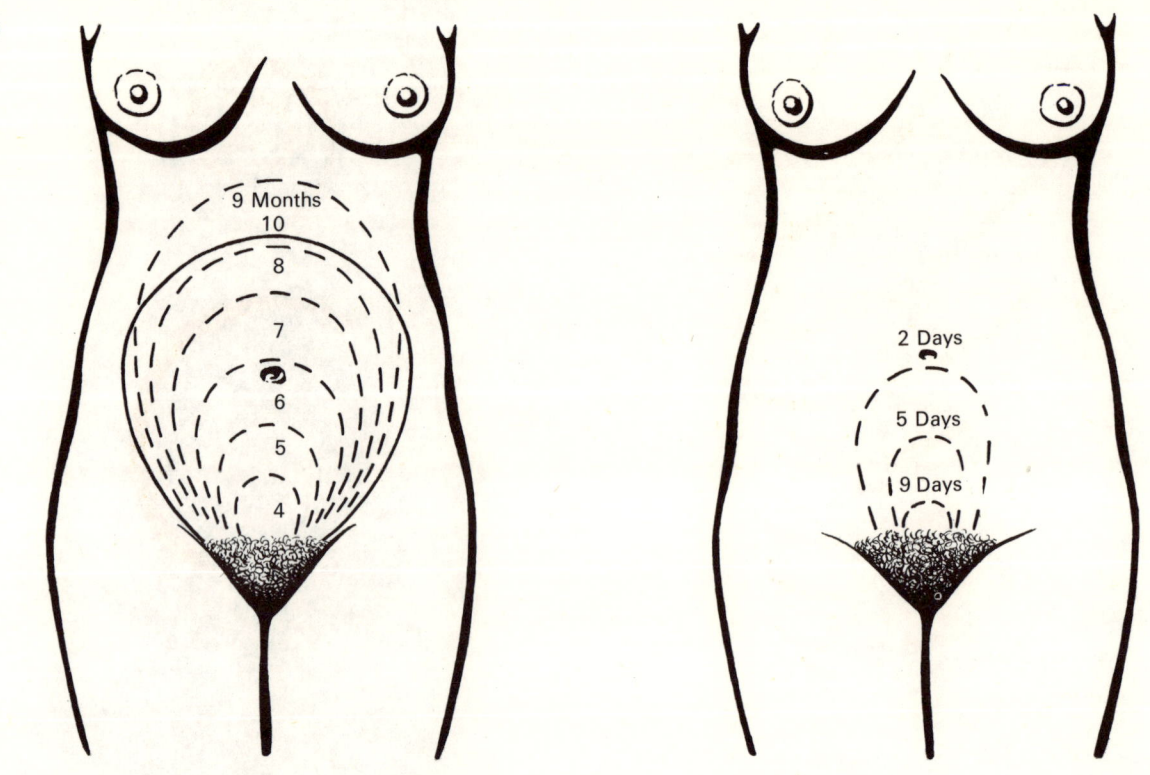

FIG. 54 *Size of uterus. Left, increase during pregnancy; right, decrease after delivery.*

foetal head in the last month of pregnancy is only possible because the cervix has also become involved in the dilatation of muscle fibres.

After delivery, in which the muscle fibres have again coiled up spirally, the uterus is only about 6 inches long and scarcely reaches to the navel. During the days that follow, it rapidly recedes in size. Five days after delivery, its summit is again about halfway between navel and pubis, and 9 days after the event it can just be felt above the pubic arch. This rapid regression is possible only because the muscle spirals coil up again. They return to their initial size after a further five weeks, and the regression is promoted by suckling (through hormonal paths).

Duration of Pregnancy and Term of Delivery

The average pregnancy lasts for 282 days, reckoned from the first day of the last menstrual period. A 'month' in pregnancy is by common agreement reckoned as 28 days, so that the total number of weeks in pregnancy is 40. The usual method of calculating the end of pregnancy is to reckon three calendar months back from the first day of the last menstrual period, add one year forward and then another seven days. Allowing for the variable length of calendar months, the result is 281 to 282 days.

The actual length of pregnancy from the day of successful intercourse to delivery is shorter and averages 266 days. In other words the woman carries for 266 days. These average periods are seldom adhered to in practice (only in 3·9% of all pregnancies). In individual pregnancies the period tends to deviate by between $1\frac{1}{2}$ weeks before and $1\frac{1}{2}$ weeks after the calculated date.

Children delivered within the first to seventh months (first to twenty-eighth weeks) of a pregnancy are not viable (miscarriages or abortions). However, children born after the end of the seventh month of pregnancy (i.e. within the twenty-ninth to thirty-ninth weeks) can live with medical aid. Such births are known as premature births.

Changes in Pregnancy

With the implantation of a fertilized ovum in her uterus, the body of a woman undergoes changes affecting all her tissues. No body cell is independent of these changes, and the emotional state of the woman also undergoes profound alterations. The goal of these changes is the preparation of the woman for motherhood, for her pregnancy and delivery. Preparation for motherhood is a process regulated by the hormones and the nervous system, and all women pass through this. Motherhood itself (like fatherhood) is a mental and spiritual process not regulated by hormones or any physical factor. We will return to this at the close of the book.

Hormonal induction of preparation for motherhood is due to the pregnancy hormone secreted by the foetal trophoblast. It affects almost all the endocrine (hormonal) glands in the body through its direct and indirect effects on the ovary and the pituitary. This marked change leads to tissue alterations, to changes in the nervous system and to an alteration in the basis for all mental processes. In addition to all this, the foetus grows and needs more room and therefore displaces organs, so that these are under a double stress, for they will also be required to do extra work and perform to greater advantage.

Body changes (see fig. 55)
Although it affects almost all tissues, one of the least obvious changes is a general impregnation of the body with water. This makes the tissue structure softer, looser and more yielding. Of the 15–28 lb. increase in weight from beginning to end of a pregnancy, only about 10 to

218 12 lb. is due to the uterus and contents. The rest is mainly water and extra fat. The increase in water content in pregnancy makes the skin more tense and smoothes out the smaller wrinkles, so that the woman looks younger. Since she loses water during and after delivery, this effect does not persist.

Deposition of fat around the hips, breasts and shoulders is due to hormone action and leads to more pronounced rounding of the body contours which usually also persists after pregnancy. Even a slightly built woman looks softer and plumper, so that after her pregnancy the woman appears to have acquired a fresh and more mature type of beauty. Hence the popular conception of a first pregnancy as an aid to beauty (the first, because this is the one in which the transformation from maidenly grace to softer maturity is most marked).

Unfortunately, the normal fat deposition in pregnancy is often exaggerated by overeating. At the beginning of a pregnancy, changes in metabolism tend to cause problems of adaptation, expressed as abnormal cravings for peculiar foods or a loss of appetite, nausea and morning sickness. (The best remedy for morning sickness is to take breakfast in bed or to lie down again after breakfast.) As pregnancy progresses, there is usually an increase in appetite, which occasionally becomes ravenous, often associated with increased thirst. The expectant mother must not let this get out of control. She should certainly satisfy her hunger in reason and can eat what she wants and reject what she does not, but she does not need to eat for two persons, and in the last three or four months of pregnancy she should not give way entirely to her thirst. Otherwise, she can put on so much fat as to change her body shape completely; this is neither normal nor healthy.

Other skin changes take place. Many women notice that during pregnancy their hair grows better and lies better, and that any dandruff present disappears. Unfortunately, this effect is temporary. Usually after delivery there is a transient increase in hair loss, so that the old condition is rapidly regained. The downy hair on the face, especially on the upper lip, often proliferates, and these hairs become stronger and longer. In some cases, this overgrowth may persist after delivery. It is common for certain skin areas to darken permanently, particularly on and around the nipples, in the midline of the lower abdomen, on the external genitals and around the anus, and sometimes the whole skin may acquire a darker hue. Brown spots often appear on the skin of the face but usually disappear again some months after delivery.

A general increase in sweat gland activity frequently leads to stronger body odour. For this reason and also in order to promote skin circulation, daily washing of the whole body (not necessarily with soap, to avoid defatting of the skin) is strongly advisable. Warm baths are permitted up to the onset of delivery, provided the bath is clean, but too hot and too cold baths should be avoided. Daily care of the nipples and breasts is also valuable, including rubbing with a face flannel (not a brush), soap and water.

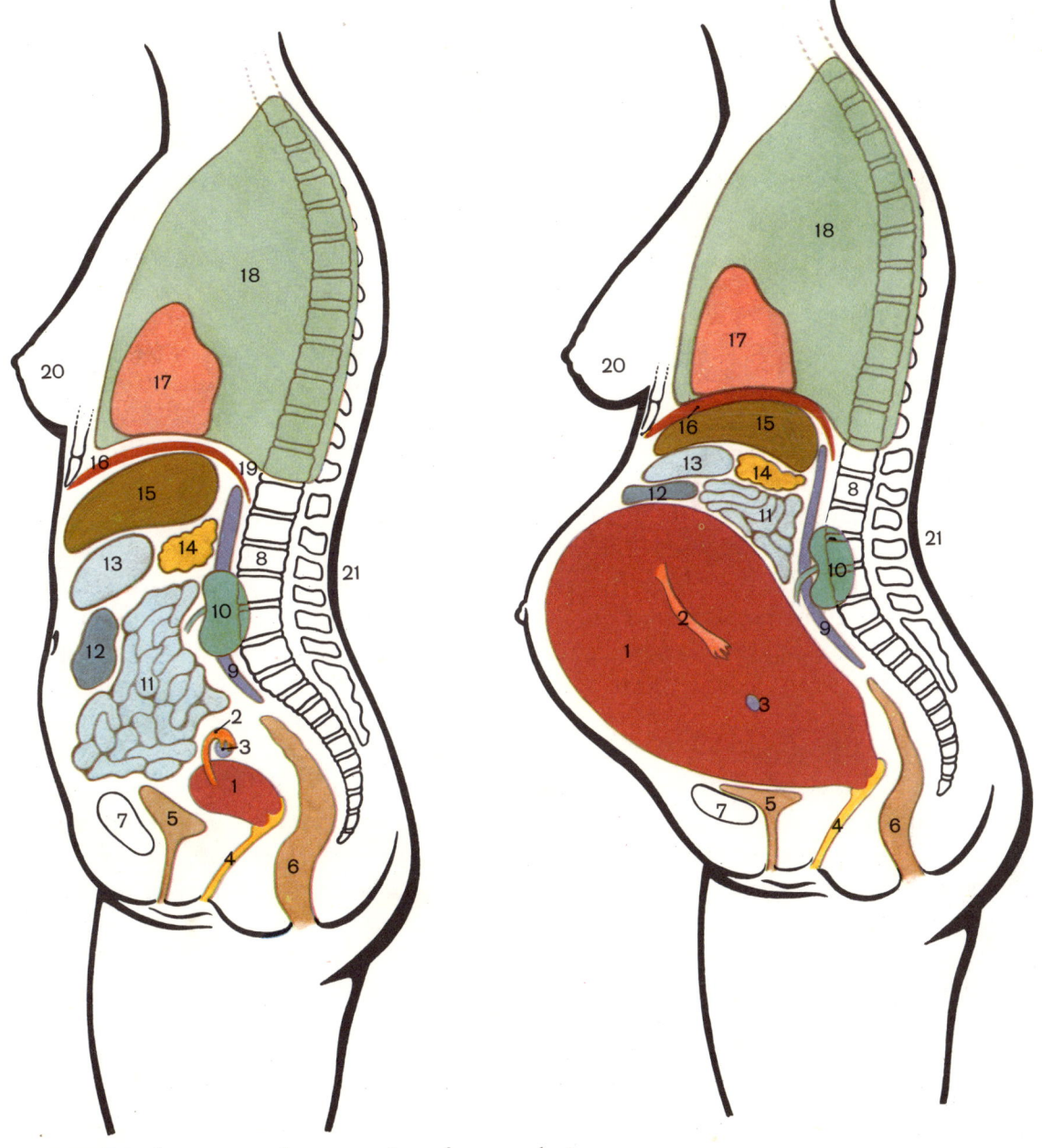

FIG. 55 *Displacement and compression of organs during pregnancy.*

*1 Uterus   2 Tube   3 Ovary   4 Vagina   5 Urinary bladder and urethra   6 Rectum
7 Branch of pubic bone   8 Vertebral column   9 Inferior vena cava   10 Kidney   11 Loops
of small intestine   12 Transverse colon   13 Stomach   14 Pancreas   15 Liver   16 Diaphragm
17 Heart   18 Lung   19 Space for lung expansion   20 Breast   21 Curve of vertebral column*

The skin of the abdomen grows to the extent required for the foetus. As a result in most women during the last three months there appear, mainly on the lower abdomen and less often over the hips, stripes or striae which shine vaguely blue and gradually turn white and pearly and wrinkled after delivery. These are permanent.

Towards the end of pregnancy the cavity of the navel becomes obliterated and the latter may actually rise above the surrounding skin; this adaptive process also recedes later.

The external genitals are affected by the general loosening up of tissue. The skin of vulva and lower vagina becomes smoother, softer, and more velvety and turns violet because blood vessels proliferate; this is one of the earliest signs of pregnancy. Thanks to this loosening of tissue, which includes the perineum and the entire pelvic floor, these organs become more flexible, so that they can stretch and let the foetus through during delivery. The ligaments holding up the bladder and rectum are also relaxed, so that they can make room for the uterus and later the emerging child. In the last stages of pregnancy the urinary bladder becomes contracted, so that the woman often has to urinate more frequently. Emptying of the bowel may also be interfered with.

Small intestine, colon, stomach, pancreas, liver, biliary tract, kidneys and ureters are all cramped for space and their muscles do less work. This means that the woman, particularly towards the end of her pregnancy, must take more frequent small meals and is liable to suffer from constipation. To relieve these digestive disturbances only mild laxatives, mostly of vegetable origin, are needed; the patient should ask her doctor about this, and not just use any laxative she happens to have. Usually the pancreas, liver and kidneys are not functionally disordered, although the kidneys in particular have more to do than usual.

To facilitate the passage of the child through the pelvic ring, all the pelvic joints become slacker during pregnancy. Since this slackening also involves the vertebral column, women with a tendency to backache or sciatica are often free from symptoms during a pregnancy. However the changes in the pelvic and vertebral joints together with the altered weight distribution due to the increasingly heavy (and in the last four weeks, forward tilted) uterus cause the pregnant woman to alter her stance late in pregnancy. This she does by hollowing her lumbar spine more, holding her head further back, and slightly raising her heels. This is the origin of the queenly gait of the pregnant woman. However the increased strain on the affected muscles can all too easily make her tired and give her pain in the lower part of the back. It is therefore helpful to wear an adjustable pregnancy girdle especially in the later months and in second and subsequent pregnancies, to avoid overstretching the abdominal wall and to assist posture.

As the breasts lay down fat they also undergo an increase in glandular tissue, and there is often a perceptible sensation of 'drawing' in this area quite soon after conception. It is therefore necessary to change the size of the brassiere several times in pregnancy to adapt it to the size of the breasts, since too much pressure on the latter may impair later breast-feeding.

Organ displacements in the abdomen raise the diaphragm, and this can make breathing more difficult and cause shortness of breath by diminishing the reserve space for ventilation. The rise in the diaphragm also displaces the heart and presses it more firmly against the chest wall, though this does not usually cause any cardiac pain or discomfort. However, the increased work on the heart during pregnancy is of some significance. The total blood volume at the end of pregnancy has increased by about $\frac{1}{2}$ to 1 litre (i.e. by about 15 to 20 per cent of the normal). This increase together with the need for an enhanced blood (and oxygen) supply to the uterus means that the stroke volume, the amount pumped out by each stroke of the heart, must rise by about 50%. There is also a gaping and loss of elasticity in the small vessels leading to the heart, so that the blood flows more slowly in the lower parts of the body and tends to stagnate there. Veins therefore become more prominent in the lower half of the body, especially on the legs, the buttocks, the vulva and the labia minora as well as the vagina itself and the anus (haemorrhoids or piles). Hence pregnant women do not like standing for long, and faint rather readily because of the stagnation of blood in their legs.

To avoid excessive superficial vein formation (though in general these veins regress after delivery, they can persist as varicose veins and lead to complications during pregnancy and afterwards) the pregnant woman is advised against wearing tight garters (modern girdles take this into account). For walking, she should wear shoes without high heels (which will throw her off balance), and she should avoid prolonged standing. The best exercise is walking in comfortable shoes. Swimming is also good exercise and relaxation, provided stress and competition are avoided. Bathing in the sea, especially if it is rough, is unsuitable because, like competitive or strenuous sport (riding, rowing, skiing, tennis, strenuous touring, gymnastics with apparatus and light athletics), it can bring on premature labour. Cycling should only be pursued if the woman is used to it and motor-cycling should be prohibited.

Appropriate exercises for pregnant women performed regularly and properly supervised promote the flow of blood back to the heart and help to strengthen the muscles of the abdomen and the postural muscles. Pregnant women can continue to do their usual housework.

If the woman has got to travel, she should do it only during the fourth to sixth months. There is a risk that prolonged trips by car or train may, through the rhythmical stimuli, induce premature labour. With modern pressurized aircraft, there is no ban on flying.

It is essential to go regularly for medical examination during pregnancy and to obtain advice about even trivial problems. The first examination should take place after the first period or two have been missed. From then on, the woman should be seen regularly every month until the fourth month and later every 14 days up to delivery.

Emotional changes.

The emotional changes associated with the physical ones are even more complex, so that it is almost impossible to summarize them in terms applicable to most women. Every pregnancy is a profound emotional stress which is not always compensated by the joy of motherhood. The latter may be experienced as a satisfying and joyful fulfilment of her womanhood, and the pleasure of thinking about her forthcoming child can make this a time of happiness and hope. In this state of mind, she will find herself able to put up with all her discomforts, even the physical ones. She will appear peaceful and balanced, concentrating on her maternal role and not responding to the usual extraneous stimuli (she is 'hatching'). However, an expectant mother may be so emotionally unbalanced that she is irritable and changeable to a high degree, and liable to excessive, sometimes uncontrollable outbursts and actions. If in addition there is conscious or unconscious rejection of the child or even a conflict of feelings, her physical discomforts and also her slumbering emotional disorders with their background in the past and perhaps into her own early childhood, may lead to serious illness.

One decisive factor in a pregnancy may be the loving care of the husband. In our culture he no longer needs to protect his wife against external perils as in the dim past, but he must assure her by his presence and actions, in word and gesture, that she is safe in his care and that he loves her dearly for herself and also as the mother of his future child. This love implies an increased awareness of the need for forbearance in sexual intimacy. The attitude of the wife towards sexual intercourse and exchange of physical caresses may vary all the way from heightened desire to relative rejection. Medically speaking, marital intimacy need not be restricted during pregnancy, with the exception of the last five weeks before term. Intercourse should be abandoned during these five weeks as well as the five weeks after delivery, because it has been shown that it may seriously endanger the health of the woman (infection after delivery).

Even if a modern woman takes a husband as a partner and not as a protector, and participates in his troubles and worries, she will need during her pregnancy to depend on his care and his strength, and she will be glad of his comforting presence and support. If she can show her husband how much she needs him, so much the better, for this will help him to learn how to be a father.

Childbirth

The Events in Labour

Childbirth or labour includes all those events which lead to the delivery of the child from its mother's body.

The onset of labour.
On an average, labour begins after 282 days from the first day of the last period. At this point the child has come to term; its development has advanced so far that it is now able to continue life separated from its mother. The cause of the onset of labour lies in a change in hormone structure. During pregnancy the placenta secretes, apart from pregnancy hormone, increasing amounts of follicular hormone or oestrogen identical with that secreted as the ovum matures in the ovary. This oestrogen by the end of pregnancy has put the uterus in a state of increased readiness for muscle contraction. The hormone which actually triggers off the muscular contractions is called oxytocin and is formed in the posterior part of the pituitary. It cannot however exert its effect as long as pregnancy hormone and luteal hormone are being formed. Only when this barrier falls, and these hormones are no longer being secreted by an ageing placenta, can oxytocin act upon a uterus primed by oestrogen. The uterus responds by muscular contractions or *labour pains*, and attempts to expel its living contents. But the organs forming the birth canal must first be dilated; these include the cervix, the cervical os, the vagina, the vaginal entrance, the perineum and the pelvic floor. These gradually dilate one after another under the influence of increasing uterine contractions.

Position of the baby during labour
The first contractions are often perceived by the woman a week or so before term as mild, relatively rhythmical and repeated niggling pains in the abdomen, associated with lower back pain, which sometimes may be the sole feature. There may be days between pains.

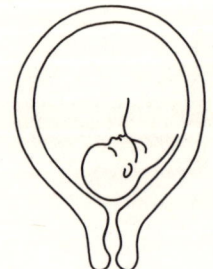

FIG. 56 *Foetal head ready for engagement.*

← Even pressure of uterus on foetal piston

Yielding of piston leads to pressure on cervix and os and opens them up

Downward suction

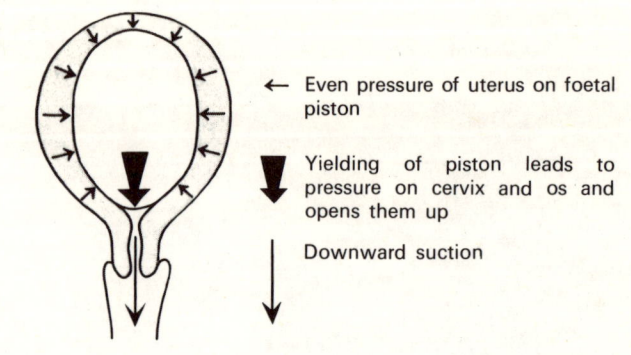

FIG. 57 *Beginning of birth canal dilatation.*

These are the so-called false pains and they serve for adjustment of the foetal position. The uterus straightens out and forms a hollow cylinder, which is the best geometrical shape to withstand the enormous forces generated during labour and to propel the foetus into the narrow birth canal. In 96% of all labours the child's head emerges first (cephalic presentation) and in 94% it is the back of the head or occiput which appears first, while in the other 2% some other part of the head shows first. In 3% of all labours the child's buttocks or breech appears first (breech presentation), and only in 1% does the foetus lie transversely and complicate labour technically. The events of labour described below apply to the usual cephalic or head presentation.

Opening up the birth canal
After the uterus has straightened and settled down, and the child's head has engaged itself in the pelvis (see fig. 56), the birth canal begins to dilate or open up. The first contractions are often very irregular at the onset and may not be noticed. As the canal opens the plug of mucus which closes off the cervix is expelled, mixed with some blood. This will be noticed by most women. Midwives call it a 'show'. With the expulsion of the plug the uterus comes into contact with the outside world, and both mother and child are now exposed to greater risk of infection. There may be as much as several days between the show and actual delivery, but a woman who has noticed a show should lose no time in calling her midwife or informing the hospital. This should also be done if regular contractions begin. The opening up of the birth canal is a complex activity.
1. Thanks to the peculiar arrangement of muscle fibres in the uterus, their contraction exerts a uniform overall pressure on the child. The latter gives way to this pressure by following the path of least resistance, the cervical canal, and exerts its own pressure on this causing dilation of the cervical canal and the external os. The lesser pressure outside the uterus acts as a suction apparatus and draws the child downwards via its presenting part, the head (fig. 57). This suction causes a soft lump to form on the scalp, known as the caput

FIG. 58 *Dilatation of cervical canal.*

1 Mucus plug still in place
2 Discharge of mucus and blood as a result of cervical stretching

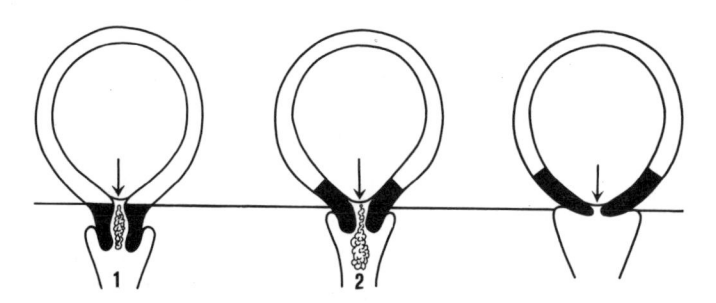

succedaneum (see fig. 62), for the child's skin is still loose and is elevated by suction with entry of some tissue fluid into the space underneath. This caput, which somewhat deforms the scalp of the newborn, soon returns to normal.

2. Because the muscular contractions of the uterus are not uniform but run as waves from above downwards, this being helped by the muscle arrangements in the cervix, contraction of the spirals leads to active dilatation of the cervix in support of (1).

3. The elastic but firm attachment of the uterus to the bony pelvis also ensures that the muscular effort directs the child downwards.

Under the influence of these forces (1 to 3) the canal opens up in stages. First, the cervical canal is dilated and taken up into the cavity of the uterus (fig. 58). Then the external os is

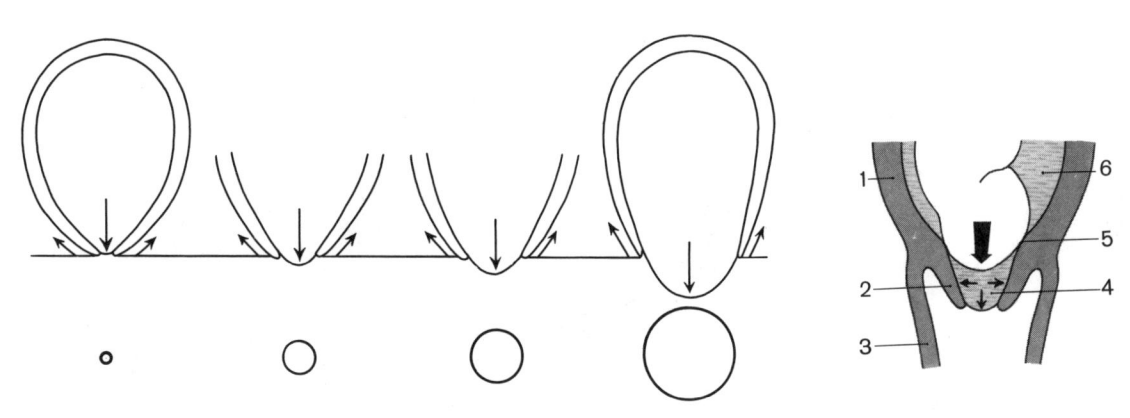

FIG. 59 *(left) Dilatation of cervical os.*

The uterus is drawn up over the foetus. The external os is therefore dilated (circle) and the foetus simultaneously expelled

FIG. 60 *(right) Transmission of forces during dilatation of the os.*

1 Uterus   2 Vaginal portion of uterus   3 Vagina   4 Fore-waters   5 Valvular plug
6 Rest of amniotic fluid

226 dilated (fig. 59) by the action of the presenting part of the child surrounded by its bag of waters. When the head passes into the narrow birth passages, it closes them off, separating off that part of the amniotic fluid lying ahead of the scalp from the rest and pushing the sealed off part before it. This bag of waters is turned into a firm cushion by the force of the following head, and dilates the passages with greater ease than the presenting part itself would (fig. 60).

If internal pressure in the bag of waters becomes too great, the membranes (amnion and chorion) enclosing the fluid will rupture and the fluid will gush out. Midwives say: 'the waters have broken', referring to the membranes enclosing the bag. If this happens the woman must call the midwife immediately or go straight to hospital. Even if the waters have broken for some other reason earlier in labour, continuing supervision will be needed from then on, since the child is now in contact with the outer world for the first time.

In some rare cases the bag of waters may not rupture in labour and the child will be born with its membranes intact (particularly likely if the child is small and the woman young and

FIG. 61 *Diagram of birth canal with tubal prolongation of soft tissue.*

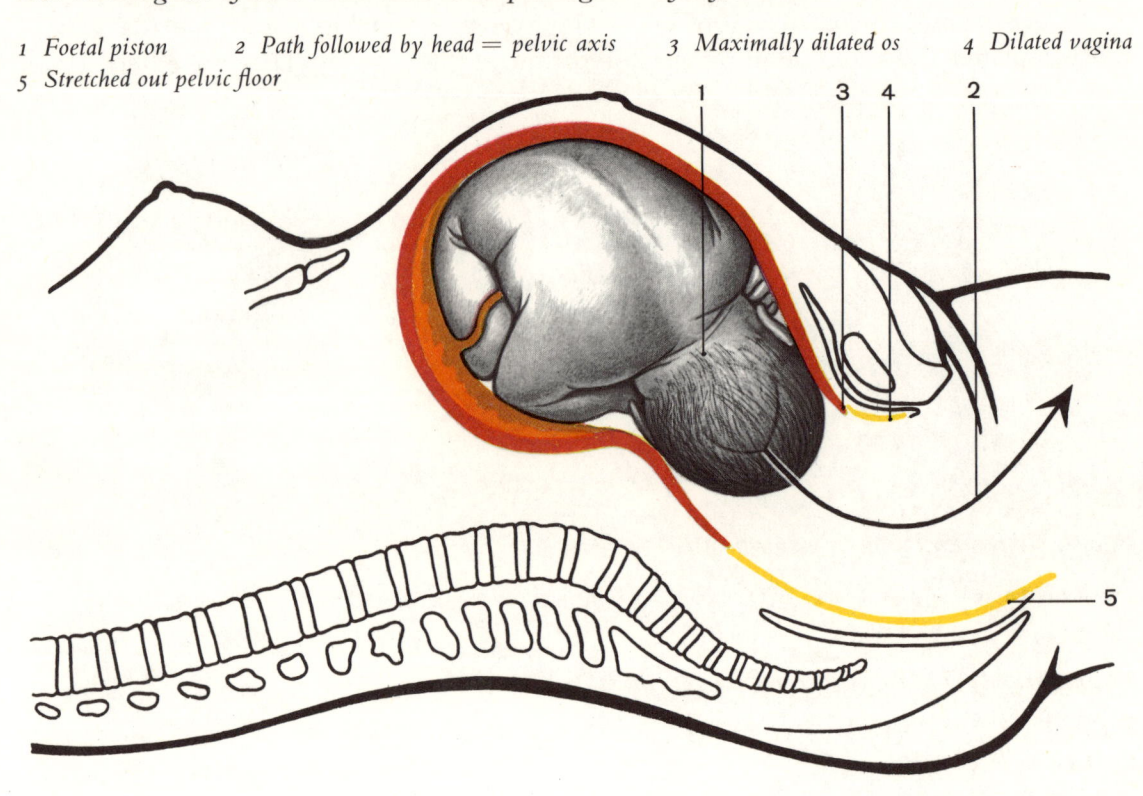

1 *Foetal piston* 2 *Path followed by head = pelvic axis* 3 *Maximally dilated os* 4 *Dilated vagina*
5 *Stretched out pelvic floor*

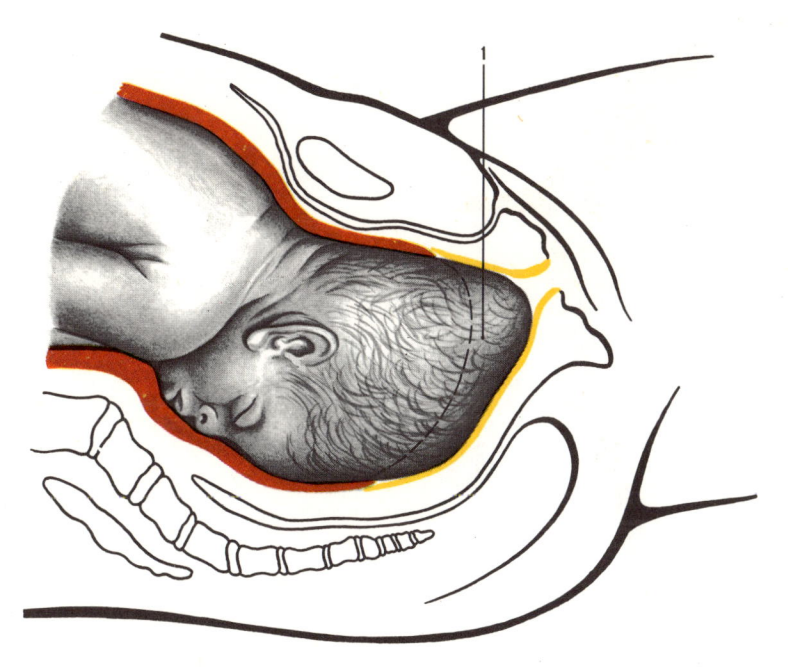

FIG. 62 *Advance of foetal head through birth canal.*

1 Caput succedaneum

with a history of several labours at short intervals, so that her birth passages offer no great resistance). This is known as being born in a caul, and the amniotic sac must then be opened up at once to allow the child to breathe.

The external genitals dilate when the child enters the period of expulsion (the second stage) and the mother begins to bear down with each contraction. Figure 61 shows diagrammatically this stage of labour from full dilatation of the os to the end of the second stage, during which the pelvic floor dilates until the vagina becomes a tubal prolongation of it. In Figure 62 the progress of the child's head through the canal and its caput are shown.

Pelvis and labour

Before describing the second stage in detail, we must turn our attention to the bony pelvis (fig. 63). The space of the so-called true pelvis surrounded by bone has a complicated shape, but we will not go into all the details. Seen from above, from which direction the child will enter, the inlet of the pelvis has its greatest diameter transversely, about 13 to 13·5 cm. The cavity below the inlet is more or less round and tapers again at the outlet below. Its maximum diameter is about 12 to 12·5 cm. At the outlet the largest diameter is no longer transverse but in the front to back axis and is about 11 cm. during labour. At the end of pregnancy the joints of the pelvis and spinal column have been loosened up by hormone action, so that the lowest segment of the column, the coccyx, can stretch and help to widen the outlet from a normal 9 to 11 cm.

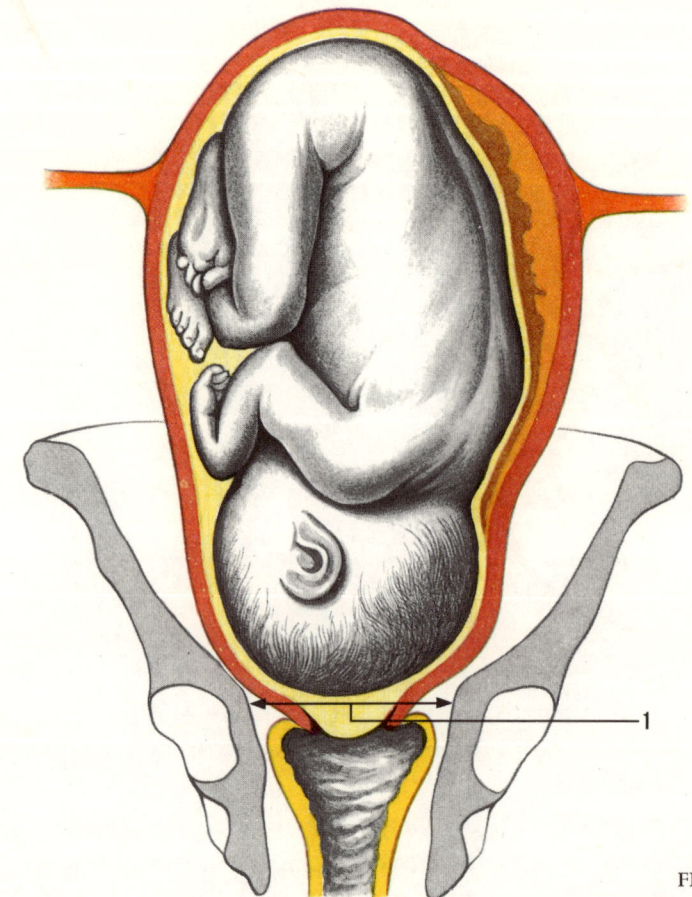

FIG. 63 *Inlet of pelvis (1) and foetus.*

If we recall that these measurements do not represent the real amount of space available to the passenger since there are also thin soft parts in between, and that the child's head measures about 11·5 cm. from forehead to occiput and is not very plastic at birth, it becomes clear that the child's head must rotate on its axis during expulsion if it is to take advantage of the maximum diameters of the pelvis. Figure 63 (early phase of first stage) shows diagrammatically that with a cephalic presentation the head will not pass through the pelvis sideways but must rotate. The shoulders and hips of the child are of course almost as broad as its head, but they deform more readily and can therefore pass through the bony pelvis more easily. As they pass through the appropriate diameter of the pelvic outlet with the shoulders in the front to back axis, the newborn head will rotate again (figs. 68 and 69). It should be noted that the inherited shape of the child's head (long or short head) has an effect on the type of labour.

Stage of expulsion

In the second stage of labour which begins after the cervix is fully dilated, the *stage of expulsion* (fig. 64), the woman must make use of her other body muscles as well as the uterine ones. The stimulus for her to do so arises from the change in character of her contractions at this time. They now give her a sensation similar to that when passing a stool and make her want to bear down. Her legs are forced apart, her hands seek something to hold on to, and her abdominal muscles tense up. Her diaphragm is forced down by deep inspiration and prevented from rising again by pressure from the larynx. Thus the intra-abdominal pressure is increased and involuntary muscular pressure in the uterus raised threefold. It is important at this time to control progressive slackening and relaxation of the pelvic floor muscles, for the child forces itself powerfully against the pelvic floor to dilate it. Most women from highly developed cultures do not know how to manage this relaxation correctly. Not infrequently they tense up through fear and not only resist the progress of labour but actually increase their pains; this of course makes them even more tense with succeeding contractions. For this reason, doctors and others (in Britain, workers with the National Childbirth Trust) have introduced courses for pregnant women in which they learn appropriate exercises designed for relaxation, correct breathing and bearing down. If the woman is also

FIG. 64 *Beginning of stage of expulsion (muscle forces).*

A Branch of pubic bone   *B* Urinary bladder and urethra   *C* Perineum   *D* Rectum and anus
E Vertebral column (coccyx)
1 Uterus with contracted muscles during a 'pain'   *2* Relaxation of pelvic floor (delivery with minimal pain)
3 Abdominal press   *4* Diaphragmatic press

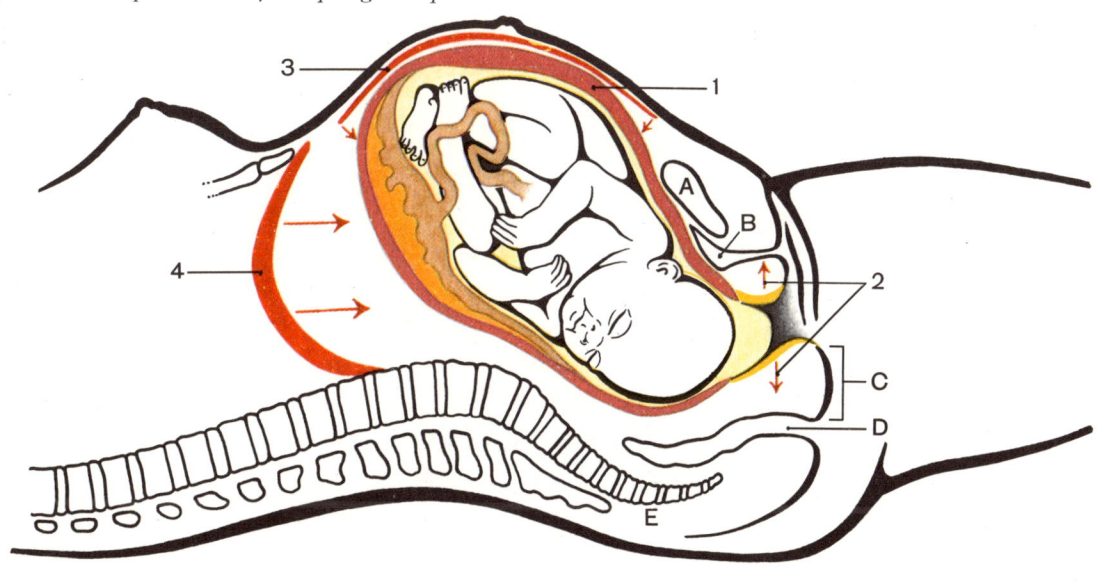

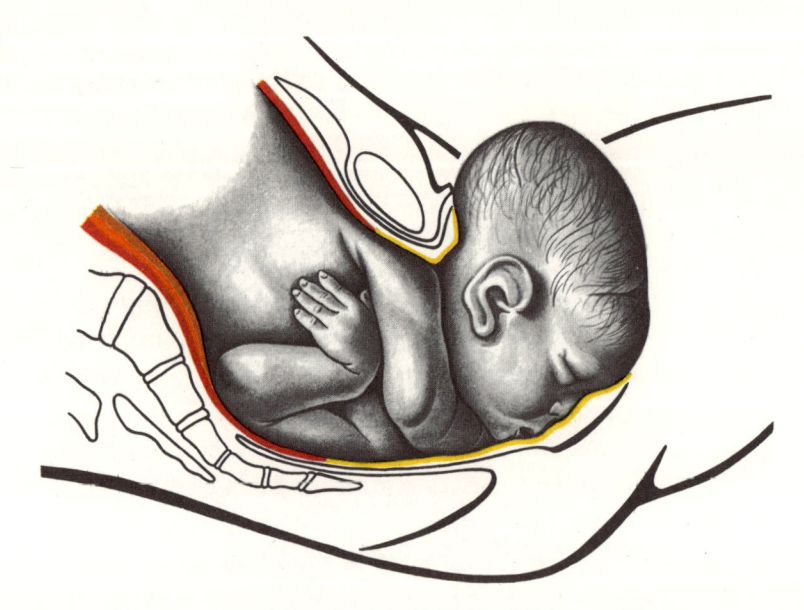

FIG. 65 *Passage of head through soft parts: the occiput is born.*

taught about the emotional side, she can learn to practise rhythmical contraction of the abdominal muscles and relaxation of the pelvic floor and so make her subsequent labour easier. This relaxation technique, formerly incorrectly called 'painless labour' but more correctly 'labour with maximal comfort', is becoming increasingly popular, and in most cases it renders local or general anaesthesia during labour superfluous. It also makes it possible for the woman to experience the whole process of becoming a mother in full consciousness. This technique is best incorporated in a course between the fourth and sixth months of pregnancy, after which the woman can continue to practise it until she comes to term.

Figure 65 shows the moment when the head is 'crowned' and the body is beginning to leave the mother, After the head has appeared, the shoulders and the rest of the body are usually delivered rapidly and more easily. The rest of the amniotic fluid is also expelled.

Figures 66 to 69 are drawn from film stills and depict the significant stages of an actual birth as seen by midwife and helpers. In Figure 68 the chest is shown compressed in the narrowest part of the canal. Mucus is flowing out of the respiratory tract through the nose by this compression. The head is about to rotate, with the face towards the mother's right thigh, because the shoulders are turning through the narrowest part of the pelvis. In Figure 69 the abdomen is compressed in the narrowest part of the canal. Mucus from the stomach and oesophagus therefore flows out through the mouth. The enormous dilatation of the external genitals is clearly shown, and their function as a soft-part tubal prolongation of the birth canal.

These pictures should help understanding of the text and also give women a positive

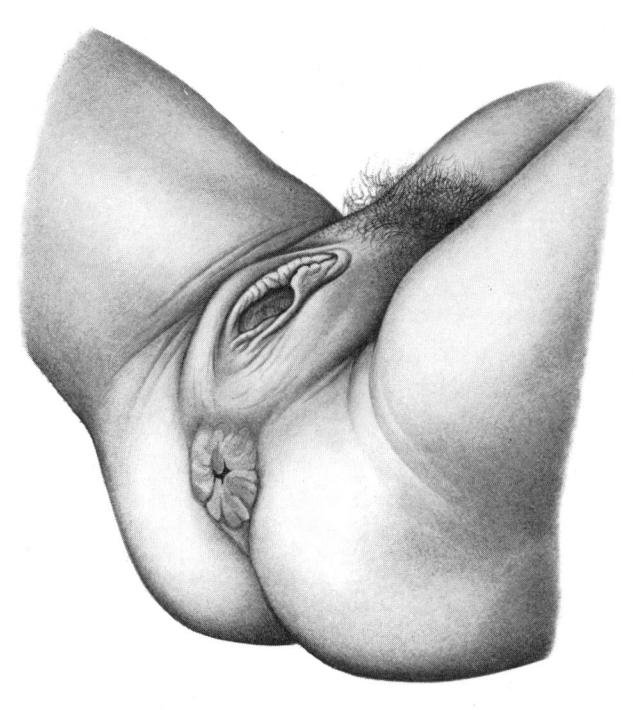

FIG. 66 *The child's head is appearing in the vaginal entrance.*

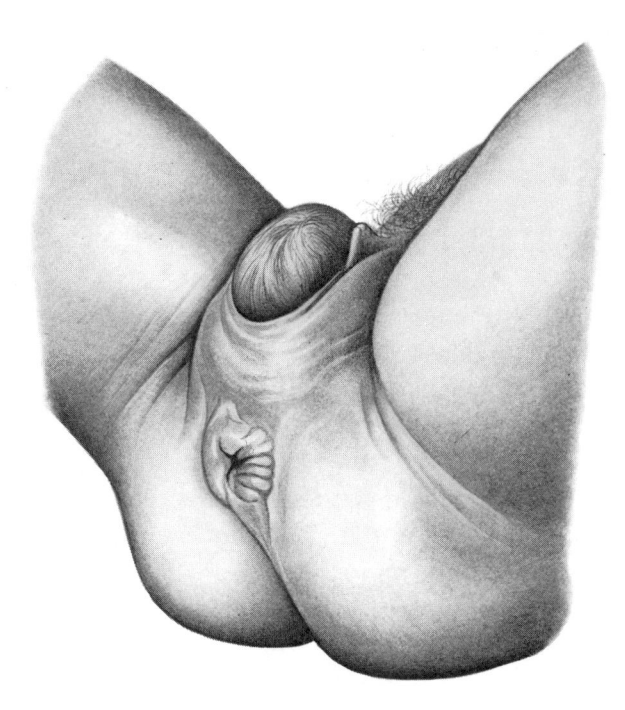

FIG. 67 *The head is 'crowned' in the entrance.*

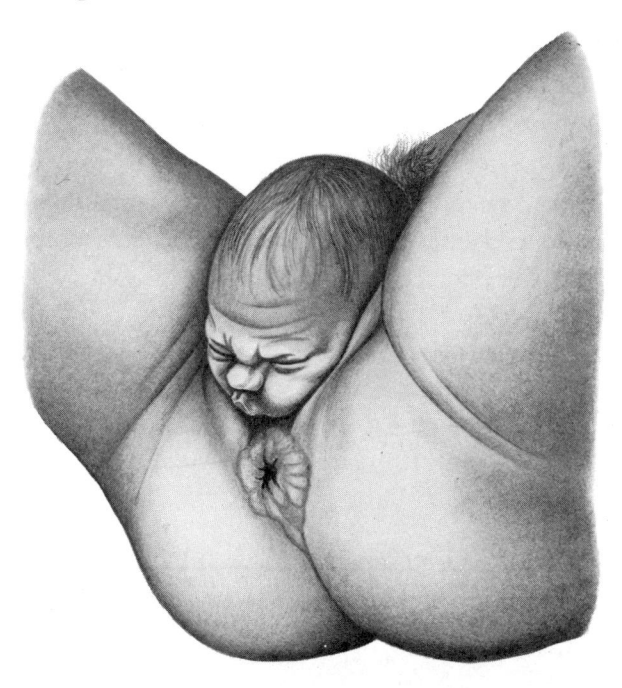

FIG. 68 *The head has been born as far as the chin.*

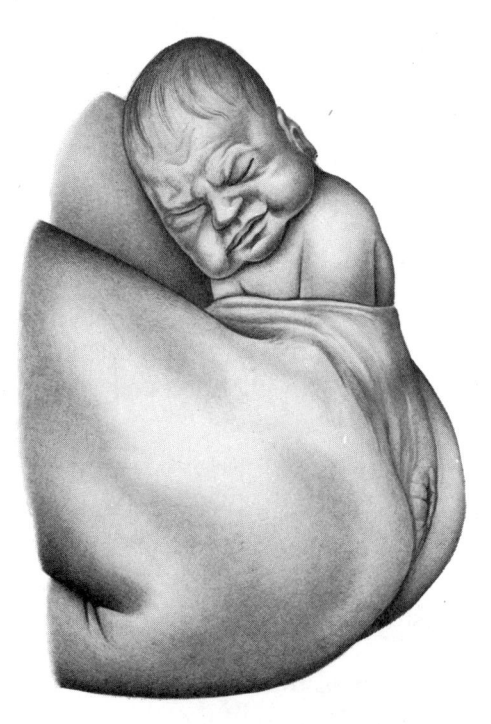

FIG. 69 *The shoulders are born.*

attitude to the progress of their own labours. Many husbands express the wish to be present at their wife's delivery. There are a number of human and physiological grounds in favour of this, but there are also some objections, discussion of which would take us too far (see p. 237). These pictures of the final phase of delivery can convey a better idea of this than the rapidly changing events actually witnessed at a delivery, but they cannot of course replace the feeling of having been present at the birth of one's own child.

Episiotomy (perineal section)
The moment at which the child's head leaves the vagina is of some significance for the perineum, which has gradually become thinner and thinner as it stretches during labour. It may become overstretched and tear; such a tear takes some time to heal and for normal perineal function to be restored. If therefore the usual protection of the perineum by the midwife's or doctor's hand, preventing too stormy a passage of the head, looks as if it will not be sufficient, a scissors cut in the perineum may be deliberately made to reduce tension (episiotomy). A straight cut is not painful because the skin nerves have been rendered insensible through stretching, and it heals more rapidly and with less complications than a tear. An episiotomy is carried out nowadays on about one in three women in their first labour (primiparae) and one in five of all later labours (multiparae). Even a series of episiotomies carried out at different labours are not detrimental to later pregnancies, although the perineum in older women becomes less elastic and more rigid and therefore more liable to tear.

Caesarean section
Where the pelvis is too small to let the child through, a condition the doctor will have confirmed by measurement long before delivery, or where there are other obstructions to labour or it is necessary to end a pregnancy before term, for example in cases of Rh incompatibility, the child can be delivered by caesarean section. Under anaesthesia, the lower abdominal wall and lower part of the uterus are opened and the child together with its membranes and the placenta is extracted. The uterus and abdominal wall are then closed again. Another pregnancy after the uterus has returned to normal and after a further waiting period is possible and permissible. However, a maximum of three caesarean sections is advisable, because the solidity and elasticity of a uterus which has been repeatedly opened and stitched up again tends to diminish. As a rule, after a third section the woman should be sterilized (see p. 124 ff.) to prevent further pregnancy.

Labour contractions
The rhythmical, initially weak but towards the end of labour increasingly powerful uterine contractions are known as pains. They first cause the child to assume a convenient presenta-

Pains of engagement   15–20 min. intervals

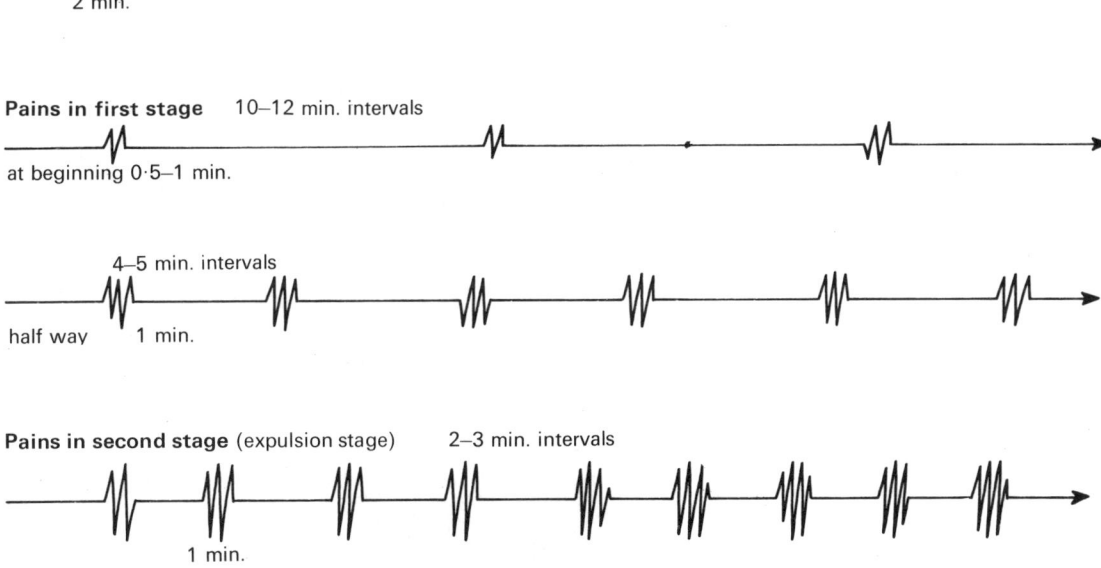

2 min.

Pains in first stage   10–12 min. intervals

at beginning 0·5–1 min.

4–5 min. intervals

half way   1 min.

Pains in second stage (expulsion stage)   2–3 min. intervals

1 min.

FIG. 70 *Overall view (schematic) of contraction activity.*

tion for delivery, then they cause the birth canal to dilate up, then they expel the child, and finally they remove the membranes and the placenta from the uterus. In accordance with these different functions, contractions vary during labour in strength, frequency and duration. Figure 70 gives a survey of the course of labour. This schema is only a generalized one, for there are many major personal variations. At any point the contractions of labour may be arrested for internal or external reasons, the situation then requiring medical supervision (the height of the spikes shown in Figure 70 is of purely diagrammatic significance).

The child's first breaths
After the child has left its mother's body, it is laid between its mother's legs for a moment and then held on high with the legs uppermost. This avoids the possibility of its sucking the mucus from its mouth and nose deeply into the respiratory tract when it takes its first breaths.

The changed pressure differentials outside the body impair blood flow within the gelatinous umbilical cord; the placenta has been damaged by the uterine contractions and can no longer carry out its functions. The first reflex breath the child takes inflates its lungs and increases the blood flow through them. As a result, pressures and circulation in the heart and the child's chest alter, so that from now on it can supply its own oxygen through breathing.

234

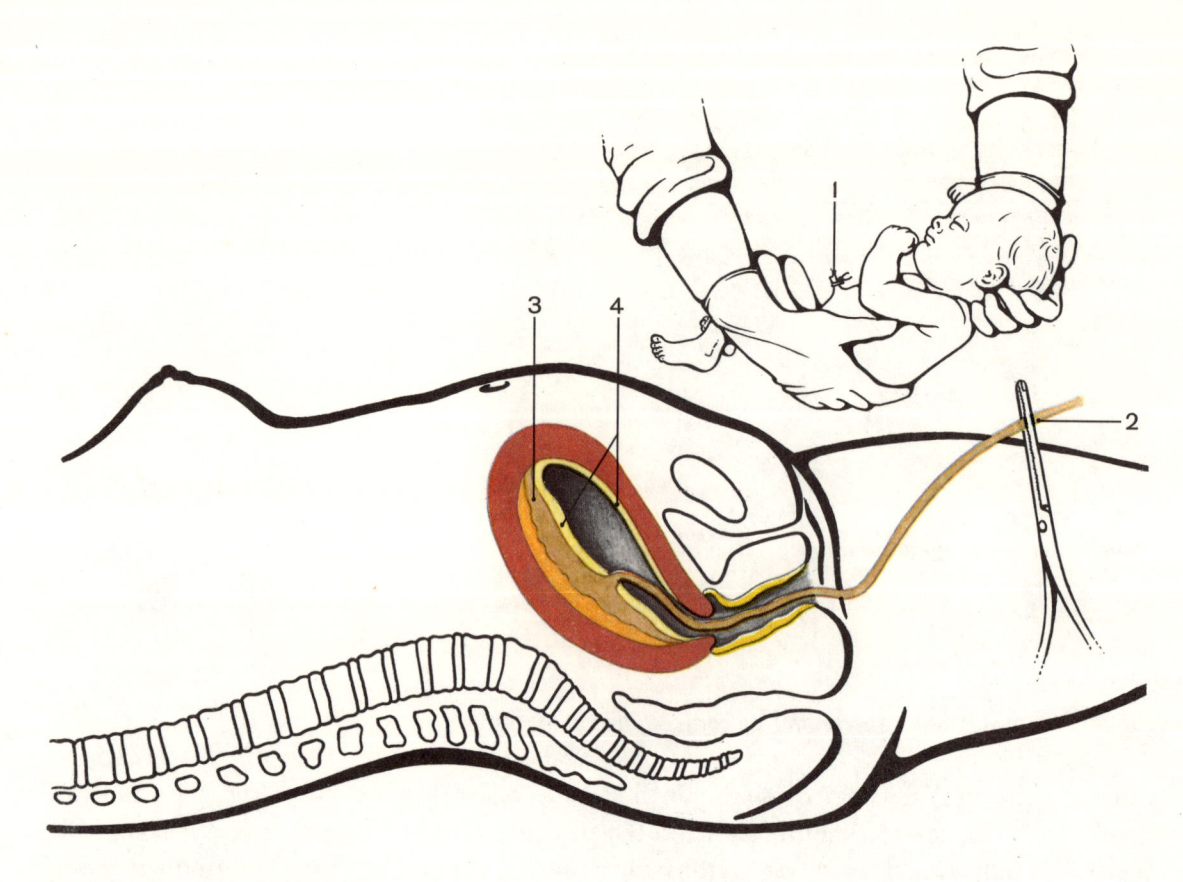

FIG. 71 *The cord tied off.*

1 Tied off stump of cord on baby
2 Clamped off cord, still in communication with 3 and 4
3 Placenta in uterus which has already contracted down
4 Membranes of foetus

Cutting the cord
After breathing has been established, the child is again laid between the mother's legs and the cord is tied off and cut. Up to now, the child has remained connected directly with its placenta, and through this with its mother. The cord is severed about a hand's breadth from the child's navel. Clamping off the cord and then tying it off prevents outflow of blood from the placenta and the child's navel. The further toilet of the cord stump can be carried out later by the midwife. It is at present more important to cover up the child after the stress of its birth. Figure 71 shows a child with the cord cut.

The after-birth
The remains of the coverings of the child, its placenta and the rest of its umbilical cord, are

still in the uterus and birth passages. These remnants are known as the after-birth. Within a few minutes of the birth of the child, the uterus begins to contract again, and thus to diminish the size of the area by which the placenta is attached to the uterus. The placenta begins to separate, through its maternal portion, and some maternal blood vessels are thereby opened. Bleeding results but should not exceed about a quarter of a litre (under half a pint), for the contractions of uterine muscle arrest haemorrhage by pressing together the walls of the opened blood vessels. A small remnant of the maternal mucosal portion stays in the uterus and is expelled later in the puerperium. Under the pull of the separated portions and with the help of the woman's abdominal muscles, the placenta moves downwards and with it come the coverings or membranes of the child, so that finally the placenta with the remains of the umbilical cord and the membranes turned inside out is expelled about a quarter of an hour after the birth of the child. The midwife or doctor examines the placenta to ensure that it has all come away; if not or if there are any other disorders of this, the third stage of labour, medical aid is required.

Duration of labour

Labours vary greatly in length, for they depend on the strength and effectiveness of the contractions as well as the active cooperation of the woman during the expulsion period. The duration also depends on the size of the child and the distensibility of the birth passages, and finally on the resistance to distension of the pelvic floor at the perineum. It has been clearly shown that women who have learned during their pregnancy how to use their abdominal muscles and relax their pelvic floor muscles take less time over their delivery. This minimises the possibility of injury to the child through too long a labour. There are however racial differences in length of labour.

In general, a woman is delivered more rapidly after she has had one child, for birth passages that have been dilated once or more offer much less resistance. The age of the woman also affects the length of labour, especially during first labours, because as she grows older her tissues lose some elasticity and capacity to loosen up. Women who are over 30 years old at their first delivery are known as 'elderly primiparae'. Comprehensive statistics have yielded the following data for duration of labour in persons with a normal occipital presentation; it must however be remembered that a labour either in a primipara or a multipara may last less than one hour or more than 48 hours.

Length of labour	Primipara	Multipara
Commonest value	9 hrs.	$4\frac{1}{2}$ hrs.
Half of all labours are over by	12 hrs.	$7\frac{1}{2}$ hrs.
Average value	14 hrs.	9 hrs.

About one hour of the difference between first labours and others is due to the length of the second stage in primiparae. In multiparae a few pains are often enough to complete this stage.

Precipitate birth implies the precipitate expulsion of the child at the end of the second stage; this may tear the umbilical cord. Such an event in our culture signifies that the woman either is totally ignorant of the processes of labour (and in particular unaware of the signs of imminent labour) or has taken pains to conceal her pregnancy and delivery. It should not be confused with *precipitate labour*, which is commoner in multiparae, in whom a few powerful pains may sometimes suffice to expel the child. In these cases, the woman almost always has the chance to lie down and avoid the child's being ejected on to the floor, even if she is too late to warn the midwife or doctor.

The end of pregnancy marks another hormonal adjustment in the female body. Production of pregnancy hormone stops rather abruptly, and this affects all the other hormone systems and is not without its effects on the woman's mood.

The Emotional Experience of Delivery

Even the healthiest woman begins to find her physical discomforts tedious by the end of pregnancy, and existing harmony between mother and her unborn child may be upset by her desire to get rid of this burden by labour. There is a struggle, often unconsciously, between the two conflicting tendencies, to retain the child and to bring it into the world. The ambiguity of this is expressed in many fears and anxieties about delivery itself, and not uncommonly leads to emotional upset of the process of birth. Whereas the woman should let nature take its course in the first two processes of delivery, engagement of the head and dilatation of the birth passages, in the second stage of expulsion she must undergo major physical and mental stresses. Overcoming the discomfort of distension of the pelvic floor and her anxieties needs great effort and self-control.

Every delivery is an effort both in the physical and the mental sense. It is a task which the woman cannot refuse when her time comes (her choice was made at conception). If she adopts a positive attitude to the task she will experience her labour as a major effort but without serious pain. If however she looks on this as part of a woman's fate which she would gladly avoid as the price of motherhood, delivery will be an emotionally painful event for her internal attitude of rejection of her lot as a childbearing woman will undoubtedly bring on muscular counteraction. We know that a blow on a tense muscle is much more painful than one on a relaxed one. The periodic thrust of the child's head and its powerful impact on the muscles of the pelvic floor can be roughly compared to such a blow. If the pelvic muscles are relaxed and contract only during a contraction to let the child out steadily and not precipitately, then the woman will certainly be aware of the great distension of the muscle ring but the discomfort associated with the distension will be submerged in the effort of active bearing down and the knowledge that progress is being made.

This process in the phase immediately before delivery lasts only a few minutes and is a unique mental and physical state which no male can properly appreciate. At this high point of delivery a state is reached which recalls orgasm. The exhaustion is gradually permeated by the woman's joy at her achievement. It is an achievement of which she can be justly proud, and her pride will enable her to forget her exertions relatively quickly. It is therefore of the highest importance for a woman to bring her child into the world while fully conscious. Her exertions, which are never entirely painless, are a necessary component of delivery; without this experience her pride in her own performance cannot be fully awakened, the experience of delivery soon fades, and the relationship between performance and result (the child) may be disturbed.

Let us not be misunderstood. This has nothing to do with the drama of the Biblical curse and the phrase 'in sorrow thou shalt bring forth children' (*Genesis* 3.16), or with rejection of aids to childbirth. It is simply a protest against the frivolous use of anaesthetics and sedatives that rob the woman of this important experience, an experience she might have had with careful emotional and physical preparation for labour, including relaxation and exercises. Preparation for labour removes the woman from an unnecessary and vicious circle between anxiety and its associated self-created pain.

Anxiety is not abolished but help is given to overcome it by sensible and voluntary collaboration during labour. The 'normal' pains are not abolished but the woman has learned to accept them as necessary and to avoid making them worse. She can now experience her delivery consciously and affirmatively. From such an experience she is ideally placed to give her personal attention fully to the newborn child and to make that first decisive contact (decisive for the child's later life) of affirmation, care, love and recognition.

The false dramatization of the Biblical curse on the occasion of the expulsion from Paradise has been the cause in the 'Christian' west of a false attitude to birth which has persisted for centuries. The correct translation of the word ETZEV in the original Hebrew text is *effort* or *stress* or *work*, and the phrase implies that labour is an effort. Translation as *pain* stems from a moral scale of values on the part of the translator, as was customary at that time. Nowhere else in the Bible is the word ETZEV translated as *pain*. The Biblical statement that the woman will bear her children with effort is nothing extraordinary but is the equivalent of the curse laid on the male, by which he will have to work his way through the world 'in the sweat of his brow'.

The stress and exertion of childbirth distorts the facial expression at the height of physical and mental tension (note the parallel to the facial distortion of orgasm). This is the unconscious reason why some women do not want their husbands present at the delivery.

Only a very deep relation of trust, such as is not usually established early in a marriage, makes it possible to bear the sight of such a distortion of the face of one's beloved. Many women fear, with some justification, that they will no longer appear lovable to their husband if he has once seen them in the throes of labour. The usually advanced motive of aesthetics is mostly only secondary or a camouflage.

The Puerperium

When the after-birth has been delivered the lying-in period or puerperium begins. It comprises the period during which the changes of pregnancy regress, and lasts for four to six weeks. In the forefront of the regressive changes stands the uterus, which rapidly contracts down by powerful 'after-pains' in the first days after delivery. Suckling the child helps this regression. During this time the endometrium also heals up. The remains of the maternal portion of the placenta are expelled, partly as rags of tissue, together with the blood clot which has reliquefied and the tissue water. This leads to a discharge of *lochia*, which at first is copious and watery-bloody, then brown, then pale, and finally by the end of the second week a dirty creamy-yellow. It dries up entirely by four to six weeks, after gradually getting lighter in colour, more watery and less in amount but is scarcely noticeable after 14 days. Renewal of the endometrium runs parallel with this. However this is complete and normal only when the wall of the uterine cavity has been healed and all the blood vessels which were needed in pregnancy to ensure conveyance of blood to and from the foetus have completely regressed. This has taken place by about three months after delivery.

Restoration of the endometrium is dependent on the reawakening of ovarian activity, for the ovaries soon take up their old cycle. In many women but by no means all, menstruation does not occur during breast-feeding. Absence of menstruation, due to the fact that the endometrium is still not functioning fully (see above), must not be taken as indicating inability to conceive, for a fertilizable ovum may be present; after every delivery the couple must realize that a new pregnancy can occur after any intercourse taking place after the five weeks puerperal recovery period. The first menstrual period is as a rule longer and heavier than normal, and the first cycles after delivery tend to be irregular. It is not uncommon to find that after a delivery the timing of menstruation has changed, so that the previous basis of calculation of fertile days must be altered. Reconstruction of the cervix, its os and its mucus plug proceed essentially faster, one reason why sexual intercourse can be permitted so soon. The external os, which was rounded and dimpled before pregnancy, is now a transverse slit.

Not many of the other changes of pregnancy remain. The aperture between the labia gapes a little. The water loading of tissues disappears, the excess water deposited during pregnancy being excreted through the kidneys in the urine and through the skin by sweating. Hence the skin needs extra care. Abdominal muscles recover their tone, being helped by a graduated course of exercises during the puerperium and by a new girdle.

In general, the lying-in woman should be treated with forbearance and not exposed to excessive physical or other stresses. If labour has been uncomplicated, she can in general leave her bed for a short while after 8 to 10 hours. Most hospitals discharge the patient after 8 to 10 days. Working women should not return to work for eight weeks after their delivery.

Thanks to better hygiene and modern treatment methods, the once dreaded puerperal fever, due to infection of the wound area in the uterus, has lost its terrors and hardly plays a part now. Any stagnation or inflammation in veins that have formed during pregnancy can also be successfully treated now. However, the woman's physical well-being should be closely watched over, and the doctor called in good time if anything is amiss.

Breast-feeding

Attitude of the Mother to Breast-feeding

With the first recession of her exhaustion after the exertions of labour, the mother begins to turn her whole attention to the child and its needs. One essential element in this attention is the satisfaction of its hunger.

The newborn takes its first natural nourishment at the human breast, and originally the female breast was significant only as a symbol of this process. Girls with well developed breasts were thought to promise well as mothers able to provide adequately for their child, although we now know that there is no constant relation between the external size of the breasts and their capacity to produce milk. In modern times the breast has also been seen as a sign of feminine charm; it now receives conscious attention from the male, apart from its unconscious connotations of giving and of providing security. This point of view will not be discussed here (see the remarks on female erogenous areas on p. 153 ff.).

Breast-feeding not only means putting the child to the mother's breast but also a special emotional relationship to the mother and a particular physical contact between mother and child during suckling. The mother also experiences something which fills her with pleasure. This first contact between mother and child must not be underrated, and cannot be replaced by anyone else. We have pointed this out earlier in the book.

If possible the child's staple diet during its first three months after birth should consist only of mother's milk. Breast-feeding should be limited to nine months, because the child by then will urgently need other nutrients not contained in mother's milk.

Structure and Function of the Female Breast

Glandular tissue of the breast
In the sexually mature woman the breast consists essentially of a somewhat flattened hemi-

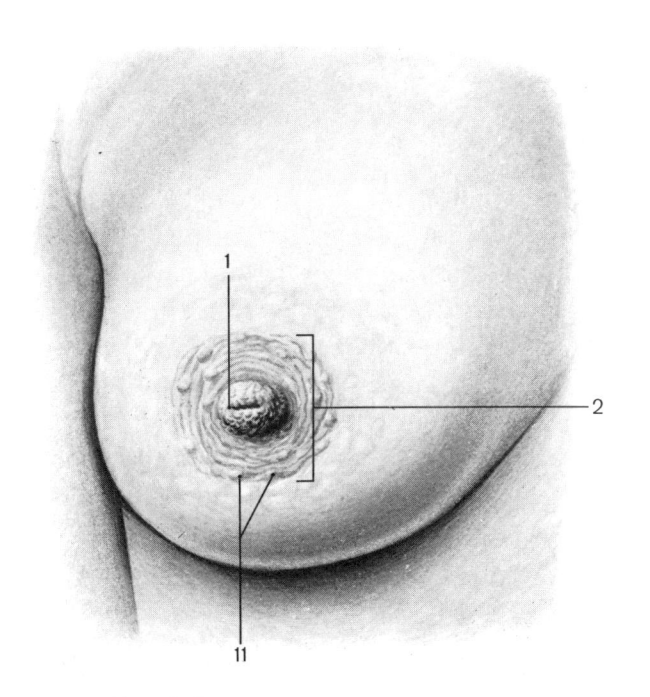

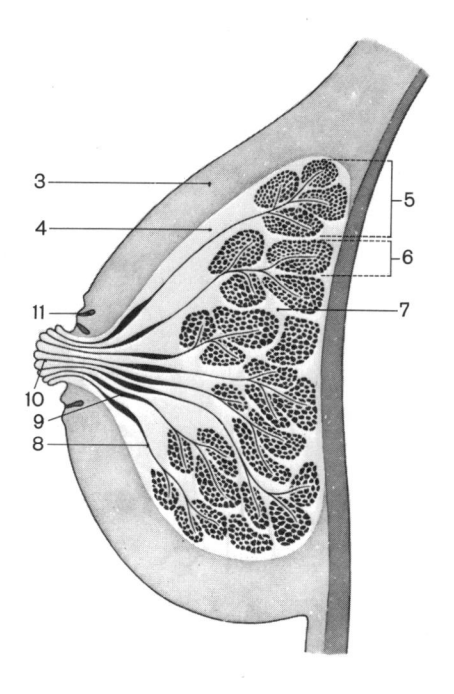

FIG. 72 *Female breast.*

1 Nipple   2 Areola   3 Skin fat   4 Glandular lobe   5 Single glands (total of 15–24)
6 Small glandular lobules   7 Fat between gland lobules   8 Milk (lactiferous) duct   9 Ampulla of duct   10 Opening of milk duct   11 Montgomery's gland

spherical mass of glandular tissue (see fig. 72) with 15 to 24 irregularly shaped lobes separated to varying extents by fat and connective tissue; each lobe is composed of small lobules. Each of the lobes has a single and separate milk (lactiferous) duct which widens out just before its end into an ampulla for collecting milk and opens into the nipple by a fine aperture. The number of these apertures (15 to 24) corresponds to the number of lobes. The glandular tissue is embedded in the skin fat and lies upon the major chest (pectoral) muscle, so that deep breathing or raising or lowering the arm can change the shape and situation of the breast.

The nipple and areola
The nipple lies in the middle of a rounded pigmented zone, the areola, and is bright pink (only in women before pregnancy) to dark brown in colour. During pregnancy the nipple and areola turn dark brown. Because it has an elastic and muscular system, the nipple can respond by erection to external physical or mental stimuli. This opens up the apertures of the milk ducts.

On the areola there is a variable number of small fine elevations due to sebaceous skin glands (Montgomery's glands) as well as fine scent glands. The external form and size of the breast do not permit any conclusions about the size and functional capacity of the gland, because the glandular tissue may be completely replaced by fat and connective tissue.

Development of the breasts
Development of the breasts (see fig. 73) begins under the influence of oestrogen from the ovary, and therefore depends on follicle maturation and the beginning of sexual maturity. Oestrogen and corpus luteum hormone together are responsible for development of the milk duct system. Hence the breast develops in girls only at puberty. Yet every ovulation cycle has an effect which is felt by some women as a transient sensation of tension in the breasts (after rupture of the follicle and at the beginning of the luteal phase). When an increased amount of the sex hormones is secreted by placenta and ovary during pregnancy, the breasts enlarge. Primiparae not infrequently notice a sensation of fullness and tension in their breasts within two or three weeks of conception, even before they have missed a period; the breast signs may draw their attention to other and later indications of pregnancy.

The breasts can be seen to increase in size, but milk is not formed during the pregnancy. It is only after the stimuli to growth have ceased (two or three days after delivery, when the remains of the pregnancy hormone from the placenta are secreted) that the pituitary begins to release a special lactation hormone which has been prepared and stored during pregnancy. Milk production is stimulated by this hormone in association with others from the thyroid and adrenal cortex.

Breast-feeding
Maintenance of milk production during breast-feeding depends essentially on the sucking and chewing of the child at the breast and on the mental attitude and readiness of the woman to breast-feed (see fig. 73). If the breast is not stimulated by sucking or the woman is consciously or unconsciously unwilling to breast-feed, milk production soon falls off.

Most women are aware of the beginning of milk production after delivery (the milk coming in). The breasts are tense and swollen, because of suddenly increased blood supply to them. Increase in milk secretion follows this. During pregnancy, the breasts secrete a very nutritious sticky yellow type of milk called colostrum, which is available immediately after delivery and suffices to satisfy the child's needs until milk production proper starts on about the third day after delivery, steadily rising in the first weeks and months provided the child empties the breast each time it feeds.

The child should be put to the breast first about 24 hours after its birth. The mother will soon find out that her child is able to suckle quite quickly if she pushes the nipple deeply enough into its mouth between its toothless gums. The sucking reflex is inborn in every child, but sucking is not the whole story. The following sequence of events takes place. First

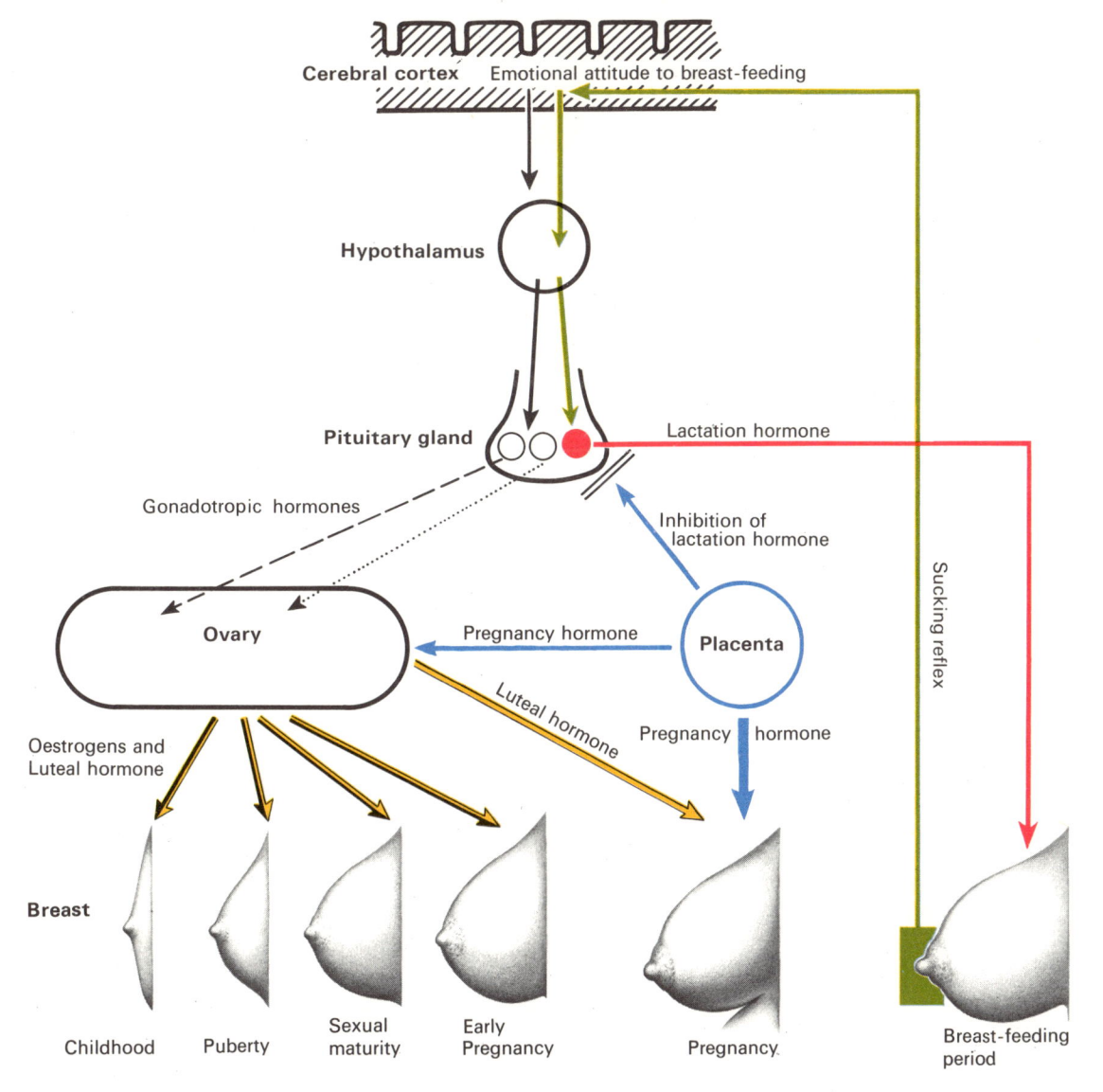

FIG. 73 *Development of breast and process of breast-feeding.*

the child encloses the nipple with the sucking pads of its mouth and thus closes it off together with its own oral cavity from the outer air. It then produces with its tongue a low pressure cavity within the mouth (sucking). So that its cheeks are not sucked in as well, they are provided with a particularly firm fatty pad. Finally, the child presses its jaws into the back part of the nipple and thus forces into its mouth the milk it has sucked into the milk ducts. It does not let go of the nipple after this but pushes its tongue forward again, manipulates and moistens the nipple and begins again. The newborn therefore both sucks and chews.

The child should be put to the breast between 7 a.m. and 9 p.m. at intervals of about $3\frac{1}{2}$ hours, a total of five times a day; the right and left breasts may be used at alternate feeds. On the first day it should get about a third of an ounce (10 grams) a feed, and then during the next ten days about an extra third of an ounce per feed each day. The subsequent quantities of milk depend on the way the child is thriving. In general, a healthy breast-fed child needs about 2 to $2\frac{1}{2}$ ounces of breast milk per pound body weight per day. Usually the child takes about five minutes to imbibe the first half of its feed, and then another ten minutes for the rest. The first milk it gets each time is poor in fat and the last has the richest fat content the breast can offer. The child should not remain at the breast more than 20 minutes. Longer suckling and chewing will lead to cracked nipples, which are liable to inflammation. Moreover, the child will get tired. If the breast is not emptied by the infant, it must be artificially pumped dry to avoid stagnation and inflammation. Feeding can be supplemented from the beginning of the fifth month, and the child weaned at the latest in the eighth or ninth month.

Weaning and breast regression
When the child ceases to be put to the breast (weaning), milk production usually dries up pretty quickly because of the absence of a stimulus. The lobules empty so that the breast returns almost to its pre-pregnancy state. The empty spaces within the breast are mostly filled by relatively firm fat and connective tissue.

In the climacteric, further regressive changes in the breasts appear as a result of failure of the cyclical hormone secretion by the ovaries; at first the tissue deficiency is made good by fat and connective tissue, but later compensation fails and the breasts wither.

Separation of the Child from the Mother

Breast-feeding and the associated close relationship between mother and child are important, and the separation from the maternal breast associated with weaning is equally significant. This is the second step the child has taken into the outside world. Weaning shows the mother once more that her child must separate himself from her to follow his own development and go his own independent way.

This event calls our attention again to the facts of fatherhood and motherhood. Every child born into a marriage is a disturbing element from the start. This is however not perceived at first because the child uses its elementary powers to draw the attention of both father and mother to itself. As the child becomes more independent, the parents begin to see the situation more clearly, for its claims conflict with the claims the parents make on each other and on the shape of their relations. Husband and wife, father and mother, have to learn anew to accept this limitation on their personal lives. This is easier with the second and third children, because they have some experience in overcoming the problems, but the problem is always present and permeates their whole life whatever the age of the children. Even when children have long left the parental home and become father and mother themselves, the limitation can be felt and needs to be accepted consciously.

To be a father or a mother demands the giving of help and care to the child, and also assistance to his development, as well as a continuing renunciation of one's own ideas and wishes.

We have seen that marriage and parenthood have a reciprocal effect on each other, and both are a venture in cooperation. Marriage remains an independent partnership of man and woman for life within the social order, apart from the problems of parenthood. In the Biblical sense it is 'one flesh', one body which can grow and strengthen, fall ill and recover. Quite apart from parenthood, a married couple need to make a constant mutual endeavour to keep their marriage physically and mentally sound. There are crises in every marriage, and to overcome them is one of the tasks a man and a woman take on when they decide to marry. Human society and its institutions should be prepared to offer help in this, for all of us are dependent on one another and on the existence of intact marriages.

Glossary

AMNION: a thin transparent membrane lining the amniotic cavity of the foetus and secreting fluid in which the latter is cushioned against outside stimuli.

ANUS: the lower opening of the alimentary canal or intestine.

AREOLA: the circular area around the nipple. In the female it is first pink then brown.

BAG OF WATERS: the part of the amniotic cavity which precedes the presenting part of the foetus in early labour, and eventually ruptures and expels its contents.

BARTHOLIN'S GLAND: a gland on either side of the vaginal opening, said to help lubricate the vagina during intercourse.

BASAL TEMPERATURE: body temperature measured with the subject still at rest after a night's sleep.

CAREZZA: a system of contraception in which intercourse is prolonged much beyond the normal without ejaculation.

CERVIX: the lower narrower part of the uterus containing a canal opening into the vagina.

CHORION: the most external covering of the foetus, serving for protection and nutrition and forming with the amnion the 'membranes' which rupture during labour.

CHROMOSOME: the body within the cell nucleus which contains the genes or hereditary factors.

CILIA: threads or hairs attached to cell surfaces and serving by their waving to propel objects outside the cells, as in the fallopian tubes.

CLITORIS: the smaller female equivalent to the penis, highly sensitive and erectile.

COITUS: sexual intercourse.

COITUS INTERRUPTUS: a misnomer for coitus abruptus in which intercourse is arrested before ejaculation, the latter taking place outside the vagina.

CONTRACEPTIVE PILL: a pill taken by mouth during most of the menstrual cycle to upset the normal hormone balance and thus prevent conception. Both oestrogen and progesterone types of compound are used in different doses and combinations; their action is complex and still controversial, but they are the most reliable method of contraception yet developed.

CONTRACTIONS: these are the contractions of the uterine muscle immediately before and during labour. Their object is to use the foetus as a battering ram to dilate up the passages through which it must go to reach the outer world, and later to push the foetus out, followed by its after-birth. Even later, further contractions stop the lining of the uterus from bleeding. They are also known as 'labour pains' though the amount of pain varies greatly.

COPULATION: coitus, sexual intercourse.

CORONA RADIATA: a collection of cells which surround the ovum as it emerges from the ovary.

CORPUS CAVERNOSUM: one of two columns of erectile tissue forming part of the penis or associated with the clitoris.

CORPUS LUTEUM: the yellow body which forms at the site of a follicle after the latter has burst and let its ovum go. Persists in pregnancy because it is needed to secrete a hormone.

CORPUS SPONGIOSUM: a single column of erectile tissue lying below the two corpora cavernosa in the penis and containing the urethra.

COWPER'S GLAND: a gland lying on either side of and below the male urethra and discharging a secretion into the latter.

EJACULATION: discharge of semen during male orgasm.

Premature e.: ejaculation very early in sexual intercourse or even before insertion of the penis.

EMBRYO: the human being which develops immediately after fertilization of an ovum by a spermatozoon; after 8 weeks or so, it is called the foetus.

ENDOMETRIUM: the mucosa or lining layer of the uterine cavity.

EPIDIDYMIS: a corded structure attached behind the testis, serving to store spermatozoa.

EPISIOTOMY: a cut deliberately made in the perineum to avoid a more ragged tear in the latter during labour.

EROGENIC or EROGENOUS: applied to areas of the body where contact arouses sexual stimulation.

FALLOPIAN TUBE: a tube running from the ovary to the uterus on either side and conveying the spermatozoa and ovum towards each other.

FERTILIZATION: union of the nuclei of spermatozoon and ovum within the latter.

FIBROIDS: benign tumours growing in the wall of the uterus in women late in their reproductive period of life.

FOETUS: the developing baby in the uterus before birth. It is also usually termed the embryo up to about the eighth week of life within the uterus.

FOLLICLE: the bag containing fluid which forms around an ovum early in each menstrual cycle, expands and finally bursts, discharging its ovum about half way between menstrual periods. It also secretes follicular hormone or oestrogen.

FRENULUM: in the male, a band under the glans penis attaching the prepuce and extremely sensitive; in the female, a similar band lying below the clitoris.

FRIGIDITY: failure of sexual arousal in the female.

GENE: a unit of heredity transmitting a character and situated at a definite place in a chromosome.

GERM CELL: that type of body cell whose function is to reproduce the person.

GERMINAL LAYERS: the entire foetus is formed from three germinal layers of cells: ectoderm, mesoderm, and endoderm.

GLANS PENIS: the soft rounded end of the penis.

GONADOTROPIC: acting on the gonads, or sex glands (testes and ovaries). Applied particularly to hormones secreted by the pituitary, and by the placenta during pregnancy.

HORMONE: a chemical messenger made by an endocrine gland and discharged into the circulation.

HYPOTHALAMUS: that part of the brain lying underneath the cerebral hemispheres and above the pituitary, with which it is closely connected.

IMPLANTATION: the implantation or embedding of the fertilized ovum in the wall of the uterus.

IMPOTENCE: inability in the male to carry out sexual intercourse.

IMPREGNATION: the act of rendering someone pregnant.

INGUINAL CANAL: the canal in the lower abdominal wall which permits passage of the seminal duct in the male.

INSEMINATION: introduction of semen into the uterus.
Artificial i.: introduction of semen without intercourse, either from a husband or a donor.

IUCD: intrauterine contraceptive device. Any object introduced into the uterus (ring, loop, bow, spiral out of plastic, metal, nylon, etc.) to prevent conception, or rather implantation of the fertilized ovum in the uterus.

LABIA: the lips which enclose the female genitals. There are two pairs, an outer or major and an inner or minor.

LOCHIA: the fluid discharged from the vagina in the days following birth.

MALFORMATION: abnormal or defective formation of a part of a foetus.

MENARCHE: the onset of menstruation in adolescent girls.

MENOPAUSE: the cessation of menstruation at the end of reproductive life in a woman.

MENSES: the monthly discharge of blood plus endometrium from the vagina during a woman's reproductive age.

MUTATION: a permanent transmissible change in character of an offspring which makes it different from its parents.

OCCIPUT: the back of the head, which usually appears first when the baby is born.

OESTROGEN: a hormone which will reproduce the changes seen in the first half of the menstrual cycle. The naturally occurring one, oestriol, is secreted by the ovary and sometimes called 'follicular hormone'. It prepares the uterine bed for the fertilized ovum to lie in.

OOCYTE: an immature ovum.

ORGASM: the climax of excitement during sexual intercourse.

OS, CERVICAL or EXTERNAL: the mouth or opening of the cervical canal into the vagina.

OVARY: a paired organ lying to either side of the uterus and containing the ova; it also secretes sex hormones.

OVULATION: the discharge of the ovum from its follicle in the ovary about midway between two menstrual periods.

OVUM: literally the egg or female germ cell.

PARAPHIMOSIS: retraction of a tight prepuce with inability to release it forward.

PELVIC FLOOR: the barrier consisting of muscles and ligaments which holds up the contents of the pelvis and opens up to let the infant through at birth.

PELVIS: the lower part of the trunk, bounded by the hip bones or pelvic bones and the sacrum and coccyx. Divided arbitrarily into false pelvis and true pelvis, the latter being the lower, narrower part totally enclosed by bone.

PENIS: the male organ of copulation.

PERINEUM: the area between the back of the vagina and the front of the anus. It stretches enormously during labour and may tear.

PESSARY: an object introduced into the vagina in order to: (1) administer a drug; (2) support the uterus; (3) oppose a mechanical or chemical barrier to spermatozoa. (3) includes caps which fit over the cervix, and diaphragms which close off the entire vault of the vagina.

PETTING: sexual play leading to orgasm in both parties but without actual sexual intercourse.

PHIMOSIS: tightness of the foreskin preventing retraction behind the glans penis.

PITUITARY GLAND: a regulating gland lying in a bony cavity at the base of the brain and secreting a number of hormones which cause other glands to function; in particular, it secretes FSH (follicle-stimulating hormone) which causes the ovarian follicle to secrete and LH (luteinizing hormone) which causes the ruptured ovarian follicle to form a corpus luteum.

PLACENTA: an organ consisting of maternal and foetal tissue intimately connected to promote exchanges of nutrients and waste matters between mother and foetus.

POLAR BODY: when primitive ova or oocytes mature they divide twice, and form more mature ova plus small polar bodies.

POTENCY: the ability of the male to carry out sexual intercourse.

PREPUCE: foreskin, the skin tube covering the glans penis in the uncircumcised penis at rest.

PRESENTATION: the commonest type of presentation of a foetus is that in which during labour the head emerges first (cephalic presentation); less common is a breech presentation in which the baby's buttocks appear first.

PROGESTERONE: the luteal hormone secreted by the ovary in the second half of the menstrual period. It ensures that the uterine mucosa will develop further after oestrogen has started development off.

PROSTATE GLAND: a gland lying just below the male urinary bladder, surrounding the urethra and contributing a secretion to the semen.

PUBIC: associated with the pubic bones, which unite the two halves of the pelvis in front.

PUERPERIUM: the lying in period after a woman has given birth.

RECTUM: the last few inches of the alimentary canal just above the anus.

REFLEX: the simplest type of stimulus-response model in the body, mediated by the spinal chord.

RHESUS FACTOR: a blood factor found in rhesus monkeys and a certain proportion of human beings. Its presence or absence in parents may in some circumstances lead to injury to a foetus.

RHYTHM METHOD: a method of contraception based on the menstrual rhythm, either by calculating a safe period or by assessing the time of ovulation by temperature measurements.

SCROTUM: the bag of skin containing the testes.

SEBACEOUS GLAND: a gland secreting sebum, a fatty substance lubricating the skin.

SEMEN: the secretion discharged by the male on orgasm and containing sperm cells, secretion from the prostate and contributions from other glands.

SEMINAL DUCT: the canal which conveys semen from the epididymis to the urethra.

SEMINAL VESICLE: one of a pair of bags attached to the back of the bladder and opening into the seminal duct.

SEMINIFEROUS TUBULE: one of the much folded tubes which make up most of the testis.

SMEGMA: the cheesy material secreted under the prepuce of the uncircumcised male.

SPERMATOGONIUM: the most primitive forerunner of the male sex cell. It divides into primary and secondary spermatocytes, then spermatids and finally spermatozoa.

SPERMATOZOON: the mature male germ cell which fertilizes the female cell or ovum.

SPHINCTER: a ring-like muscle closing an opening.

SPINAL CORD: that part of the central nervous system contained within the vertebral column.

TESTIS: the male sex gland which produces the spermatozoa.

TROPHOBLAST: that part of the embryo which is concerned with maintenance of its nutrition in the uterus.

UMBILICAL CORD: the cord attaching the foetus by its navel to the placenta or afterbirth and containing blood vessels and jelly.

UMBILICUS: navel, or site of former attachment of the individual to its placenta.

URETHRA: the tube running from the urinary bladder to the exterior and conveying urine in both sexes and semen also in the male.

UTERUS: a hollow organ which contains and nourishes the embryo before birth.

VAGINA: the female canal extending from vulva up to cervix and receiving the penis in intercourse.

VILLUS: a finger-like protrusion from a membrane which serves to increase the surface area available for exchanges across the latter.

VULVA: the external genital area of the female including the labia, clitoris and vestibule of the vagina.

YOLK SAC: a bag lying outside the embryo and attached to its primitive gut.

A Select English Bibliography

There is a vast literature on sex and marriage available in English today. The books here suggested are particularly suitable for teachers, social workers, ministers, counsellors, and others who have to deal with problems of sexual relationships.

STAFFORD-CLARK David, *Psychiatry Today* (Baltimore: Penguin, 1952)
A standard popular description of modern psychiatry, free from extreme views.

STORR Anthony, *The Integrity of the Personality* (Baltimore: Penguin, 1963)
A Jungian analyst presents for the educated layman a general psychiatric account of the maturation of human personality.

BOWLBY John, et al., *Child Care and the Growth of Love* (Baltimore: Penguin, 1953)
One of the first to emphasize the harm done by separation of young children from their mothers, this book offers advice which can help prevent much emotional illness in later life.

MOTTRAM Vernon H., *The Physical Basis of Personality* (New York: Penguin, 1944)
Includes an extended account of the basis of human heredity.

HADFIELD James A., *Childhood and Adolescence* (Baltimore: Penguin, 1962)
An experienced psychiatrist provides an excellent account of the psychodynamics of growing up.

WALKER Kenneth M., *The Physiology of Sex* (New York: Penguin, 1940)
A surgeon long connected with marriage guidance gives a readable account of the biological and sociological aspects of sex.

WALKER Kenneth M., and Owen WHITNEY, *The Family and Marriage in a Changing World* (Mystic, Connecticut: Verry, 1965)
The last of a series of Dr Walker's books on various features of sexual relationships.

WRAGE Karl, *Children—Choice or Chance* (Philadelphia: Fortress, 1969)
Dr Wrage's practical little manual on controlling conception.

NIXON William C. W., *Childbirth* (London: Duckworth, 1955)
An obstetrician's detailed description of pregnancy and labour.

WALLIS Jack H., *Sexual Harmony in Marriage* (New York: Roy, 1965)
Written out of a long career in marriage counselling and the training of counsellors.

JONSSON G. and L., *Can Two Become One?* (Philadelphia: Fortress, 1965)
A husband–wife conversation points to the central joys and problems facing married couples.

RUBIN Isadore, and Lester A. KIRKENDALL, *Sex in the Adolescent Years* (New York: Association, 1968)
A straightforward book on sex instruction for young people, written for parents, teachers, clergy and all who are concerned with youth work.

BRACHER Marjory, *Love, Sex, and Life* (Philadelphia: Fortress, 1966)
Geared directly to the needs and language of the teenager.

THIELICKE Helmut, *The Ethics of Sex* (New York: Harper and Row, 1964)
A section from the major work of a distinguished professor of theological ethics.

Index

Note: Figures in italics denote illustrations.

Abdomen, as centre of child's life, 49
Abortion, ethics of, 176
Adolescence, 61
Adoption, explanation of, to child, 50
Adrenal cortex, 98
Affection, striving for, 44
After-birth, 234
Ageing, dignity of, 158
Alcohol, effect of, on hereditary factors, 171
    placental transport of, 207
Aloofness, childhood causes of, 44
Amnion, 226, 246
Anaemia of the newborn, 210
Anatomy, male and female, 79
Anus, 246
Areola, 241, 246
Artificial insemination, 113, 248

Bartholin's gland, *107*, 108, 246
Birth, precipitate, 236
Birth canal, 224, *226*
Bladder, urinary, *93*, *94*
Blood supply, mother-foetal, 205
Body build, *78*

Body odour, in pregnancy, 218
Breaking of waters, 226, 246
Breast(s), *241*
    development, 242, *243*
    glandular tissue, 240
    mature, 82
    in pregnancy, 220
    in pre-menstrual period, 134
    regression, 244
Breast-feeding, 244
    attitude of mother towards, 240
    in sex education, 30
    timing, 244
Breast milk, 242
Breath, first, of the newborn, 234

Caesarian section, 232
Cancer, 89, 189
Cap, cervical, 185
Caput succedaneum, 224–5
Carezza, 182, 246
Caul, 227
Cavernosa clitoridis, 108
Cell complexes, 165
Cerebrum, 97
Cervix. *See under* Uterus
Chastity, definition, 154, 177
Child, independence of, 211

    separation from mother, 244
Childhood, sex education in, 19
Children, sleeping in parents' bedroom, 33
Chorion, 226, 246
Chromosomes, 160 *et seq.*, 246
    crossing over, 162
    maturation division, 161
    pairing (conjugation), 162
    schema for sex cells, 167
Cilia, 246
Circumcision, 89
Climacteric, 127, 136, 156
    male, 157
Clitoris, *106*, 108, 246
Coccyx, *94*
Coitus. *See* Sexual intercourse
    abruptus, 181
    interruptus, 173, 181, 246
Colostrum, 242
Conception, 173
    post-delivery, 238
    timing, 174
Condom, 183
Conscience, shaping of, 35
Contact, striving for, 36
Contraception
    apparatus, 183
    bases of, 175

chemical agents, 186
combination of method and agent, 187
information on, to pubertal children, 51
methods, 174
pills, 135, 189, 246
safe period, 178
Contractions, 232, 246
Copulation. *See* Sexual intercourse
Cord, spinal, 250
umbilical, 234, 250
Corona radiata, 118, 123, 247
Corpora cavernosa, 93 *et seq.*, 247
female, *107*, 108
Corpus luteum, 119, 247
in preganancy, 194 *et seq.*
Corpus spongiosum, 93 *et seq.*, 247
Cowper's glands, 92, *93*, 94, 247
Criticism, in sex education, 41
Crossing over (of hereditary factors), 162

D factor in rhesus incompatibility, 208 *et seq.*
Delivery, emotional experience of, 236
Deoxyribonucleic acid (DNA), 161
Devotion, mutual, and sexual intercourse, 151
Diaphragms, 185
Digestive disturbances in pregnancy, 220
Digestive system, in embryo, 200
Disease, hereditary, 171
Disillusion, following infatuation, 66

DNA (deoxyribonucleic acid), 161
Don Juan complex, in adolescence, 62
Douche, vaginal, 185, 186
Down's disease (mongolism), 169
Drugs, placental transport of, 207
Dwarfism, 169

Ectoderm, 198
Education, and generation gap, 17
sex. *See* Sex education
Ejaculation
definition, 247
mechanism, 95
onset, preparation for, 57
premature, 104, 247
sperm count in, 103
Embryo, 194, 196, 201, 247
Emotion, restraint of, in childhood, 44
Emotional development, at adolescence, 61
Endoderm, 199
Endometrium, uterine, 113, 125, *126*, 247
Engagement period, 73
Environment, desexualized, 71
Epididymides, 87
Epididymis, 91, 93 *et seq.*, 247
Episiotomy, 232, 247
Erogenous zones, 80, 152, 247
in man, 154
in woman, 153
Exhibitionism, 45

Fallopian tubes, 105, 110 *et seq.*, 123, *124*, 247

Family planning, 117. *See also* Contraception
methods, 178
Family in society, 15
'Father's girl', 47
Fertilization, definition, 167, 247
Fetishism, 61
Fibroids, 247
Foam, contraceptive, 186
Foetus
advance of head through birth canal, *227*
birth, *231*
definition, 247
development, 201
false maternal claims on, 211
false paternal claims on, 212
food supply, 204
head ready for engagement, *224*
independence and dependence, 211
and mother, relation between, 203
presentations, 224, 249
Follicle, 247
primary, 116, 119
rupture, *117*, 118, 175
Follicular hormone. *See* Oestrogen
Foreskin, *88*, 89. *See also* Phimosis
Fourchette, 108
Frenulum, 89, 247
Frigidity, 110, 247
FSH, 98, 129

Generation gap, 17, 21
Genes, 160 *et seq.*, 169, 247
Genitalia
of boys (external), 80, *81*, 90

female, 105
    erectile tissue, *107*
    external, *106 et seq.*, 220
    internal, *105*, 110 *et seq.*
  of girls (external), 80, *81*
  male, 87
    external, 82, 87, *88*, *94*
    front aspect, *93*
    internal, side aspect, *94*
Germ cells, 247. *See also* Ovum; Spermatozoa
Germinal layers, 247
Giving, in sex education, 39
Glans penis, *88*, *89*, *93*, *94*, 247

Hair distribution, 79, 82
Harmony of body and mind, need for, 45
Heart, in pregnancy, 221
Hereditary substance, *161*, *162*
Hermaphrodites, 168
Hernia, inguinal, 92
Home
  influence of, in adolescence, 72
  role of, in sex education, 28
Homosexuality, environmental basis for, 60
Hormone(s)
  definition, 97, 248
  follicle-stimulating, 98, 129
  follicular. *See* Oestrogen
  gonadotropic, 136, 144, 248
  interstitial-cell-stimulating, 98
  luteal. *See* Progesterone
  luteinizing, 98, 129, 131
  oestrus, 145
  pituitary, 97, *98*, 128
  pregnancy, 195 *et seq.*, 217
  for prevention of ovum maturation, 135, 187
  regulation of menstruation, 128, *131*
Hymen, *106*, 109, 111 *et seq.*
Hypothalamus, 97, 248
Hysterectomy, orgasm following, 118

ICSH, 98
Identification of child with parent, 46
Implantation, definition, 248
Impotence, 103, 248
Impregnation, 173, *174*, 248
Infant(s)
  reaction to parental emotions, 25
  sleeping with parents, 33
Infatuation, 66
Infectious disease, maternal: effect on foetus, 207
Infertility in marriage, 103
Inguinal canal, 92, 93, 248
Inguinal hernia, 92
Inheritance, 159
  social, 164
Insemination, definition, 248. *See also* Impregnation
Intrauterine contraceptive device (IUCD), 185, 196, 248
Irradiation, 'aimed', 170
IUCD (intrauterine contraceptive device), 185, 196, 248

Jaundice of the newborn, 210
Jellies, contraceptive, 186

Labia, *106*, 107, 248
Labour, 223
  contractions, 232, 246
  duration, 235
  expulsion stage, *229*
  onset, 225
  relaxation-breathing exercises, 229
Lactic acid, 115
Levitical marriage laws, 46
Lochia, 238, 248
Love
  definition, 67
  first, 65
  striving for, 43
LSH, 98, 129
Luteal hormone. *See* Progesterone
Lutein, 129

Malformation, foetal, 207, 248
Man, anatomy, 87–104
Marriage
  early, 73
  forced, 70
  Levitical, 46
  mixed, 68
  partner choice, 68
  preparation for, and adolescence, 61
  with relatives, 171
  responsible, concept of, 177
  in society, 15
  'weekend', 155
Masochism, 61
Masturbation, 46, 58, 72
  anxiety, 25
  danger of disapproval of, 138
  in development of sex life, 138
  origin of sinful connotation, 46
  in puberty, 139

Maternal pride, 212
Maturation, physical, 57
Maturity, definition, 61
Meiosis, 160
Memories, influencing reflexes, 145
Menarche, 126, 133, 135, 248
　　emotional experience of menstruation at, 133
Menopause, 127, 136, 248
Menses, 248. See also Menstruation
Menstrual calendar, *128*
Menstrual cycle, 127
　　anovulatory, 132
　　calculation, 132
Menstruation, 125
　　disorders of, 127
　　emotional aspects, 133
　　hormone regulation of, 128, *131*
　　onset, 54
　　　　preparation for, 57
Mesoderm, 198
Milk, breast, 242
Mittelschmerz, 118
Models, in sex education, 63
Modesty, 31, 84
Mongolism (Down's disease), 169
Monogamy, explanation of, to adolescents, 65
Mons veneris, *106*, 107
Montgomery's glands, 242
Mother and foetus, relation between, 203
'Mother's boy', 47
Muscles, uterine. See Uterus: muscles
Mutations, 169, 248
Mutuality, 42

Naming of child, 203
National Childbirth Trust, 229
Necking, 72
Nervous system, 142 *et seq.*, 200
Nicotine, placental transport of, 207
Nipples, 242
Norms, social, and sex education, 63
Nudism, 32
Nudity in the family, 29
　　modesty and, 31
Nudity in the home, 85
Nutrition organs, in embryo, 200

Obesity in pregnancy, 218
Occiput, *230*, 248
Oedema of the foetus and newborn, 210
Oestrogen, 129 *et seq.*, 248
Onanism, 46
Oocyte, 162, 248
Orgasm, 148, 248
　　clitoral, 116
　　following hysterectomy, 114
　　mental attitude and, 148
　　speeds of attainment, 150
　　vaginal, 110, 116
Os. See Uterus: cervical os
Ovaries, 110 *et seq.*, 116, 248
　　follicle rupture, *117*, 118
　　function, and menstruation, *130*
　　function and pregnancy, *195*
Ovulation, 248
Ovum, 119, 248
　　cell division, *192*, *193*
　　external lifespan, 119
　　fertilization, 191
　　forms, *120*
　　maturation, 120, *121*
　　　　compared with that of spermatozoon, *122*
　　and inheritance, 159, *163*
　　psychological influences, 179
　　mature, 122, *123*
　　mechanism of uptake, *118*
　　numbers, 116
　　transport, and fallopian tube, *123*, *124*
Oxytocin, 225

Paedophilia, 60
Pains, false, 223
Pains, labour, 232
　　origin of term, 237
Papilla, 109
Paraphimosis, 90, 248
Parenthood, responsible, concept of, 177
Paternal pride, 213
Pelvis, 248
　　floor, 248
　　inlet, and foetus, *228*
　　in labour, 227
Penis, 81, 87 *et seq.*, 93, *94*, 249
　　erectile tissue, 93, *94*, *95*
　　hygiene, 89
　　section, *95*
Perineum, *106*, 107, 249
Perversion, information on, to pubertal children, 52
Pessaries, 184, 186, 249
　　intrauterine, 185
Petting, 72, 140, 249
　　as form of contraception, 181
Phimosis, 89, 90, 249
Pills, contraceptive, 135

Pituitary gland, 97, *98*, 249
Pituitary hormone
    regulation of menstruation, 128
Placenta, 204, 207, 234, 249
Plasma, in inheritance, 164
Pleasure, bodily, in puberty, 58
    sexual, in sex education, 23
Polar body, 249
Polarity, definition, 13
Possession, striving for, 38
Potency, 249
Pregnancy, 191
    attitude of parents towards, 31
    beginning of, *194*
    body changes, 217, *219*
    changes in, 217
    children's share in, 30
    displacement and decompression of organs in, *219*
    duration, 216
    emotional changes in, 222
    explanation of, to children, 49
    husband's role in, 222
    multiple, 119
    post-menopausal, 175
    suitable interval between, 31
    twin, binovular, 119
    uterine muscles and, 214
Pregnancy hormone. *See* Hormone(s): pregnancy
Premarital encounter, 69
Pre-puberty, state of, 54
Prepuce, 249. *See also* Foreskin
Presentation. *See under* Foetus
Privacy, need for, 85
Progesterone, 129 *et seq.*, 195, 249
Prolapse, uterine, 112
    vaginal, 115

Proliferation phase, of uterine endometrium, 130
Promiscuity, cause of, 62
Prostate gland, 92, *93*, *94*, 249
Prostitution, 63
Protein units, in hereditary substance, 161 *et seq.*
Puberty, 54 *et seq.*
    crises in, 56
    definition, 54
    emotional tensions in, 54
    sex education for, 51
    sexuality in, 56
Pubis, *94*
Pudenda, 105
Puerperium, 238, 249

Radiation injury, to hereditary material, 169
Rectum, 249
Reflex(es), 249
    affected by memories, 145
    copulatory, 144
    in sexual stimuli, 142
    spinal reflex arc, *143*
Renunciation, and adaptation to society, 17
Reproduction
    asexual, 165
    responsibility for, 24
    sexual, 165
Responsibility, and sexual intercourse, 175
Rhesus factor, 207, 249
    hereditary mechanism, *207*
    possible combinations, *209*
Rhythm method, of contraception. *See* Safe period
Role(s), definition, 14
    linked, *16*
Rupture, 92

Sadism, 61
Safe period, 178
Safety, need for, 43
Scrotum, 87, *88*, *93*, *94*, 249
Sebaceous gland, 249
Secretions
    education on, 25
    of female external genitals, 108
Secretory phase, of uterine endometrium, 130
Self-assertion, in childhood, 42
Self-confidence, in childhood, 43
Self-criticism, 41
Self-delimitation of infants, 32
Semen, 249
    in artificial insemination, 113
    ejaculation, 95
    maturation, 98 *et seq.*
Seminal cells, 91
Seminal ducts, 92, *93*, *94*, 249
    physical characteristics, 102, *103*
Seminal emission, onset, 54
Seminal vesicles, 92, *93*, *94*, 249
Seminiferous tubule, 97, *100*, 250
Separation, of child from mother, 244
Sex
    childhood theories of, 22
    determination, *166*, 167, 200
    early questions on, 21
    timing, 28
    familiarity with, in childhood, 27
    self comprehension in childhood, 24
Sex cells, 165
    precursors, in embryo, 199
Sex characteristics, awareness of,

in children, 45
Sex characters, *78*, 80
   adult, 82, *83*
Sex education, 18
   from animal and plant example, dangers of, 23
   answering children's questions, 48
   atmosphere in, 21
   bases of, 35
   in childhood, 19
   definition, 19
   erroneous, in childhood: consequences, 35
   home as right place for, 28
   models and social norms, 63
   nursery school role in, 53
   obstacles to, 19
   in pre-puberty and puberty, 56
   primary school role in, 53
   religious influence on, 20
Sex knowledge, sharing of, in childhood, 29
Sex life, 137
Sex organs, *78*
   arousal of interest in, 80
   male, internal, 91
   nomenclature, 26, 81
Sexual development, deviations in, 60
Sexual deviation in adolescence, 62
Sexual disturbances in adolescence, 62
Sexual drive, awakening of, 58
Sexual intercourse
   abstention from, as method of family planning, 178
   childhood witness to, of parents, 34
   duration, 155
   during pregnancy, 196
   explanation of, to pubertal children, 51
   forms, 154
   frequency, 154
   in later years, 157
   positions, 115, 155, 183
   premarital, incidence, 63
   responsibility and, 175
   'Spanish', 183
Sexual reactions, 142
Sexual relationships, erotic, in children, 45
Sexual satisfaction, striving for, in children, 45
Sexual stimuli, 142
Sexuality, 76
   differences, 79
   in later life, 156
   in puberty, 56
Sheath, 183
Skeletal system, in embryo, 200
Skin changes in pregnancy, 218
Smegma, 89, 250
Social forms, 13
Social inheritance, 164
Society and the adolescent, 64
Sperm cells. *See* Spermatozoa
Spermatocyte, 162
Spermatogonium, 250
Spermatozoa, 250
   aids to mobility, 92
   duration of development, 102
   effect on, of alcohol, 171
   life span, 102
   maturation, 98 *et seq.*
      compared with that of ovum, *122*
      and inheritance, 159, *163*
   number per ejaculation, 103
   physical characteristics, 102
   route, 91
Sphincter, 250
Spinal cord, 250
Sponges, contraceptive, 186
Status, striving for, 40
Step-children, explanation of origins, 50
Sterilization, 102, 124, 176
Stimulus, response to, 144, *146*
Striae, abdominal, 220
Sucking process, 242

Tablets, contraceptive, 186
Taking, in sex education, 39
Tampons, contraceptive, 186
   sanitary, 125
Temperature, basal, 180, 246
   chart, in calculation of 'fertile' period, 132, 180
Tenderness, striving for, 43
Testes, 87, 93 *et seq.*, 250
   undescended, 88
Testicles. *See* Testes.
Tetrad formation, of chromosomes, 162
Toddlers sleeping with parents, 33
Toxins, placental transport of, 207
Transvestism, 61
Trophoblast, 196 *et seq.*, 250
Twin pregnancy, binovular, 119, 193

Umbilicus, 250
Urethra, 87, *88*, 93 *et seq.*, 250
Uterus, 105 *et seq.*, 111 *et seq.*, 250
   cervical canal, dilatation, *225*
   cervical os, dilatation, *225*

cervix, 113, 246
    mucus plug, 113, 173, 174, 224
functions, 113
mucosa. *See* Endometrium, uterine
muscles, and pregnancy, 214
    structure, *215*
in the puerperium, 238
size, changes in, 215, *216*
tilting and kinking, 113, *114*

Vagina, 105 *et seq.*, 114, 250
Vaginal entrance, *106*, 109
Vaginismus, 110
Vasa deferentia. *See* Seminal ducts
Vascular system, in embryo, 200
Villus, 250
Voyeurism, 45
Vulva, 81, 250

Weaning, 244

Weight increase in pregnancy, 217
Will, development of, in childhood, 41
Woman, anatomy, 105–36
Womb. *See* Uterus

Yolk sac, 250
Youth groups, in sex education, 70

Zoophilic inclination, 60